Treatment of
EARLY DIABETES

ADVANCES IN EXPERIMENTAL MEDICINE AND BIOLOGY

Recent Volumes in this Series

Volume 111
HORMONES AND ENERGY METABOLISM
Edited by David M. Klachko, Ralph R. Anderson, and Murray Heimberg

Volume 112
OVARIAN FOLLICULAR AND CORPUS LUTEUM FUNCTION
Edited by Cornelia P. Channing, John M. Marsh, and William A. Sadler

Volume 113
PARKINSON'S DISEASE –II: Aging and Neuroendocrine Relationships
Edited by Caleb E. Finch, David E. Potter, and Alexander D. Kenny

Volume 114
FUNCTION AND STRUCTURE OF THE IMMUNE SYSTEM
Edited by Wolfgang Müller-Ruchholtz and Hans Konrad Müller-Hermelink

Volume 115
DYNAMICS OF ARTERIAL FLOW
Edited by Stewart Wolf and Nicholas T. Werthessen

Volume 116
MODULATORS, MEDIATORS, AND SPECIFIERS IN BRAIN FUNCTION
Edited by Yigal H. Ehrlich, Jan Volavka, Leonard G. Davis, and Eric G. Brunngraber

Volume 117
STEROID HORMONE RECEPTOR SYSTEMS
Edited by Wendell W. Leavitt and James H. Clark

Volume 118
CELL SUBSTRATES: Their Use in the Production of Vaccines and Other Biologicals
Edited by John C. Petricciani, Hope E. Hopps, and Paul J. Chapple

Volume 119
TREATMENT OF EARLY DIABETES
Edited by Rafael A. Camerini-Davalos and Bernard Hanover

Volume 120A
KININS – II: Biochemistry, Pathophysiology, and Clinical Aspects
Edited by Setsuro Fujii, Hiroshi Moriya, and Tomoji Suzuki

Volume 120B
KININS – II: Systemic Proteases and Cellular Function
Edited by Setsuro Fujii, Hiroshi Moriya, and Tomoji Suzuki

Treatment of EARLY DIABETES

Edited by

Rafael A. Camerini-Davalos
and
Bernard Hanover

Diabetes Center
New York Medical College
New York, New York

PLENUM PRESS • NEW YORK AND LONDON

Library of Congress Cataloging in Publication Data

International Symposium on Early Diabetes, 4th, Algarve, 1978.
Treatment of early diabetes.

(Advances in experimental medicine and biology; v. 119)
"Sponsored by the Diabetes Center of New York Medical College."
Includes index.
1. Diabetes – Congresses. I. Camerini-Dávalos, Rafael A., 1916- II. New York Medical College, Flower and Fifth Avenue Hospitals. Diabetes Center. III. Title. IV. Series.
RC660.A1I59 1978 616.4'62'06 79-16121

DOI 10.1007/978-1-4615-9110-8

Proceedings of the Fourth International Symposium on Early Diabetes,
sponsored by the Diabetes Center of New York Medical College,
held in Algarve, Portugal, November 7–11, 1978.

MyCopy version of the original edition 1979

A Division of Plenum Publishing Corporation
227 West 17th Street, New York, N.Y. 10011

Preface

To obey the precepts of therapeutic rationality, we should avoid treating the "effect" when there is a way to attack the cause. But what is the cause of diabetes?

Diabetes is a molecular disease, that is, a disease in which important cellular components are seriously impaired. Eventually, the activities or the products arising from the impairment find expression in various ways, finally culminating in the abnormalities of diabetes.

How early is early enough to attempt to delay this sequence of events? What will provide us with the basis to explore ways and means of halting the progression of the pathological process? What are the new approaches for the treatment of early diabetes?

The Fourth International Symposium on Early Diabetes, sponsored by the Diabetes Center of the New York Medical College, held in Algarve, Portugal in November 1978, from which this book evolved, attempted to answer some of these questions.

A list of the participants, including their affiliations, will be found preceding the index.

Rafael A. Camerini-Davalos

Acknowledgments

To our *sponsors*, U.S.V. Pharmaceutical Corp., Pfizer Pharmaceuticals, Ames Company, Hoechst, Frankfurt; *supporters*, Boehringer, Manheim, Laboratoires Servier, Nordisk Laboratory, The Upjohn Company, Eli Lilly and Company, F. Hoffman La Roche; and *contributors*, Bayer A. G. Leverkusen, McNeil, Novo Research Institute, ICI Belgium, Hope for Diabetics Foundation, New York, we express our appreciation for the financial support which made possible the Fourth International Symposium on Early Diabetes.

THE ORGANIZING COMMITTEE

Rafael A. Camerini-Davalos, M.D.
Stefan S. Fajans, M.D.
Norbert Freinkel, M.D.
J.J. Hoet, M.D.
Ernst Pfeiffer, M.D.

Contents

ENZYME INHIBITORS

MECHANISM OF ACTION OF ORAL COMPOUNDS

LONG TERM TREATMENT WITH ORAL COMPOUNDS

Animals

Humans

EARLY DIABETES. CONCEPT. TERMINOLOGY

R. A. Camerini-Davalos *

Can the art of predictive medicine anticipate the development of diabetes? Early diabetes is the period in life before fasting hyperglycemia (overt diabetes). In Fig. 1, we represent different levels of blood sugars. In the natural history of those predisposed to overt diabetes on genetic basis, the progression of the disease (increase in severity), if slow, would allow us to distinguish two stages: the first, with still normal blood sugars (first stage of early diabetes in Fig. 1); the second, with already abnormal blood sugars (second stage of early diabetes in Fig. 1) and finally, the "diabetic" level.

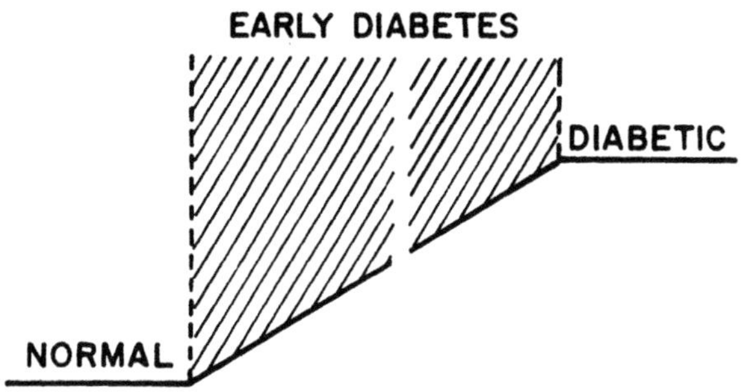

Fig. 1. Schematic representation of the 2 stages of early diabetes.

How early is early enough to attempt to delay the progression of the disease, or perhaps even prevent the abnormalities? Not at the stage of carbohydrate dysmetabolism,"by the time the carbohydrate abnormality manifests itself in terms of an abnormal glucose tolerance test, the damage has already been done. If we are to be of any help, we must work in a far earlier stage of the disease" (Conn) (1). If hyperglycemia, or even a barely significant abnormality of the glucose tolerance test, is a late event in the development of diabetes, what is before?

If disease is any deviation from the normal in form, function and/or chemistry of the body, then every disease, diabetes in our case, consists of abnormalities of these elements in varying degrees, proportions and importance. In the previous definition, hyperglycemia may not be present, but if other "deviations from the normal" can be *consistently* shown *before* hyperglycemia in those predisposed to it, that stage should be considered part of the disease.

THE PRE-HYPERGLYCEMIC PERIOD

What metabolic aberrations exist to produce a large baby, while the carbohydrate tolerance of the mother remains normal for another 10, 20 or even 30 years? Why is hyperplasia of the islet of Langerhans present in the fetal pancreas of the child, while the blood glucose of the mother remains normal?

We now know that these are some of the "abnormalities" inherited with the diabetic predisposition. They occur before hyperglycemia, during the "phase of dynamic resistance to diabetes" (2) the euglucemic stage of diabetes of Williams (3), which we call prediabetes.

Prediabetes means before diabetes, and was applied for the first time in 1927 by Marañon to signify the stage before hyperglycemia (4). Foglia used the term in 1944 (5). The term has been arbitrarily defined as the condition of those persons who are predisposed to hyperglycemia, but in whom no abnormalities of carbohydrate metabolism is demonstrable. From the definition, it is clear that the end of this stage is marked by the first detectable abnormality of carbohydrate metabolism. But when does it begin?

If conception marks "the beginning" of the disease, how early in life is the disease trend manifested? Even in those highly predisposed to diabetes on genetic basis, there is a period in life where the "dynamic resistance" is so effective that no abnormalities can be detected with our present capabilities and where diabetes can only be suspected on a genetic basis. Jackson (6) called this first stage without abnormalities "suspected prediabetes." (Fig. 2). The second, with abnormalities, we recognize as prediabetes.

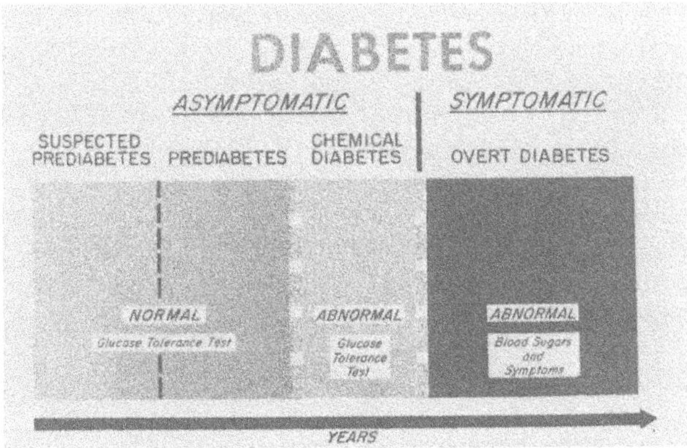

Fig. 2. Natural history of diabetes.

POSITIVE FINDINGS IN PREDIABETES

If disease in a person or in a population is testimony of failure, we need to use the concept of predisposition to heed the signs of incipient failure. But, in those predisposed to hyperglycemia, what are the biochemical hormonal and/or histological abnormalities which we must be able to find consistently in a given case, which would entitle us to call, prospectively, a patient prediabetic?

In persons with a greater diabetic potentiality (suspected prediabetics), studies have been conducted in the period of life up to the first abnormal glucose tolerance test. Many "deviations from the normal" have been found by us and other investigators. Some are shown in Table 1.

In spite of these findings and our advance in the knowledge of diabetes, no continuous systematic study has been attempted over the years on suspected prediabetics. How can we deny the possibility of making the diagnosis of prediabetes when we haven't really tried it? It has been known for a long time that there are persons with greater diabetic potentiality, and now we know that many abnormalities can be found in them. Probably the time has come to investigate in a significant number of suspected prediabetics for a sufficient number of years *all* the parameters found abnormal by different investigators (and some new ones), before we conclude that it is not possible to make the diagnosis of the pre-hyperglycemic stage, regardless of the term used for that period. There are many disease entities where a positive

TABLE 1. Positive findings in prediabetes.

MICROANGIOPATHY	
Thickened muscle capillary basement membrane	(7) (8) (9)
Abnormal monocrotic pulse wave	(10)
Nailbed aneurysm-like knobs	(11)
Microaneurysm in the conjunctiva	(in 10)
Microaneurysm in the retina	(in 10)
Increased mesangial area	(in 10)
HORMONAL DYSRHYTHMIA	
Decreased serum immunoreactive insulin levels (in Caucasian)	(in 12)
Decreased serum immunoreactive insulin increments at 30'	(in 12,13)
Increased serum immunoreactive insulin increments at 30' (in Pima Indians)	(14)
Increased serum glucagon levels	(in 10)
Non-suppression of glucagon during OGTT in twins	(15)
Decreased insulin/glucagon molar ratio	(16)
Higher growth hormone levels	(in 10 and 12)
OTHERS	
Increased intrahematic glycolysis	(17)
Increased serum sialic acid levels	(in 10)
Decreased replicative life-span of fibroblast	(18)

diagnosis is based on more than one or two abnormalities. Perhaps, for prediabetes, we may need 3, 4 or even more. Which ones?

NATURAL HISTORY OF DIABETES

The four stages, from suspected prediabetes to overt symptomatic diabetes (Fig. 2), are not necessarily progressive in a forward direction, but the condition may revert to earlier stages (as from chemical diabetes to prediabetes), and this may take place without change in body weight or treatment. In fact, during the early stages, diabetes must be regarded as a "fluid" condition which can progress or revert, depending upon different factors (Fig. 3).

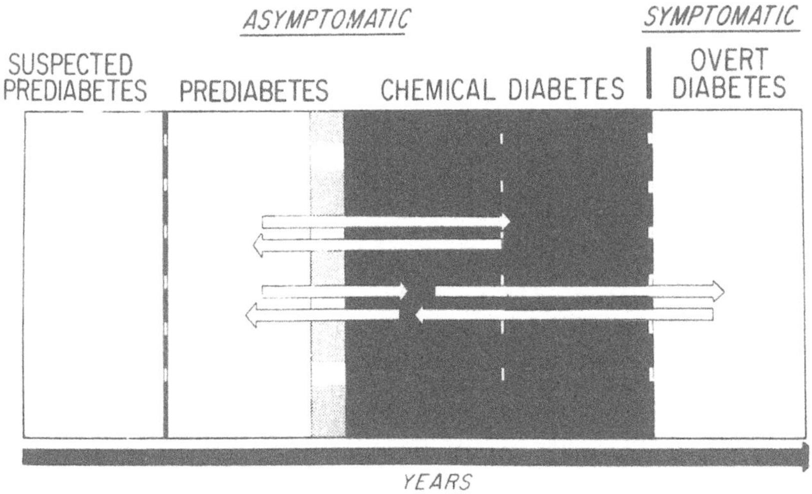

Fig. 3. Progression and/or regression in diabetes.

TABLE 2. Terminology in diabetes.

<table>
<tr><th colspan="3">ASYMPTOMATIC</th><th>SYMPTOMATIC</th></tr>
<tr><td colspan="2">POTENTIAL

POTENTIAL ABNORMALITY OF GLUCOSE TOLERANCE

PREVIOUS ABNORMALITY OF GLUCOSE TOLERANCE</td><td>LATENT

SUBCLINICAL

IMPAIRED GLUCOSE TOLERANCE

GESTATIONAL DIABETES</td><td>TYPE I
INSULIN-DEPENDENT DIABETES
JUVENILE ONSET DIABETES (JOD)

TYPE II
NOT INSULIN-DEPENDENT DIABETES
MATURITY ONSET DIABETES (MOD-MODY)</td></tr>
<tr><td>SUSPECTED PREDIABETES</td><td>PREDIABETES</td><td>CHEMICAL DIABETES</td><td>OVERT DIABETES</td></tr>
<tr><td colspan="2">Pre-Hyperglycemic</td><td></td><td></td></tr>
</table>

Table 2 shows the terminology proposed by the international work group convened by the NIH in 1978 at the top, and the one used by us at the bottom. We added the prehyperglycemic stage (to include both suspected prediabetes and prediabetes), since we found, lately, wider acceptance for this term.

CLINICAL SIGNIFICANCE

Aside from the significance that the recognition of the prehyperglycemic (prediabetic) stage has for research, can we accept that this has an important place in our daily work with patients? Is this stage the beginning of the disease? Is this part of what should be considered early diabetes? As we will show later, in a 12 year follow-up of 62 non-obese, non-treated prediabetic Caucasians, 20-45 years of age, 30 (48%) developed abnormality of the oral glucose tolerance test, and 8 (27%) overt diabetes.

Accepting that by the time the carbohydrate abnormality manifests itself, the damage has already been done (Conn) (1), the diagnosis of diabetes at the prehyperglycemic (prediabetes) stage of early diabetes will provide us with a basis to explore ways and means of halting the progression, or perhaps induce the regression, of the pathological process. Identification of risk factors (probably multifactorial), acting on the progression of diabetes, and longitudinal assessment of feasibility, safety and effectiveness of risk-factor modification seems a valuable approach to prevention.

REFERENCES

1. *Conn, J.W. (1970) in Early Diabetes. eds. R.A. Camerini-Davalos and H. Cole. Ac. Press. New York, p. 259.*
2. *Conn. J.W. and S. Fajans (1961). Am. J. Med. 31, 389.*
3. *Williams, R.H. (1970) in Early Diabetes. eds. R.A. Camerini-Davalos and H. Cole. Ac. Press. New York, p. 259.*
4. *Marañon, G. (1927). Novak, Budapest.*
5. *Foglia, V.G. (1944). Rev. Soc. Arg. Biol. 20, 21.*
6. *Jackson, W.P.U. (1962). Diabetes, 11, 334.*
7. *Camerini-Davalos, R.A., et al. (1979). J. Clin. End. Met. 48, 251.*
8. *Siperstein, M.B., et al. (1968). J. Clin. Inv. 47, 1973.*
9. *Aronoff, S.L., et al. (1976). Abstract 1st Int. Symp. on the Biology and Chemistry of Basement Membranes. Phila, Penn. p. 8.*
10. *Camerini-Davalos, R.A., et al. (1970) in Diabetes Mellitus: Theory and Practice. M. Ellenberg and H. Rifkind. McGraw-Hill, New York. p. 508*
11. *Camerini-Davalos, R.A., et al. (1977) in Insulin and Metabolism, ed. J.S. Bajaj. Excerpta Medica. Amsterdam, p. 147.*
12. *Johansen, K., et al. (1974). Metabolism 23, 1185.*
13. *Oppermann, W., et al. (1979) in Treatment of Early Diabetes, ed. R.A. Camerini-Davalos and B. Hanover. Plenum Press, New York p. 177.*
14. *Savage, P.J. (1979) in Treatment of Early Diabetes ed. R.A. Camerini-Davalos and B. Hanover. Plenum Press, New York p. 13.*
15. *Day, J.L. and Anderson, J. (1973). Clin. End. 2, 211.*
16. *Tiengo, A., et al. (1978). Acta Diab. Lat. 3-4, 143*
17. *Castillo-Olivares, J., et al. (1973). Diabetes 22: 6, 466.*
18. *Goldstein, S., et al. (1978). Science 199, 781.*

EARLY STAGES OF DIABETES: DEFINITIONS AND PRESENT CONCEPTS

S. S. Fajans*

Definitions are necessary in devising a classification of various types of diabetes mellitus and stages in the evolution or natural history of the disease(s). Definitions and classifications are useful if they can be applied uniformly to various forms and stages of diabetes so that investigators can compare data derived from studies in similarly defined populations groups. In the past, definitions of the stages of the disease have varied between different investigators and in different countries. In April of 1978, the National Diabetes Data Group of the National Institutes of Health convened an International Work Group in Bethesda in the hope of devising a uniformly acceptable classification and terminology of diabetes mellitus. Although the outcome of these deliberations did not deal specifically with early diabetes mellitus, I will try to incorporate some of the definitions proposed at this meeting, and to be published soon, in the attempt to present and define up-to-date concepts of early diabetes mellitus. I should mention at the onset that some of the terms accepted for classification of idiopathic diabetes mellitus and other categories of glucose intolerance are compromises and not ideal solutions.

Why are we interested in recognizing early diabetes? There are two main reasons. In the first place, the only way to find the underlying basic etiological and pathogenetic mechanisms that lead to clinical diabetes is to study the disease in its earliest possible forms. Secondly, the only way to apply effective prophylactic measures is to find the genetic defects which characterize a predisposition to the diabetic state and to identify the environmental factors which initiate or cause further progression of the biochemical, physiological and pathological abnormalities of the disease.

Before proceeding with an attempt at discussing definitions for early diabetes, we must have an understanding of 1) the heterogeneous nature of primary or idiopathic diabetes and 2) the natural history of the various forms of the disease. Excluded from a definition of primary or idiopathic diabetes is glucose intolerance associated with certain conditions and syndromes such as diabetes secondary to pancreatic disease, secondary to endocrine disease or hormone administration, drug-induced carbohydrate intolerance, the large number of chromosomal and genetic syndromes associated with glucose intolerance, and finally, the rare cases of diabetes associated with severe insulin receptor abnormalities or defects. Another possible exclusion would be glucose intolerance associated with hyperlipidemias.

In defining the heterogeneity of idiopathic diabetes we must recognize two large groups of patients which differ from each other in genetic background and in the superimposed environmental factors which precipitate the disease. The first group is insulin-dependent, ketosis-prone diabetes. It is also called juvenile-onset *type* diabetes, abreviated as JOD, or Type I diabetes. The second large group is not-insulin-dependent, ketosis-resistant or Type II diabetes. This is also known as maturity-onset *type* diabetes of middle age or older populations (MOD) and maturity-onset *type* diabetes of the young (MODY). Although there is clear-cut evidence for further heterogeneity within both types of diabetes, I will not discuss these subclasses further at this time.

There are at least five lines of evidence that these two major types of diabetes differ from each other genetically. These lines of evidence, reviewed previously (1), are: 1) differences in familial patterns of inheritance, 2) characteristic findings of histocompatibility antigens or HLA patterns in JOD but not in MOD, 3) differing incidence of diabetes in identical twins of JOD and of MOD diabetics, 4) evidence for cell-mediated immunity and 5) of circulating islet cell antibodies in JOD but not in MOD. These two types of diabetes appear to differ from each other also in the environmental causes which precipitate the disease. At the present time the best theory is that viral infections leading to an autoimmune process precipitate the disease in the majority of patients with insulin-dependent diabetes, while the most important environmental factor leading to not-insulin-dependent diabetes is excessive caloric intake leading to obesity.

Let us now return to an attempt at the definition of "early diabetes". This may be facilitated by considering what is not early diabetes. First, we will discuss insulin-dependent diabetes mellitus. Obviously, ketosis-prone diabetes is not early diabetes even at first recognition, since it is associated with ketosis and fasting hyperglycemia. The same is true for the pre-ketotic stage, since it is associated with fasting hyperglycemia - it is overt diabetes. By prospective testing of asymptomatic siblings of insulin-dependent diabetics, abnormalities of glucose tolerance uniformly accepted as characteristic of diabetes may be found. If test results fall below these criteria for interpretation of the glucose tolerance test, but above glucose levels accepted as indicating normal glucose tolerance test, such patients would be classified as having "impaired glucose tolerance". In either case, one could accept such patients with abnormal or impaired glucose tolerance as having early diabetes because they progress rapidly (usually within two years) to overt diabetes. Other characteristics of JOD, in addition to glucose intolerance, may be found in such individuals. These patients may have the same characteristic HLA type as their diabetic family members, and they may have circulating islet cell antibodies (ICA).

The period of time or stage before the development of an abnormal glucose tolerance test or an impaired glucose tolerance test in an identical twin of a JOD patient would have been defined as prediabetes by our nomenclature or potential diabetes by the W.H.O. nomenclature in the past. (2) These terms were used to identify the interval of time from conception until the demonstration of abnormal or impaired glucose tolerance in an individual predisposed to diabetes on genetic grounds. This period can be identified only retrospectively. The term proposed at the NIH meeting for this stage is "potential abnormality of glucose tolerance". "Potential abnormality of glucose tolerance" can be suspected to be present in individuals who have an increased probability of developing diabetes on genetic grounds, such as in some nondiabetic identical twins of JOD diabetic patients or in some offspring of JOD patient who is also a sibling of a JOD. The likelihood of a genetic predisposition to diabetes is firmer if the nondiabetic individual shares histocompatibility antigens identical to those of his diabetic first-degree relative. If islet cell antibodies (ICA) are detected during this stage, the likelihood of this individual developing diabetes is even greater. If ICA are present, the assumption may be made that superimposed environmental factors such as viral infection may have caused islet cell damage leading to an autoimmune process. Since diabetes does not develop until there is the superimposition of an environmental factor on a genetic predisposition, the term prediabetes is not appropriate to label a genetic predisposition alone.

Let us proceed to the second large group of idiopathic diabetes, namely not-insulin-dependent diabetes, ketosis-resistant diabetes, Type II diabetes, or MOD or MODY. If there is fasting hyperglycemia, even if asymptomatic, it is not early diabetes. Let us take the patient who has abnormal or impaired glucose tolerance with a normal fasting level of plasma glucose. If this patient progresses to fasting hyperglycemia rapidly, the stage during which an abnormal or impaired glucose tolerance test was present could be designated as early diabetes. But what if the progression to fasting hyperglycemia takes two decades? I would like to give two examples.

Patient A.S. is an individual who had abnormal glucose tolerance on routine testing at age 10, and repeatedly thereafter, but did not develop fasting hyperglycemia until age 28. Patient G.G. was 16 years old when impaired glucose tolerance test was first found because routine glucose tolerance tests were performed on her and family members because of a strong family history of diabetes. She developed fasting hyperglycemia 19 years later. She had delayed and low insulin responses to administered glucose. Both patients come from families with MODY and vascular disease. Is the period of 18 years of abnormal or impaired glucose tolerance early diabetes? This depends on whether our definition of early diabetes is made on the basis of a biochemical abnormality alone without considering the duration of glucose intolerance.

What if there is an abnormal glucose tolerance test which does not progress to fasting hyperglycemia? A few would say that this is not diabetes. An example is patient B.V. in whom there has been no progression of glucose intolerance for 25 years. This patient has other evidence of abnormalities characteristic of the diabetic state such as muscle capillary basement membrane thickening. She comes from a family of four generations of MODY some members having had vascular disease. If the first abnormal glucose tolerance test and the glucose tolerance test after 25 years are similar, are we dealing with a quarter of a century of early diabetes? If we designated only the first abnormal test as indicating early diabetes, how do we know that abnormal glucose tolerance might not have been present 15 years earlier in this asymptomatic patient. Abnormal glucose tolerance test were found at ages 17 years in her two sons. The earliest stage certainly would have been from conception to the first recognition of abnormal glucose tolerance since we are dealing with a genetically-determined disease. But this stage, formerly called prediabetes and now called potential abnormality of glucose tolerance, can be recognized only retrospectively, since we still lack a reliable marker for the disease. Note that "potential abnormality of glucose tolerance" is no improvement on the term "potential diabetes" in this context.

In summary, the definition and characterization of "early diabetes" is most difficult even if we insist on the presence of an abnormal glucose tolerance test or impaired glucose tolerance test as a marker for early diabetes. Under these circumstances, early diabetes can be easily defined in patients who will be insulin-dependent diabetics because of their usual rapid progression. On the other hand, in patients with not-insulin-dependent diabetes, the definition of early diabetes is difficult because of the nonprogressive or slowly progressive nature of the disease. Since the recognition that a genetic predisposition alone does not lead to diabetes under all circumstances but that superimposed environmental factors are necessary, we should not designate a genetic predisposition to diabetes as early diabetes.

REFERENCES

1. *Fajans, S.S., et al., (1978). Diabetes 27, 1112.*
2. *Fajans, S.S., et al., (1974). In: Diabetes: Proceedings of the 8th Cong. IDF, Excerpta Medica Int'l. Cong. Series No. 312, Malaisse, W.J.& Pirart, J., Eds., Amsterdam, 329.*

Supported in part by U.S. Public Health Service Grants AM-00888, National Institute of Arthritis, Metabolism and Digestive Diseases and by grants from The Upjohn Company, Kalamazoo, Michigan and Pfizer, Inc., New York, New York.

PREDIABETES IN THE PIMA INDIANS

P. J. Savage*, R. F. Hamman, and P. H. Bennett

The Pima Indians, an American Indian tribe with the highest known prevalence of ketosis-resistant diabetes mellitus, have participated in a longitudinal study of diabetes and related conditions for over a decade (1). They offer a unique opportunity to study the changes associated with the development of diabetes.

METHODS

Studies have been conducted among the residents of the Gila River Indian Community, primarily Pima Indians with some admixture of the closely related Papago tribe. An attempt has been made to examine all residents of the community five years of age and older. Approximately 88% of the eligible population has had at least one examination which includes a medical history, physical examination and a 75 gm oral carbohydrate tolerance test which is performed without regard to age, weight, time of day or time since last meal.** Two hours later venous blood is obtained for measurement of plasma glucose concentration by the ferricyanide method.

The effect of the presence or absence of parental diabetes upon glucose tolerance and the degree of obesity has been examined in a subgroup of 1261 offspring, 5 to 24 years of age, whose both parents had glucose tolerance tests. Body mass index (weight/height) was utilized as a measure of obesity in subjects over the age of 24 years. (2) Because of difficulties in interpretation of the body mass index in growing subjects, the percent of desirable weight was determined as a measure of obesity in 5-24 year old subjects (3).

For studies of factors leading to the development of diabetes, subjects were considered non-diabetic if two hour plasma glucose

**Dexcola, Ames Laboratories, Tarrytown, N.Y.

levels were less than 200 mg/dl and they had no history of use of hypoglycemic medications. A two hour plasma glucose greater than or equal to 250 mg/dl was considered diagnostic of an incident case of diabetes. The area between 200 and 250 mg/dl was excluded in this analysis since during a period of follow-up, some of these subjects spontaneously improved while glucose tolerance deteriorated in the majority. In assigning a diagnosis to parents for the studies of the offspring, a two hour plasma glucose level of greater than or equal to 200 mg/dl was considered diagnostic of diabetes. These definitions have been selected after consideration of the previously described bimodal character of the distribution of logarithms of the two hour plasma glucose levels in Pima adults. Two hour plasma glucose concentrations between 200 and 250 mg/dl fall between the two distributions and thus contain a mixture of subjects from both groups (4).

A smaller number of subjects characterized on the basis of parental diabetic status were admitted to the Clinical Research Unit of the Phoenix Indian Medical Center for studies of glucose, insulin and glucagon responses to oral and intravenous glucose and to arginine infusion, and studies of the binding of insulin to circulating mononuclear cells. This smaller number had two hour plasma glucose levels in response to oral glucose of less than 140 mg/dl. They were classified, on the basis of parental glucose tolerance, into genetic normals and genetic prediabetics. Serum insulin was measured by a double antibody method, plasma glucagon by the method of Unger using antiserum 30K. Binding of ^{125}I-insulin to circulating mononuclear cells was measured as described by Bar (5) with results standardized for the percentage of monocytes in the preparation. Monocytes were quantified by the non-specific esterase stain of Li (6).

RESULTS AND INTERPRETATION

The logarithms of the two hour plasma glucose concentrations in Pimas above the age of 25 years are distributed bimodally. Subjects in the second mode of the distribution are considered unequivocally diabetic. They are generally characterized by both fasting hyperglycemia and two hour plasma glucose levels greater than 225 mg/dl. Subjects with two hour plasma glucose levels in the first mode of the distribution are a mixture of those with unequivocally normal glucose tolerance and those with borderline or impaired glucose tolerance. Although they cannot be individually identified, within this mode are the "true prediabetics", i.e., those subjects who cannot yet be said to be diabetic but who are destined to progress to unequivocal diabetes.

Follow-up examinations of subjects in the first mode of the bimodal distribution has enabled further characterization of the prediabetic state. Of individuals 25 years of age and older who entered the study from 1965 to 1973, 1020 had two hour plasma glucose levels below 200 mg/dl. Of these, 132 had two hour plasma glucose levels at or above 250 mg/dl upon subsequent examination and were considered to have developed unequivocal diabetes. Standard life table methods were utilized to obtain maximum data on risk of decompensation (7). The eight year cumulative probability of developing diabetes was calculated to be 23.7%. In addition, a binary multiple linear regression model was used to adjust simultaneously for multiple variables, in addition to duration of follow-up (8), enabling assessment of the corrected risk of decompensation for each individual factor. This analysis yielded significant associations of decompensation on follow-up examination with initial two hour plasma glucose ($p < 0.001$), the initial degree of obesity ($p < 0.001$) and a history of diabetes in one or both of the parents ($p < 0.01$).

After adjustment for confounding variables, both obesity and initial two hour plasma glucose levels greater than or equal to 140 mg/dl remained significant independent risk factors. In contrast, the contribution of family history decreased substantially, suggesting that the risk of decompensation due to diabetes in a parent is expressed, at least in part, through changes in other measured variables. In addition, combinations of the risk factors were at least additive in prediction of risk of decompensation.

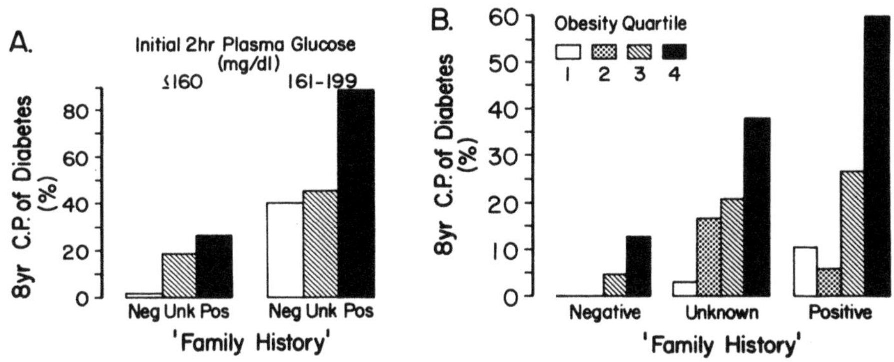

Fig. 1. A) Effect of initial 2 hour glucose level and family history and B) of obesity quartile and family history upon the 8 year cumulative probability of diabetes.

Figure 1A shows the effects of combining parental history and initial two hour plasma glucose level upon the frequency of progression to diabetes. It can be seen that within each two hour plasma glucose group the risk of decompensation was substantially increased by a history of diabetes in one or both parents. Similarly, the effect of combining obesity and a parental history of diabetes is seen in figure 1B. Again, within each obesity quartile, the risk of decompensation associated with a positive parental history is increased.

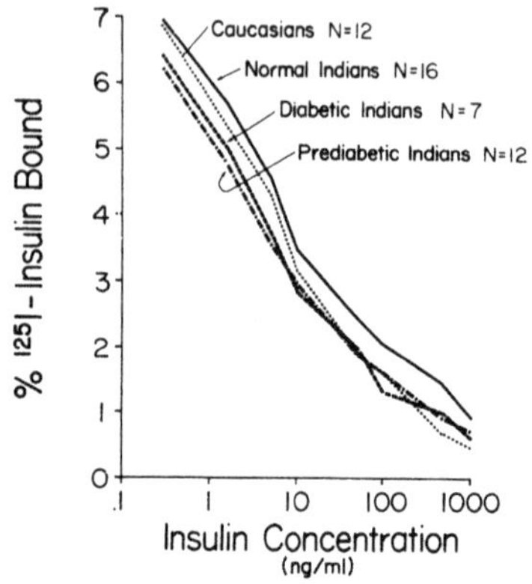

Fig. 3. Mean specific binding of ^{125}I-insulin to circulating mononuclear cells in the presence of 0 to 1000 ng/ml of unlabeled insulin in Caucasians (····), normal Indians (——), diabetic Indians (----), and prediabetic Indians (-·-·) corrected for percentage of monocytes in each subject.

In conclusion, studies of the prediabetic state in the Pima have indicated a complex interrelationship between family history, degree of obesity and the initial two hour plasma glucose level. It appears that diabetes in the parents may contribute to the development of diabetes by initially predisposing the subject to obesity which is followed, after some period of years, by the development of impaired glucose tolerance. Unexplained hyperinsulinemia has also been demonstrated in the Pimas. It appears that further studies to elucidate the relationship of hyperinsulinemia to the development of obesity may extend our understanding of the earliest changes occurring in subjects predisposed to the eventual development of diabetes.

ACKNOWLEDGEMENTS

We wish to thank the Pima Indian patients who volunteered for this investigation, together with Ms. Judy Brown, Linda Phillips, and Mary Barham for technical assistance, and Ms. Jean Koopman and the nursing staff of the Phoenix Clinical Research Section, and Ms. Janet Clark for secretarial assistance.

REFERENCES

1. *Bennett, P.H., (1976). in Recent Progress in Hormone Research, Greep, R.O. ed., Academic Press, N.Y., 333.*
2. *Keys, A., et al., (1972) J. Chron. Dis. 25, 329.*

while mean glucose levels of offspring of mixed parentage have remained similar to those of the offspring of non-diabetic parents. In this age group the difference in mean percent desirable weights (Figure 2D) has increased ($p < 0.05$) and mean percent desirable weights of subjects with mixed parentage are intermediate between those of the genetic normals and the genetic prediabetics. If the subjects with mixed parentage are combined, mean percent desirable weights of these subjects differ significantly ($p < 0.05$) from those of subjects with two normal parents.

Frequency distributions of logarithms of two hour plasma glucose levels were examined in 5-14 and 15-24 year old offspring to look for evidence of bimodality. In the 5-14 year old subjects there were no obvious differences in distributions based upon parental classification. In the 15-24 year old subjects differences in the frequency distributions became apparent. The lowest distribution is made up of subjects with two non-diabetic parents. In subjects with two diabetic parents the distribution of plasma glucose levels is skewed to the right and median values are elevated. In addition, the appearance of a small percentage of outliers probably represents the first detectable evidence of development of bimodality in the distribution of glucose levels.

To investigate the prediabetic state further subjects with unquestionably normal glucose tolerance (two hour plasma glucose levels less than 140 mg/dl on an OGTT) who had two parents with unequivocal diabetes or individuals who had two parents over age 45 years with two hour plasma glucose levels less than 160 mg/dl were compared to each other and to overtly diabetic Pimas and to Caucasians with normal glucose tolerance and no family history of diabetes (9). Results of both oral and intravenous glucose tolerance tests and of arginine infusion tests have demonstrated both fasting and stimulated hyperinsulinemia in the non-diabetic Indians compared to Caucasians of a similar degree of obesity ($p < 0.01$). No detectable abnormalities in glucagon secretion were found in the prediabetic state (10).

Figure 3 shows binding of ^{125}I-insulin to circulating mononuclear cells. No differences were apparent among genetic normal and prediabetic Indians, diabetic Indians or normal Caucasians suggesting that abnormalities in binding are not a primary determinant in the pathogenesis of diabetes in the Pima. Nevertheless, the levels of insulin binding found in the Indians occur in the presence of fasting insulin levels twice those of the Caucasians ($p < 0.05$). This suggests that hyperinsulinemia in the Pima may be secondary to either an abnormality in circulating insulin or to a post-receptor resistance to the action of bound insulin.

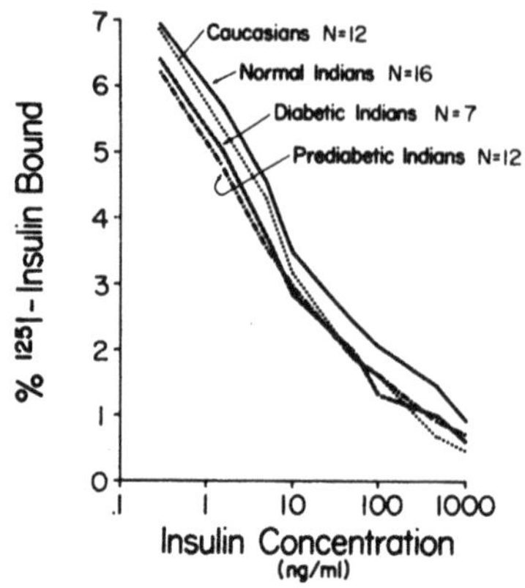

Fig. 3. Mean specific binding of ^{125}I-insulin to circulating mononuclear cells in the presence of 0 to 1000 ng/ml of unlabeled insulin in Caucasians (····), normal Indians (——), diabetic Indians (----), and prediabetic Indians (-·-·) corrected for percentage of monocytes in each subject.

In conclusion, studies of the prediabetic state in the Pima have indicated a complex interrelationship between family history, degree of obesity and the initial two hour plasma glucose level. It appears that diabetes in the parents may contribute to the development of diabetes by initially predisposing the subject to obesity which is followed, after some period of years, by the development of impaired glucose tolerance. Unexplained hyperinsulinemia has also been demonstrated in the Pimas. It appears that further studies to elucidate the relationship of hyperinsulinemia to the development of obesity may extend our understanding of the earliest changes occurring in subjects predisposed to the eventual development of diabetes.

ACKNOWLEDGEMENTS

We wish to thank the Pima Indian patients who volunteered for this investigation, together with Ms. Judy Brown, Linda Phillips, and Mary Barham for technical assistance, and Ms. Jean Koopman and the nursing staff of the Phoenix Clinical Research Section, and Ms. Janet Clark for secretarial assistance.

REFERENCES

1. *Bennett, P.H., (1976). in Recent Progress in Hormone Research, Greep, R.O. ed., Academic Press, N.Y., 333.*
2. *Keys, A., et al., (1972) J. Chron. Dis. 25, 329.*

3. *Recommended Dietary Allowances. (1964). Publication 1146. Rpt. of Food and Nutr. Board. Wash., D.C., Nat'l. Res. Council, Nat'l. Acad. of Sci.*
4. *Rushforth, N.B., et al., (1971). Diabetes 20, 756.*
5. *Bar, R.S., et al., (1976). J. Clin. Invest. 58, 1123.*
6. *Li, C.Y., et al., (1973). J. Histochem. Cytochem. 21, 1.*
7. *Cutler, S.J. and Ederer, F. (1958). J. Chronic. Dis. 8, 699.*
8. *Feldstein, M.S. (1966). J. R. Stat. Soc. 129, Ser. A, Part 1, 61.*
9. *Aronoff, S.L., et al.(1977). Diabetes 26, 827.*
10. *Aronoff, S.L., et al.(1976). Diabetes 25, 404.*

Supported in part by National Institutes of Health Contract N01-AM-6-2219.

THE PROGNOSIS OF INSULIN DEPENDENT DIABETES MELLITUS AND THE IMPORTANCE OF SUPERVISION

T. Deckert* and M. Larsen

The aim of this study was to determine whether metabolic control, treatment of complications, education and social support have really been of benefit to our juvenile diabetic population.

One thousand four hundred fifty-one insulin-dependent diabetics (797 men and 654 women) with onset before the age of 31, and prior to the year 1953, admitted between 1933 and 1975, were studied. This group comprised about 18% of all patients in Denmark. We tried to follow this group either until death or until 1/1/76. Onset is defined as the year in which diabetes was diagnosed. Twenty-six were diagnosed before insulin first came into use in Scandinavia in 1923. All but 13 (9 females and 4 males) were treated with insulin, mostly twice daily. Forty-four (3%) of the 1451 patients could not be traced. The remaining 1407 patients were followed until death (654 patients, 46.4%) or until 1/1/76 (753 patients).

Morbidity was evaluated during the year before death, or in the case of survivors, in 1973, partly on the basis of information from our own case records, and those from other hospitals (153 cases), partly by written inquiries (49 cases) and personal interviews and examinations (62 cases). The following factors were analyzed: Visual acuity: impaired vision = unable to read the daily paper without a magnifying glass. Blindness = vision 6/60. Renal function, impaired renal function = serum creatinine persistently 2.0 mg/100 ml (measured by the Jaffe method), or blood urea persistently 60 mg/100 ml (measured as per van Slyke). Proteinuria = Albustix or Heller positive (50-100 mg protein/1000 ml urine) for more than one year. Cardio-vascular functions: the presence of gangrene, amputation below-knee or above knee, objective evidence of previous or present stroke with limb paralysis, objective evidence of myocardial infarction (typical ECG changes combined with pyrexia, chest pain and/or elevated glutamic-oxalacetic acid transaminase, or findings at autopsy).

For assessing survival two parameters were used: 1) duration of diabetes, 2) relative survival, i.e., survival in relation to the general population of the same age and sex. This calculation was based upon the comparable mortality rated/1000 for the total population of Denmark given in the Danish Year Books of Statistics (Statistisk Arbog).

To describe the duration of survival, decrement analysis were used (1), and for comparison of the two decrement curves, Gehan's Wilcoxon test was used (2,3). The prognostic importance of supervision was studied: 1) by comparing survival with frequency of out-patient visits during the first 20 years of diabetes, and 2) by comparing domicile to survival, since the only diabetic center in existence between 1932 and 1953 was located in the Copenhagen area. Domicile was divided into greater Copenhagen, urban areas outside Copenhagen and rural districts.

All the patients in the study on supervision had been admitted to the hospital within the first fifteen years of their diabetes (n = 1060). One group (n = 537) did not have further contact with the out-patient clinic after the first admission. The second group (n = 162) had one to six contacts at the out-patient clinic during the first 20 diabetic years, the third group (n = 205) had 7 to 42 contacts at the out-patient clinic, and the fourth group (n = 156) had 43 to 156 contacts at the out-patient clinic during the first 20 years of diabetes.

RESULTS

Fig. 1 shows the importance of the duration of diabetes to survival. Almost 50% of the patients had died after 30 years of diabetes, irrespective of whether the diabetes had developed during the age range 0-10, 11-20, or 21-30. Only diabetics with diabetes onset between 0 and 10 years of age had a significantly longer survival. The relative survival is shown on figure 2a. At the time when only 10% of the age and sex-matched background population had died, about 60% of the diabetic population had succumbed. Patients whose diabetes had begun between the ages of 0 and 10 years had a significantly worse relative survival than patients with diabetes onset between 11 and 20, or 21 and 30 years (Fig. 2b). Compared to age and sex-matched non-diabetics, diabetic females did not have a better survival than diabetic males.

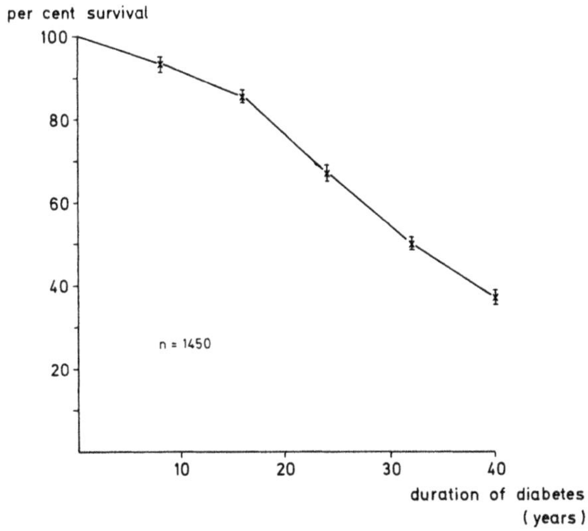

Fig. 1. *Percent survival (mean ± standard deviation) of 1450 juvenile diabetics with diabetes onset before 1953. Whole study population; age at onset.*

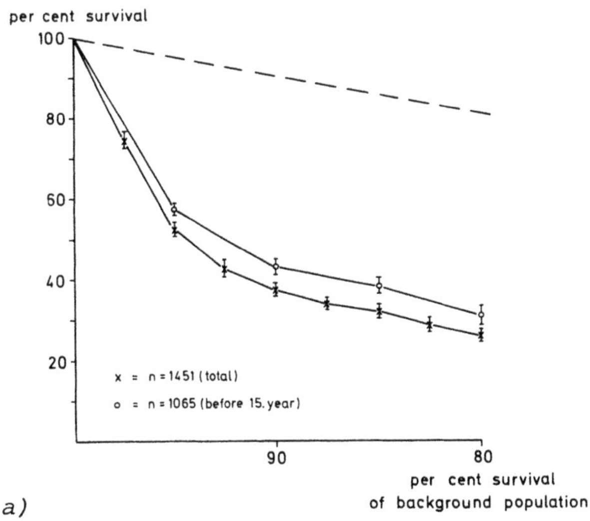

a)

Fig. 2. *Percent survival (mean ± standard deviation) of 1451 juvenile diabetics compared to the percent survival of age and sex matched non-diabetics taken from the Danish Statistical Year Book. Survival of the non-diabetic population is shown by the dotted line.*

a) Whole study population and patients who have been seen at the Steno Memorial Hospital during the first fifteen years of diabetes

b) According to age at onset

Survival was decreased by the development of proteinuria (Fig. 3). Although patients without proteinuria in the course of 40-50 years of diabetes had a mortality about twice that of sex and age matched background population, the mortality among diabetics with persistent proteinuria was about eight times.

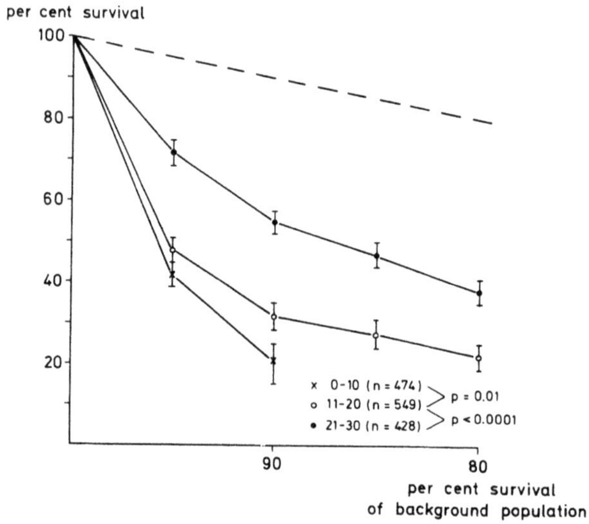

Fig. 2b

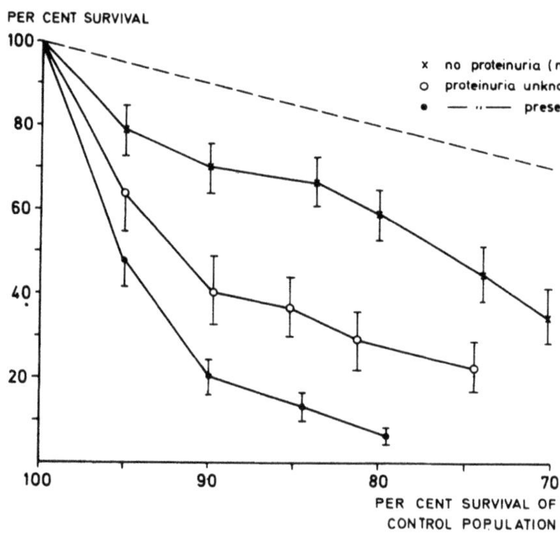

Fig. 3

Fig. 4 illustrates the importance of supervision at the out-patient clinic. Patients with frequent visits during the first 20 years of diabetes had a significantly better prognosis than patients with few visits. Patients who contacted the hospital within the first fifteen years of diabetes and who were domiciled near the hospital had a significantly better survival than patients living far away, despite the fact that rural residents live longer than Copenhagen residents (Fig. 5). Serious end-stage diabetic complications occurred earlier and more frequently in patients with less than 20 visits to the out-patient clinic during the first 20 diabetic years, than in patients with more frequent visits to the out-patient clinic (Table 1).

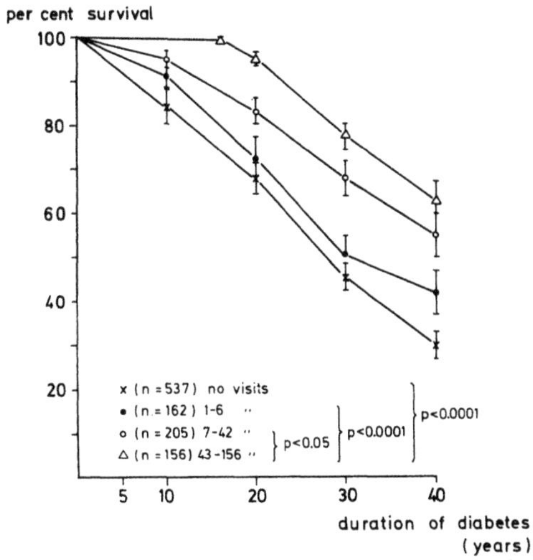

Fig. 4. *Percent survival (mean ± standard deviation) of four groups of juvenile diabetics until more than 40 years after onset of diabetes. The patients were admitted to the Steno Memorial Hospital within 15 years from the onset of diabetes and had frequent (7-42 visits and 43-156 visits), sporadic (1-6 visits) or no visits at the hospital during the first 20 years of diabetes. Duration of diabetes, all patients included.*

Fig. 3. *Percent survival (mean ± standard deviation of 307 juvenile diabetics with diabetes onset before 1933, compared to the percent survival of age and sex matched non-diabetics (dotted line). Group 1: patients who did not develop proteinuria until 1973; Group 2: patients who developed proteinuria before 1973; Group 3: (in between) patients in whom development of proteinuria before 1973 was unknown; Group 1/2: $p < 0.0001$; Group 1/3: $p < 0.0001$; Group 2/3: $p < 0.0005$.*

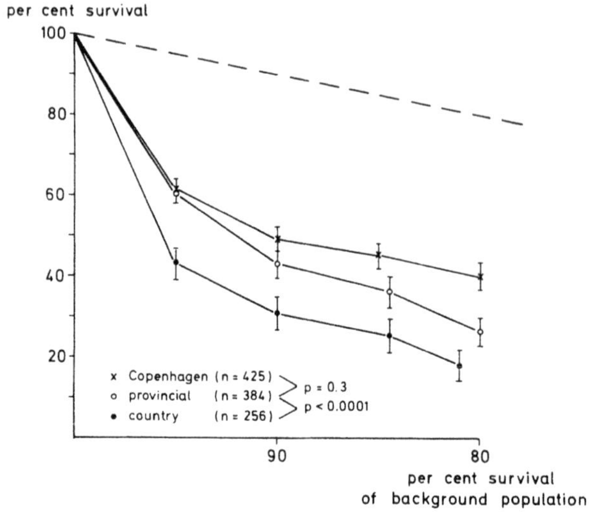

Fig. 5. Percent survival (mean ± standard deviation) of 3 groups of juvenile diabetics living in Copenhagen, provincial towns or in rural districts. The patients were admitted to the hospital during the first 15 years of diabetes. Comparison with age and sex matched non-diabetics. Survival of the non-diabetic population is shown by the dotted line.

Table 1

	FREQUENT CONTACT N = 51	SPORADIC CONTACT N = 67
DIABETES DURATION (YEARS)	40 ± 9	32 ± 10
BLINDNESS (PER CENT)	12	29
AMPUTATION/GANGRENE	10	15
CEREBRAL VASCULAR INSULT	6	12
PROTEINURIA	28	47
UREMIA	16	35
MYOCARDIAL INFARCTION	29	18

CONCLUSIONS

Duration and quality of life are considerably reduced in insulin-dependent diabetic patients, but regular metabolic supervision, education of the patients, and social support can reduce the prevalence of severe late diabetic complications and prolong life by about 10 years.

REFERENCES

1. *Kaplan, E.L. and P. Meier (1958). J. Am. Statist. Anoc. 53,475*
2. *Gehan, E. (1965). Biometrica 52, 203*
3. *Aalen, O. (1979). Ann. Statist. (In Press)*

DISCUSSION

G. M. REAVEN: *Dr. Savage, in the patients who begin to develop differences in the two hour postprandial sugars, your 15-24 age group, are there more obese? What are their insulin levels and have you tried to reduce their weights to see what happens to their abnormalities?*

P. SAVAGE: *The group which deteriorates at the youngest age tends to be more obese. The insulin levels are high in some of these individuals. We haven't been able to follow all of them. We have dieted only a few of the individuals and they seemed to respond quite nicely to diet.*

N. FREINKEL: *Dr. Savage, do you notice any difference in the offspring when you have one diabetic parent, such as diabetic mothers with normal fathers vis a vis diabetic fathers with normal mothers? I'm thinking specifically of intrauterine environment.*

P. SAVAGE: *I didn't mention it, but one of the things we've noticed is that the offspring of a diabetic mother and non-diabetic father, 15-24 years of age, are heavier than the offspring of the diabetic father and the non-diabetic mother. Therefore, one of the things we should look into is whether or not obesity at birth, possibly related to maternal diabetes, leads to heavier children and more likely deterioration at earlier age groups.*

N. FREINKEL: *Do you have any data with regard to insulin secretory potential, etc., as a function of intrauterine environment?*

P. SAVAGE: *We don't have any data on that at the moment.*

J. BARBOSA: *Dr. Savage, what kind of correlation do you find between obesity and insulin levels in these patients? Also, do you measure the insulin several times on a prospective basis to see if this is a persistent or fluctuating phenomenon?*

P. SAVAGE: *The correlation between fasting insulin levels and degree of obesity is about .6 to .7, which I think is reasonably comparable to what has been seen in other racial groups. However, there is a hyperinsulinemia in the Pimas which doesn't seem to be accounted for by the degree of obesity. As far as sequential insulin levels are concerned, the data hasn't been fully analyzed, but they do appear to be hyperinsulinemic on multiple examinations. The hyperinsulinemia, from some cross-sectional data, appears to develop around the time of puberty.*

J. A. RULL-RODRIGO: *Dr. Savage, have you tried to correlate insulin levels with some special foodstuff in the diet, as high content of carbohydrates?*

P. SAVAGE: *We have. We don't have complete information on that yet, but there were some dietary surveys of the Pimas early in the study. The basic finding was that the percentages of protein, carbohydrate and fat were similar to that of the U.S. population, although the total caloric intake of Pima adults was increased by a couple of hundred calories per day. The one striking difference which was noted was that the source of protein differed; there was a higher percentage of protein obtained from vegetable sources.*

R. CAMERINI-DAVALOS: *We found bimodality when we determined the muscle capillary basement membrane in our genetic prediabetics. Dr. Savage also found what appears to be a bimodality. In our study one group of prediabetics had basement membrane within the range of the normal population;in the other group the basement membrane was abnormal. Fifty-four percent of those with abnormal basement membrane develop chemical diabetes. It seems to us that this progression of the disease should be an indication that prediabetes is the first step. Dr. Fajans, why don't you accept now that prediabetes is a stage of the disease?*

S. FAJANS: *First of all, as far as basement membrane thickening is concerned, we've performed about 170 basement membrane biopsies now in our relatives of diabetic patients who do not have glucose intolerance. Thus far, we have not seen basement membrane thickening in those who do not have glucose intolerance. As far as your question is concerned, we once used the same definition of prediabetes which you did, but I think we are further along now since the last Early Diabetes conference. First of all, we have at least two types of diabetes, as I've pointed out. Secondly, I think, since that time, we have clarified what we've known right along, but really not crystallized in our minds, that there are both genetic and environmental factors.*

Referring back to the insulin-requiring diabetics, a sibling with the same HLA type as a diabetic is not necessarily a prediabetic. He becomes a diabetic only with a superimposition of the environmental factor.

R. CAMERINI-DAVALOS: *Steve (Fajans) I hope you realize that you didn't answer my question. I asked you what abnormalities you would like to find at the stage of prediabetes which will change your mind and accept prediabetes as a stage?*

S. FAJANS: *I think I did answer that. I don't think we can make a diagnosis of prediabetes. We said 18 years ago that prediabetes is a stage from conception to the first recognizable abnormality of carbohydrates. It's something that can be made only in retrospect. I don't think you can make a prospective diagnosis of prediabetes.*

H. LEBOVITZ: *Question-comment to Dr. Savage. I was very intrigued by the observations that there was no real change in insulin-binding to the monocytes, and I wonder if this doesn't mean that indeed the Pima Indians represent a different disease than the maturity onset diabetic patients which we see in the Caucasians? Certainly, in light of some of Dr. Reaven's and others' data, showing decreased binding of insulin to monocytes and presumably to other receptors on insulin-sensitive tissues, one would presume at least that some of the insulin resistance is due to this decrease in receptors, particularly in the Pimas, with the diabetic population being obese as it is. This would suggest that this is genetically a different disease, and therefore, that maybe all of the data which is accumulated in the Pimas is very fascinating, but really needs to be restricted to that particular kind of diabetes and, extending it even further, maybe one of the reasons we're into so much difficulty is that there is no one maturity onset diabetes, maybe there are several. Then, when one puts studies together, the standard errors are large enough to obscure differences.*

P. SAVAGE: *I think that it may very well be possible that maturity onset diabetes will eventually turn out to be a spectrum of diseases in its own right. Some of the diminished binding which has been claimed to occur in maturity onset diabetics has been associated with obesity and with elevated fasting insulin levels. The groups that I showed were basically matched, so that the Caucasians and the Pimas in the study were, within each of the four groups, relatively weight matched. We feel that some of the differences are associated with weight. Then, there is the unexplained difference of Pimas, with double the fasting insulin levels, having binding similar to the Caucasians. That's why we think there may be an interacellular of postreceptor defect which plays a role in the Pimas. However, I would guess that might also be important in a substantial number of Caucasians, or people of other races.*

K.G.H.H. ALBERTI: *I have a question for Dr. Fajans about non-Pima Americans. As you know, there has been a move to redefine glucose intolerance from the European and British Diabetic Associations that two-hour glucose level must be around 200 before one can make a diagnosis of diabetes. First, would you like to comment on how you feel about that? Secondly, what difference is this going to make in the concepts and definitions, or non-definitions, of early diabetes?*

S. FAJANS: *In my introduction, I referred to the NIH workshop which tried to redefine the stages of diabetes. The combined opinion was that diabetes should be defined with a two-hour postglucose blood sugar level at 200, and between normal and diabetic was identified as "impaired glucose tolerance", not "borderline diabetes." This is fine, because this singly distinguishes between the more and less severe glucose intolerance, rather than diabetes, as long as one doesn't forget about this group. As to others, who've simply put the dividing line at 200 and said that below 200 is normal while above 200 is abnormal, I object. We have enough evidence in cases between 140 and 200 which may not be normal.*

N. FREINKEL: *Dr. Deckert, have you had an opportunity to break down your population on the basis of multiplicity of insulin injections?*

T. DECKERT: *No, we have not done this because the tradition continued from the beginning, which means, from the 1930's, to treat the patient with insulin twice a day, and that refers to 80% of the diabetic population.*

A.S. REDDI: *Dr. Deckert, you mentioned that 40% of your juvenile diabetics had glomerulosclerosis. Was there any correlation or relationship between blood glucose control and the development of glomerulosclerosis? Secondly, did you measure other hormones, such as growth hormone, aldosterone, renin, or norepinephrine?*

T. DECKERT: *Regarding your second question, we did not measure those hormones. As to your first question, I mentioned that 40% did not develop proteinuria. There was no difference in the quality of metabolic regulation and presence or absence of proteinuria.*

HLA AND THE GENETIC ASPECTS OF THE PREDISPOSITION TO JUVENILE DIABETES MELLITUS. A FOLLOW-UP

P. Rubinstein* and N. Suciu-Foca

Information on the genetics of juvenile diabetes mellitus (JDM) has been gathered in a logical sequence beginning with the recognition of the HLA association by Nerup et al., Cudworth et al. and others (1). Shortly afterwards Cudworth and Woodrow (2) encountered a significant excess of HLA-identity among pairs of sibs with JDM and postulated the existance of (a) JDM-gene(s), mapping in or close to the HLA region. A few months later we confirmed their findings and extended them with some evidence for the recessive nature of the predisposition gene (JDM-P). We further found the penetrance to be incomplete and of a numerical value similar to the concordance rate for identical twin pairs (2). The finding of a number of intra-HLA recombinants among JDM-sib pairs permitted us to demonstrate that the susceptibility maps to the left (HLA-D side) of B/D crossovers (2) in agreement with data first gathered by the Danish group (3) and subsequently confirmed by us and others that the association of JDM-P is strongest with HLA-D and -DR.

In this communication we reviewed the information gathered in studying 78 nuclear families ascertained through at least one patient with completely clear-cut juvenile onset, ketosis-prone, insulin dependent, Type 1, idiopathic diabetes mellitus.

MATERIAL AND METHODS

Families

78 pedigrees were ascertained from the families of JDM patients. The clinical criteria used for the selection of these families were as described previously (2). 60 of the families had a single

affected sib, 16 had two and two had three. The average number of children per family was 3.48 ± 1.1 (S.D) for those with one affected and 3.38 ± 1.31 for those with two.

Testing for Genetic Markers

All members of each family were studied for the following markers:

HLA. HLA-A, B, and C antigens were tested using the conventional two-stage cytotoxicity technique with multiple reagents able to identify 18 HLA-A, 20 HLA-B and 5 HLA-C specificities. HLA-D typing was performed and analyzed as described previously (4), HLA-DR was performed with either, or both, the B-cell-enriched lymphocyte suspension technique by dye-exclusion, and with the two-color fluorescence test, exactly as described by van Rood et al. (5). For HLA-D typing, at least 2 homozygous typing cells (HTC) of each of the accepted specificities (DW1-DW11) and three others, specific for "new" antigens were used. For DR typing, twenty families were tested with the 7th Workshop reagents; the rest, with the local serum sets that permit us to identify 7 HLA-DR antigens.

Other markers of the HLA region. Bf (factor B of properdin) was typed by immunofixation after serum electrophoresis in agarose as described by Alper and GLO as in Kompf (both cited in ref. 2).

Independently segregating genetic markers. Ten blood group systems and 16 other polymorphic traits of the plasma and red cells were tested using conventional techniques. All the inheritance patterns were consistent with the hypothesis that each putative father was in fact the progenitor.

RESULTS

The Recessive Nature of JDM

Because both the HLA and JDM-phenotypes of all members in each family are known, the pattern of inheritance may be examined against the null hypothesis of independent segregation. If the propositus of each family is used as the index case, the respective sibs may be scored as sharing 2, 1 or no haplotypes with him, and as being diabetic or not. Table 1 shows the data. A significant χ^2, with $p < 0.001$, demonstrates that the inheritance of JDM is not independent from that of HLA. The same data demonstrate the lack of dominance of the JDM trait: if the condition were dominant the ratio of HLA-identical to non-HLA-identical affected sibs would not exceed 1 as discussed previously by Thompson and Bodmer and by us (refs. in 6);

it is 2.33. Furthermore, if JDM-P were a dominant trait, the risk (penetrance) for the group of sibs that share one HLA haplotype should be, on the average, 0.5 that for the group of two-haplotype-identicals: it is 0.165. The χ^2 for this difference is 6.9, with a $p < 0.01$. The penetrance for HLA-identical sibs is 0.33, down from our previous estimate of 0.5, but the difference is not significant ($\chi^2 = 2.33$).

Table 1. Inheritance of HLA and JDM by 173 sibs of 78 JDM propositi

		JDM	no JDM	
No of HLA-D	2	14	28	42
haplotypes shared	1	5	92	97
with propositus	0	1	33	34
		20	153	173

$\chi^2 = 25.8$, $p < .001$

Mapping Location of the JDM-P Gene

Evidence from three intra-HLA recombinants (one A/BD and two AB/D crossovers) previously described by us (2) established that JDM-P segregates with the BD and the D segment respectively. Because of the availability of GLO as a separate marker it would be possible to circumscribe the distance of JDM-P from HLA-D if one of two JDM sibs could be found to carry an HLA-GLO recombinant. If JDM-P mapped "outside" this interval, then the postulated pairs of affected sibs would be HLA-non-identical, barring the unlikely event of a double crossover. No such families have been found. If the affected sib pair should be HLA-identical, GLO-different, the JDM-P gene could not be farther from HLA than the GLO locus. Two families that fit this second model have been found: Gn. and Ki., one (Gn.) is shown in Fig. 1. Thus, JDM-P is not farther from HLA-D than GLO.

Furthermore, in two other families (Ge. and Di.) each with 2 affected sibs that differed in one HLA haplotype, no HLA/GLO recombination was found. Thus, if HLA/JDM-P recombination were the cause of discordant sib-pairs, the JDM-P gene would have to map "outside" the HLA-GLO interval, which is incompatible with the evidence from Gn. and Ki. families or on the HLA-A side, which is incompatible with the previously published evidence.

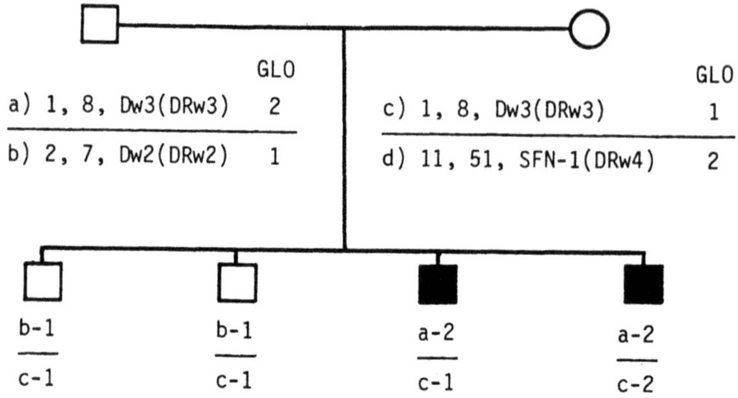

Fig. 1. The Gn. Family: an HLA/GLO recombinant placing the JDM - P gene.

Linkage Disequilibrium

Because all members of each family have been HLA-typed, it is possible to compute the linkage disequilibrium between JDM and various HLA alleles directly rather than from the population frequencies as is customary. Thus, if no disequilibrium existed, 0.5 of the times the suspected HLA allele from a heterozygous parent should be inherited by the JDM child. If significantly more than 0.5 of the time the HLA allele in question is transmitted together with JDM. the disequilibrium would be proved and its strength directly measured. For example, when DW3 was found in single dose in a parent, it was inherited by his (her) JDM child in 49 of 54 cases, instead of the expected 27 ($\chi^2 = 17.9$, $p < 0.001$; thus, 81% of the DW3 (and DRW3) haplotypes carry the JDM-P gene. Similarly, DRW4 was transmitted with JDM from heterozygous parents in 36 of 47 instances rather than in 23.5 as expected ($\chi^2 = 6.65$ $p = 0.01$). DRW4 is thus accompanied by the JDM-P gene 53% of the time. Since two different alleles are in linkage disequilibrium with JDM-P, we have investigated whether the genotypes of the JDM probands are in Hardy-Weinberg equilibrium. It has been suggested that the risk to the DRW3/DRW4 heterozygotes is disproportionately higher than that for the homozygous classes. The data are given in Table 2, which shows no deviations from the expected figures, and thus, no evidence of "overdominance".

The issue of crossing-over in the HLA region. We have reported an increase in the frequency of intra-HLA recombinations in families with JDM. Other groups are not in agreement with this suggestion, while reports from independent labs might be in agreement with it. We now have a large number of informative meioses and the data for the different intervals are shown in Table 3. Although higher, these figures are not significantly different from those generally accepted for the general population.

Table 2. Frequencies of the DRw3 and DRw4 alleles and their genotypic assortment in JDM patients

Gene frequencies: DRw3 = 0.39; DRw4 = 0.31; DRw(non-3, non-4) = 0.30

Genotypes	Expected	Found	X^2
DRw3/DRw3	11.6	13	0.16
DRw4/DRw4	7.3	10	1.00
DRw3/DRw(non-3,non-4)	17.94	17	0.06
DRw4/DRw(non-3,non-4)	14.26	11	0.75
DRw3/DRw4	18.33	16	0.13
DRw(non-3,non-4)/DRw(non-3,non-4)	6.96	9	0.57

Table 3. HLA recombination in families with JDM

Site of crossover	Number	No of informative meiosis	%
HLA-A/BD	7	440	1.59
HLA-AB/D	6	498	1.21
HLA-ABD/GLO: fathers	9	120	7.5
mothers	12	105	11.4

DISCUSSION

The material presented here has been collected from 78 fully-typed families. No effort has been made to select families with two or more affected siblings, a selection that would introduce a strong bias in the "effective" frequency of the JDM-P gene. As we have discussed before (7) selection for multiple cases increases the number of JDM-P homozygous parents, and this leads to an increase in the number of HLA haplotypes that carry the gene in that family thus increasing the likelihood that affected sib pairs will differ by one HLA haplotype. Lack of awareness of this problem may lead to erroneous conclusions, regardless of the power of the statistical tools used to analyze the data. This has been the case with a recent study (8) in which lack of correction for the "effective" gene frequency has led to the hypothesis of "loose" linkage between HLA and JDM. This hypothesis is incompatible with the data on recombination presented above and would have considerable difficulty explaining the persistence of linkage disequilibrium, which is eroded at the rate of $(1-\theta)$ per generation. Insofar as the recessive nature of the JDM-P gene is concerned: the data presented here increase the odds against the possibility of dominance, co-dominance and over-dominance. This last hypothesis was based exclusively on the relative risk estimate which, for reasons discussed elsewhere (7, and manuscript in preparation) is an inappropriate statistic when dealing with two allelic traits each of which is in linkage disequilibrium with a third one.

Our previous estimate of the penetrance for HLA-identical sibs was about 0.5, very close to that found in identical twins. The current data indicate a lower value, of about 0.33, but the difference is not significant: $\chi^2 = 2.33$. It is important to recognize that the method of ascertainment favors those families with more than one affected, since the selection stems from consultation. These estimates of the penetrance are, therefore, subject to considerable bias and should be taken as approximations. It is also likely that if environmental triggers are required for the expression of the JDM genotype, such factors may have different "strength" in families who already have JDM children than in those with genetically susceptible children but without a previous patient. Thus penetrance figures from families ascertained through probands do not necessarily apply to all JDM-P homozygous individuals.

We can use the data to compute the JDM-P gene frequency from the proportion of affected sib pairs who are HLA-identical as of the order of 0.2, very close to the figure obtained by Thomson and Bodmer (6) from data gathered by Cudworth and Woodrow. We can also extrapolate from the linkage disequilibrium data for DRW3 and DRW4 to obtain an independent estimate. Given that these two alleles in JDM patients account for 0.7 of all their HLA-DR genes and that they carry JDM-P 0.81 and 0.53 of the cases respectively, we can apply these data to the general population, where DRW3 has a gene frequency of 0.1 and DRW4 one of 0.15. If the values of linkage disequilibrium are valid for the general population, as proposed by Thomson and Bodmer (6), we can expect that DRW3-linked JDM-P has a frequency of 0.081 and DRW4-linked JDM-P one of 0.08. Considering the relative proportion of JDM-P genes not linked to either of these alleles (0.3) the expected JDM-P gene frequency would be ~ 0.23 in rather excellent agreement with our previously and independently derived estimate of ~ 0.20 (9).

A further problem in studying the genetics of JDM has been its possible heterogeneity. While it is obviously impossible to disprove that genetic heterogeneity may occur in the idiopathic form of JDM, the real question is whether a homogeneous model may account for the observed facts. So far the proportion of HLA-identity for affected sib pairs in the three main reports is as follows:

a)	Cudworth and Woodrow (cited in 6):	10/15 = 0.66
b)	Barbosa et al.(8):	21/38 = 0.55
c)	Rubinstein and Suciu-Foca (this paper)	14/20 = 0.70

The overall proportion, 45/73, has a mean of 0.62 and a standard error of 6% so that all three samples actually do not differ significantly in the proportion of HLA-identical sib pairs. Even when the two more different samples are compared, the actual difference between the proportions is only 1.1 times the standard error of the difference.

Our hypothesis is thus consistent with the overall findings of all three series and genetic heterogeneity need not be invoked so far for the explanation of these differences. Clinical heterogeneity, of course, need not be caused by genetic heterogeneity, particularly for a disease with important environmental participation.

The most important task now before us is clearly the definition of the mechanism of action of the JDM-P gene and the identification of the environmental triggers that lead to its expression.

REFERENCES

1. *Nerup, J., et al., (1977). In HLA and Disease, J. Dausset and A. Svejgaard, eds., Munksgaard, Copenhagen, 149.*
2. *Rubinstein, P., et al., (1977). N. Engl. J. Med. 297, 1036.*
3. *Thomsen, M., et al., (1975). Transplant. Rev. 22, 125.*

4. *Suciu-Foca, N., et al., (1978). Tissue Antigens 12, 94.*
5. *van Rood, J.J., et al., (1976). Nature 262, 795.*
6. *Thomson, G. and Bodmer, W., (1977). In HLA and Disease, J. Dausset and A. Svejgaard, eds., Munksgaard, Copenhagen 84.*
7. *Rubinstein, P., et al., (1978). In: Proceedings of the Symposium on the Immunology of Diabetes, Edinburgh, 1979. J. Irvine, Ed., in press.*
8. *Barbosa, J., et al., (1978). J. Clin. Invest., 61, 492.*
9. *Suciu-Foca, N., et al., (1979). Proceedings of the 7th Cong. of the Transplantation Soc., Transplant. Proc., in press.*

Supported in part by grants (AM19631 and HL09011) from the U.S. Public Health Service and by a grant from the Juvenile Diabetes Foundation.

HLA STUDIES IN DIABETICS

L. P. Ryder*, M. Christy, J. Nerup, P. Platz,
A. Svejgaard, and M. Thomsen

The inheritence of diabetes mellitus (DM) has for a long time been an insoluble enigma. Some necessary steps forward have been taken, however, by the recognition of probable genetic heterogeneity of DM. One of the main contributions of the HLA investigations in relation to DM has indeed been to provide evidence for such heterogeneity. Another important contribution has been the use of the HLA factors as genetic markers in family and population studies, permitting tests of various genetic models.

In this report, we shall give a short survey of the data on HLA in DM available at the HLA and Disease Registry in Copenhagen including some of our own recent results.

THE GENETIC HETEROGENEITY IN DM

That the disease entity "Diabetes Mellitus" is heterogeneous, is based on clinical and some genetic evidence. Attempts to subdivide the disease into separate groups have been based on clinical criteria such as age-at-onset of the disease, body weight, and the requirement of insulin treatment. Now, data from HLA studies add to this knowledge.

At the HLA and Disease Registry we have compiled the data on the frequencies of the HLA antigens in DM patients and normal controls from a variety of background populations in order to estimate the statistical association between the HLA factors and disease occurrence (1). The data are mostly from the published literature but some have been submitted directly to the registry.

We have previously noted a difference between the HLA associations in the juvenile onset DM and the maturity onset DM (2). For the purpose of further analyzing this heterogeneity, we lumped together in one class the data on juvenile and/or insulin dependent diabetes mellitus (JOD/IDD) and in another class the data concerning maturity onset diabetes mellitus (MOD). This classification is, of course, a rather crude compromise between overlapping, non-complementary criteria, but information on the patient groups made this the only practicable way of subdividing. Table 1 gives a print-out of the combined data from Caucasian populations on the HLA-B series in the JOD/IDD group, which should be compared to the combined data on MOD in Table 2. It appears from Table 1 that several HLA-B antigens are significantly and quite strongly associated with JOD/IDD. Note especially that the HLA-B8, B15 and B18 antigens occur with a considerably higher frequency in the patients than in the controls, giving an increased relative risk of disease to carriers of these antigens, while HLA-B7 apparently confers some degree of resistance.

Legend to Tables 1, 2 and 3.
HLA-associations of DM

Only data on the HLA-B series from Caucasian populations are given. For each antigen is given the number of studies taken into the calculation, the total number of patients investigated and the range of percentage positive individuals found in all the studies, analogous data on the controls, the combined relative risk, the statistical significance of the combined relative risks' deviation from 1 and, if more than one study, the statistical significance of the variation in relative risks observed in the individual studied.

A relative risk e.g. 2.56 for HLA-B8 indicates a 2.56-fold risk of the disease for individuals carrying B7 compared to those not carrying it and a significance of 2.3E-06 means that the p-value is 2.3 x 10^{-6}. For references, see (1).

Table 1

DISEASE WHO-CODE: 250.001 Juvenile and/or insulin dependent DM

HLA	NO. of studies	PATIENTS TOTAL	PATIENTS %POS-range	CONTROLS TOTAL	CONTROLS %POS-range	R.RISK	SIGNIFICANCE (r.risk)	SIGNIFICANCE (heterog.)
B 5	12	1230	0- 14	6295	9- 21	.59	2.3E-06	>.05
B 7	14	1493	3- 29	7677	3- 32	.54	<1E-10	5.6E-03
B 8	18	1785	19- 60	13349	2- 29	2.56	<1E-10	>.05
B 12	12	1154	5- 26	6295	11- 34	.79	4.8E-03	>.05
B 13	12	1154	0- 8	6295	3- 6	1.27	>.05	>.05
B 14	11	1006	0- 9	5837	0- 15	.67	1.5E-02	>.05
B 18	13	1244	5- 59	6577	5- 50	1.69	4.1E-08	>.05
B 27	12	1154	2- 14	6295	4- 14	.96	>.05	>.05
Bw15	17	1769	4- 50	13175	2- 26	2.05	<1E-10	6.2E-04
Bw16	7	540	6- 20	4992	4- 14	1.38	3.9E-02	>.05
Bw17	12	1154	0- 13	6295	2- 23	.77	>.05	>.05
Bw21	8	640	0- 12	5262	0- 13	1.37	>.05	>.05
Bw22	11	1006	0- 6	5837	1- 6	.97	>.05	>.05
Bw35	13	1170	6- 38	6364	6- 35	.70	4.4E-04	1.5E-03
Bw37	5	362	0- 3	2511	2- 4	.91	>.05	>.05
Bw38	1	100	6- 6	270	4- 4	1.55	>.05	-
Bw40	12	1154	4- 29	6295	2- 21	1.26	2.5E-02	>.05
Bw41	2	217	0- 3	1091	1- 1	2.53	>.05	>.05

Table 2

DISEASE WHO-CODE: 250.002 Maturity onset DM

HLA	NO. of studies	PATIENTS TOTAL	PATIENTS %POS-range	CONTROLS TOTAL	CONTROLS %POS-range	R.RISK	SIGNIFICANCE (r.risk)	SIGNIFICANCE (heterog.)
B 5	4	210	10- 14	2538	10- 15	1.07	>.05	>.05
B 7	4	210	4- 33	2538	3- 30	1.10	>.05	>.05
B 8	6	406	4- 37	2920	2- 29	1.43	6.1E-03	>.05
B 12	4	210	11- 38	2538	11- 28	1.00	>.05	>.05
B 13	4	210	0- 5	2538	3- 5	.96	>.05	>.05
B 14	4	210	0- 14	2538	5- 15	.99	>.05	>.05
B 18	4	210	7- 54	2538	5- 50	1.36	>.05	>.05
B 27	4	210	4- 11	2538	6- 11	1.17	>.05	>.05
Bw15	5	246	4- 30	2638	2- 18	1.46	>.05	>.05
Bw16	2	89	10- 14	2063	5- 14	1.67	>.05	>.05
Bw17	4	210	0- 21	2538	7- 23	1.02	>.05	>.05
Bw21	2	89	3- 11	2063	4- 13	1.03	>.05	>.05
Bw22	3	110	5- 7	2163	4- 5	1.53	>.05	>.05
Bw35	4	210	7- 19	2538	11- 19	.84	>.05	>.05
Bw37	1	28	0- 0	96	2- 2	.66	>.05	-
Bw40	4	210	4- 15	2538	3- 18	.91	>.05	>.05

Table 3

DISEASE WHO-CODE: 250.001 Juvenile and/or insulin dependent DM

HLA	NO. of studies	PATIENTS TOTAL	PATIENTS %POS-range	CONTROLS TOTAL	CONTROLS %POS-range	R.RISK	SIGNIFICANCE (r.risk)	SIGNIFICANCE (heterog.)
Dw2	2	115	0 - 0	422	26 - 26	0.	1.8E-06	>.05
Dw3	2	201	30 -46	510	19 - 26	2.19	1.0E-05	>.05
Dw4	2	232	48 -52	478	19 - 19	4.01	<1E-10	>.05
DRw2	2	149	0 - 7	269	22 - 29	0.24	5.0E-05	>.05
DRw3	3	199	36 -59	376	11 - 24	5.69	<1E-10	>.05
DRw4	2	76	32--58	216	16 - 28	2.84	3.5E-04	>.05

This contrasts strongly to the pattern observed in table 2 for MOD, where the only antigen showing a slightly significant association is HLA-B8, which may well be explained as an admixture of (biologically) wrongly classified patients with a late onset diabetes of JOD/IDD type. In spite of the relatively few MOD patients studied and in spite of the very rough criteria used for JOD/IDD and MOD, the difference in their association with HLA-B8 is highly significant ($p < 0.0001$).

The HLA-D (and DR) series antigens show stronger associations with JOD/IDD than their correlated HLA-B antigens do (3), and this has placed the HLA-D/-DR series in the focus of genetic studies on diabetes. Unfortunately, no HLA-D data in MOD has come to our knowledge. Table 3 gives the combined data on significantly associated D/DR antigens in JOD/IDD. The most striking finding is the repeated observation of virtual absence of Dw2 among the patients. In contrast, the Dw3 and Dw4 antigens (and the corresponding DR antigens) have quite strong positive associations with JOD/IDD.

FAMILY STUDIES

The pronounced associations between HLA-B and D/DR determinants and especially JOD/IDD has naturally led to the question of the possible existence of a diabetes-predisposing gene linked to the HLA locus on chromosome 6. The tremendous polymorphism of the HLA system itself makes it a very efficient tool to study this possibility. Further questions on the actual mode of inheritence - recessive, dominant, involving one or more loci, etc. - are more difficult to answer.

The common strategy has been to investigate the HLA-genotypes in pairs of sibs, both affected with JOD/IDD and simply counting how many parental HLA haplotypes they share. For this strategy, very general models have been developed (4). In short, if the disease in question had no relation to the HLA system (or if only normal sib-pairs had been investigated) the expectation would be that ¼ of the pairs shared 0 parental HLA haplotypes, ½ of the pairs shared only 1 haplotype and ¼ were two HLA haplotype identical by descent. If the disease susceptibility (DS) was governed by one or more loci closely linked to HLA, the above proportions ¼:½:¼ would be distorted towards an excess of two HLA haplotype sharing sibpairs, while the other two groups would have a deficit.

Table 4

Number of sibpairs with	0	1	2	shared HLA haplotypes
Data source:				
Barbosa et al.	0	9	9	18
Copenhagen study	3	10	15	28
Cudworth	1	16	23	40
Möller & Persson	0	2	6	8
Spielman & Zmijewski	0	3	7	10
Suciu-Foca et al.	1	4	9	14
Total observed	5 (4.2%)	44 (37.3%)	69 (58.3%)	118
Expected if no relation to HLA	29.5 (25%)	59 (50%)	29.5 (25%)	$\chi^2 = 77.1$ (2 df, $p < 10^{-15}$)
if dominant susceptibility .. (for the P_D giving best fit)	4.3 (3.6%)	58.5 (49.6%)	55.2 (46.8%)	$\chi^2 = 7.1$ for $P_D = 0.04$ (1 df, $p < 0.01$)
if recessive susceptibility . (for the P_D giving best fit)	6.3 (5.3%)	41.9 (35.5%)	69.8 (59.2%)	$\chi^2 = 0.38$ for $P_D = 0.30$ (1 df, $p > 0.1$)

For explanations to table 4, see text. For references see (1).

The combined data available today (Table 4) show a clearcut and highly significant deviation from the proportions ¼:½:¼, which supports the assumption of at least one DS locus closely linked to HLA, as noted by several authors.

MODE OF INHERITENCE

The general model involving one DS locus with two alleles D and d predicts that the proportions of affected sibpairs sharing no, one or two parental HLA haplotypes will depend on two sets of parameters, namely (i) the gene frequency (P_D) in the population of the DS-allele D, and (ii) the penetrances (i.e. risk of being affected) for the three possible genotypes at the DS-Locus: D/D, D/d and d/d (provided that the linkage to HLA is tight). As pointed out by Suarez (4), it will always be possible to find more than one set of values between 0 and 1 for the gene frequency and the penetrances which will fit the data completely.

However, two simple cases treated by Thomson & Bodmer (5) may be worth considering. These are the completely dominant and the completely recessive susceptibility. The completely dominant susceptibility means that individuals carrying one or two DS alleles have equal (but unknown) risk of disease (i.e. the same penetrance in homo-and heterozygotes) and individuals carrying no DS allele have negligible risk of the disease, while the completely recessive susceptibility assumes that only homozygotes for the DS allele have an (unknown) risk of the disease. In both of these cases, the expected proportions of the three classes of sibpairs are independent of the value of the penetrance and depend only on the gene frequency P_D.

Thus, for given values of the gene frequency P_D, the hypothesis of a completely dominant inheritance of susceptibility to DM governed by a locus closely linked to HLA can be tested against the data in Table 4 by a chi-square goodness of fit test. This can, of course, also be done for the completely recessive case. Fig. 1 shows a graph of the chi-square values for the two models as dependent on P_D, given the observations in Table 4. The two minimum chi-squares correspond to the gene frequencies giving the best fit to the two models. Apparently the completely dominant model is untenable with a significant minimum chi-square $\simeq 7.1$ (d.f. = 1, $p < 0.01$), while the completely recessive model gives a good fit for $P_D = 0.30$ (chi-square $\simeq 0.33$) and thus cannot be rejected on the basis of these data. The values of P_D giving an acceptable fit (e.g. at the 5% significance level) of the recessive model are rather high, between 0.2 and 0.45 which is considerably higher than found by Rubenstein et al. (6). The estimate of P_D must be taken with some reservation because most of the data will probably have a biased ascertainment.

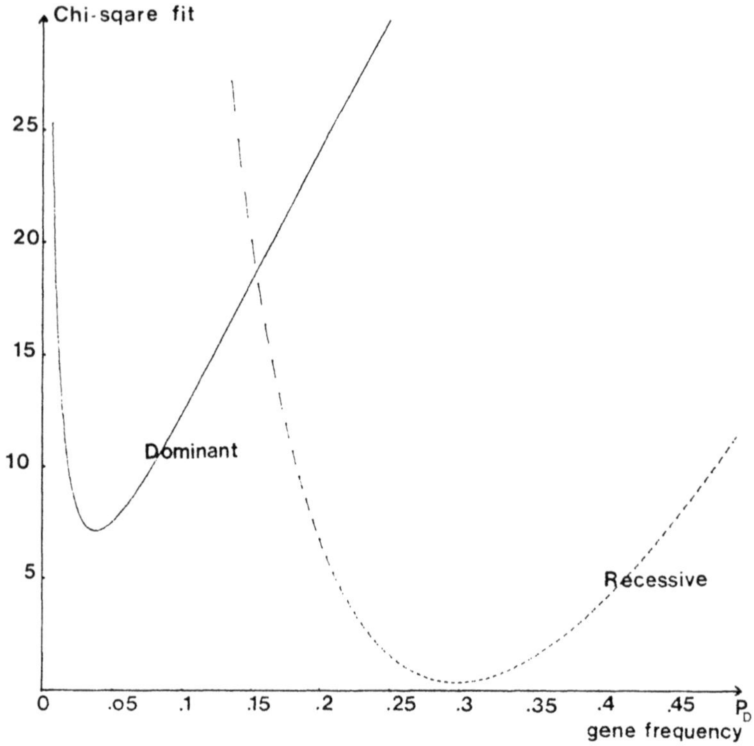

Fig. 1.

Before accepting the completely recessive model, its consequences must, of course, be studied and compared to evidence independent of the above sibpair - and - HLA data. The high DS gene frequency P_D of about 0.3, which is necessary to fit these data, corresponds to a frequency in the population of genetically susceptible individuals (P_D^2) as high as 4-20 per cent. Assuming a JOD/IDD prevalence of about 2.5 per 1000 individuals(7), this implies a penetrance as low as about 1.25- 6.25 per cent. This figure is rather far from the figures obtained in studies on the concordance rate in monozygotic twins, which gives estimates of the penetrance in the range 25-50 per cent. Moreover, the available data on the frequency of affected sibs of propositi (about 5-10%) (8) are only compatible with this model if the penetrance is about 10-25 per cent.

These discrepancies in penetrance values make of course the one locus, two allele, completely recessive model proposed by Rubinstein et al. (6) much less plausible although they probably cannot disprove it, since the data are not from exactly the same populations and are subject to statistical uncertainty.

The completely recessive model may fully explain the decreased frequencies of HLA-B7 and Dw2 among the patients by the assumption that the HLA haplotypes involving B7 and/or Dw2 very rarely (and far less frequent than expected) carry the DS-allele but instead carry the normal allele. This would be a so-called negative linkage disequilibrium between the B7 and Dw2 genes and the DS allele. The increase in B8, B15, B18 and Dw3, Dw4, would correspond to a positive linkage disequilibrium of these factors with the DS-allele. Linkage disequilibria - positive as well as negative - are well known within the HLA system itself; for example, HLA-B7 is in strong positive linkage disequilibrium with Dw2, B8 with Dw3, and B15 with Dw4.

The recessive, two-allele model is, however, incompatible with the notion of an overdominant effect of Dw3 and Dw4 (and correspondingly B8 and B15) earlier proposed by us. The overdominance means that heterozygotes Dw3/Dw4 have a higher risk of diseases than both homozygotes Dw3/Dw3 and Dw4/Dw4, while the prediction from the model would be a risk intermediate between the risks of the homozgotes. This is a crucial point not yet fully resolved, both because of insufficient data and insensitive statistical methods to test the hypothesis. Most of the data published so far show however a slight excess of the B8/B15 heterozygotes among patients with JOD/IDD. As often pointed out, it is not always possible to distinguish between a recessive inheritance and a mode of inheritance involving interaction of multiple alleles at one locus (overdominance) or of alleles at two or more loci (epistasis).

If the completely recessive model in the proposed form resists rejection when more sufficient data become available, we are left with the fact that the HLA linked, putative DS gene, as indicated by its low penetrance, only accounts for a small fraction of the factors leading to JOD/IDD. A prediction would be that the remaining factors, which may be genetic or environmental, will cause recurrent nightmares to the geneticists and epidemiologists.

SUMMARY

The studies of HLA in diabetes mellitus have strongly supported the subdivision into (at least) two genetically distinct groups: The juvenile onset (or perhaps better the insulin dependent) type DM, which shows a marked association to the HLA system, and the maturity onset type with a weak or no association to HLA. The HLA system has provided tools to test specific genetic models for the insulin dependent DM. A model involving one disease susceptibility locus closely linked to the HLA-loci and with a recessive susceptibility allele in linkage disequilibrium with some of

the HLA factors has been proposed by others. This model cannot be totally rejected on the basis of the available data, but it is made less likely, especially because it leads to very low estimates of the penetrance which is discrepant from independent estimates, based both on studies on monozygotic twins and other families. In addition suggestive but not yet conclusive evidence of an excessive risk for HLA-Dw3/Dw4 heterozygotes is in conflict with this model.

REFERENCES

1. *Third Report from the HLA and Disease Registry. Tissue Antigens (1979), in press.*
2. *Nerup J., et al., (1974). Lancet 2, 864.*
3. *Thomsen, M., et al., (1975). Transplant. Rev. 22, 125.*
4. *Suarez, B.K., (1978). Tissue Antigens 12, 87.*
5. *Thomsen, G. and Bodmer, W.F., (1977). Eds. F.B. Christiansen and T. Fenchel. Springer Verlag. 545.*
6. *Rubinstein, P., et al. (1977). New Engl. J. Med. 297, 1036.*
7. *Green, A.: personal communication.*
8. *Degnbol, B. and Green, A., (1978). Ann. Hum. Genet., Lond. 42, 25.*

The secretarial assistance of Mrs. Elly Anderson and Mrs. Janne Pedersen is highly acknowledged. This study was aided by the Danish Medical Research Council, the European Communities Medical Research Council and Nordic Insulin Foundation.

DISCUSSION

P. RUBINSTEIN: *I disagree with Dr. Ryder's conclusion on the increased risk for the DW 3, DW 4 heterozygote. This is a problem of a statistical nature. It is a question of relative risk measured when you have two alleles each of which have been previously known to be in association with increased risk. If you put the two together and compare them with the risk in people having neither of the two, of course, the risk appears to be much more increased than for either. However, as I will show you, when you do the computation from the Hardy-Weinberg law, of the possible number of such heterozygotes in the juvenile diabetic population, they are all in line in all the observations, including those from Denmark.*

J. BARBOSA: *Since disagreements and differences make life interesting, I have good news for you. I disagree with Dr. Rubinstein on a number of things. In a few minutes, I will present our data, which is really a different way of looking at the HLA as a model for diabetic genes. Our approach is that of the LOD scores, and I think that most geneticists would agree that, mathematically and statistically, it is at least as valid as Dr. Rubinstein's. I'd like to add that I'm concerned with the fact that Dr. Rubinstein seems to put a lot of emphasis on the homozygocity of parents. I believe that most, if not all, of these parents are phenotypically normal. So, it's somewhat tenuous then to assume that some of them are homozygous for the hypotypical recessive diabetic gene. On the other hand, if there is anything we can take for granted in this meeting, I would think that JIDD is genetically heterogeneous. It's very hard to accept that one single recessive gene is going to explain all juvenile insulin-dependent diabetes. Additionally, did you find only one family with a recombination between glyoxalase and the D-plus hypothetical JDH gene? If that is the case, one family would not invalidate the other data.*

P. RUBINSTEIN: *There are two families identical to this, and I showed only one slide. There are also two other families with the opposite effect, where we have two children who share only one HLA type and there is no recombination. So, in fact, you have four events which are against your idea of 13% recombination between the two. Besides, for 13% recombination, as you will probably say soon, the chance that you would still observe the linkage disequilibria is extremely small. Linkage disequilibrium disappears in time, as a function of the recombination frequency. I calculate that it would disappear in about 11 generations.*

CHAIRMAN FREINKEL: *Dr. Ryder, will you close?*

L.P.RYDER:*Yes, I'm not quite sure that it's allowed to use the Hardy-Weinberg equilibrium in a population ascertained as patients,*

when you know that the HLA factors are associated with a disease.

P. RUBINSTEIN: *That would be correct, if deviations had been found. They were not.*

L. P. RYDER: *Quite so.*

ON THE GENETIC HETEROGENEITY OF JUVENILE HYPERGLYCEMIA

J. Barbosa* and M. M. Chern

Studies of the major histocompatibility system (HLA) and of twins have strengthened the current view that juvenile, insulin-dependent diabetes (JIDD) is pathogenetically different from adult onset, insulin-independent diabetes. Even for JIDD the HLA and twin studies suggest heterogeneity.

Furthermore, a new hyperglycemic syndrome, the maturity onset type of hyperglycemia in young people (MOHY), has been identified, and some evidence suggests that it may be pathogenetically different from other known types of hyperglycemia.

Although population studies (particularly in Europeon Caucasians) have provided us with important knowledge on associations between various HLA antigens and JIDD, family studies are essential in order to test the hypothesis that genes with a role in the pathogenesis of JIDD or MOHY are linked to the HLA. This hypothetical phenomenon of genetic linkage might explain the weak associations HLA-JIDD reported before. Alternatively, these gene effects might be totally independent from those associations, and reflect a different pathogenesis. It is our purpose to present data from our family studies which suggest that juvenile diabetes is a highly heterogeneous syndrome.

JUVENILE, INSULIN-DEPENDENT DIABETES

All JIDD patients included in these studies developed the disease before age 40 and were taking insulin. The great majority were ketosis prone.

Segregation Analysis

This type of analysis is useful in suggesting modes of inheritance and penetrance levels which may be needed when performing linkage analysis. In preliminary studies of 136 families, each of which had one or more JIDD members, we could not reject most of the models fitted to the data (1). Based on the likelihood ratio criterion, the best fit was obtained with a model including approximately 50% phenocopies or sporadic cases. This agrees with twin studies. The inability to reject both autosomal dominant and recessive models supports our findings on linkage analysis described below.

Linkage Analysis

Since there was evidence from diabetic twin studies, and HLA population reports that juvenile diabetes is heterogeneous, our sampling strategy was aimed at obtaining for study families likely to harbor a) diabetes with a strong genetic component, and b) homogeneous types of diabetes within families. This strategy is, therefore, likely to select against mainly sporadic, including environmental, cases of disease. The study of families with high intrasibship prevalence of diabetes (multiple sibship or MS families), families with affected individuals in multiple generations (multiple generation or MG families), and families with concordant diabetic identical twins all meet the above criteria. The chances of sampling for JIDD cuased by genes with Mendelian modes of inheritance are maximized by studying such families. Consequently, linkage studies with the HLA can be carried out in a more straightforward manner. This approach will lead, of course, to findings that cannot be generalized to all cases of JIDD, and may apply only to identically selected diabetic families. Studies of randomly selected families with a JIDD proband for HLA linkage, however, are likely to help in evaluating the extent of the genetic heterogeneity of diabetes.

In our first studies on MD type of diabetic families (Fig. 1) we found a statistically significant association between the sharing of an identical haplotype and the development of JIDD in a sibship (2). Furthermore, about half of the patients were HLA identical (shared both haplotypes). This non-Mendelian HLA haplotype assortment confirmed a previous study from Great Britian, and suggested that one or more diabetic genes exist in the HLA area. Since our ascertainment strategy for these families would be expected to increase the likelihood of selecting for recessive disease (phenotypically normal parents, several affected sibs) we performed formal linkage analysis by the lod score method on 21 of these kindreds (3). This analysis showed that the highest total lod score (3.98) was obtained at a penetrance of 50% and for a recombination fraction of 13%. Although the test for heterogeneity was not significant, inspection of the lod scores suggested the possibility that heterogeneity may emerge if a larger sample is studied and more information can be collected on the patients. Furthermore, we found that the HLA identical sibs were significantly more concordant for age

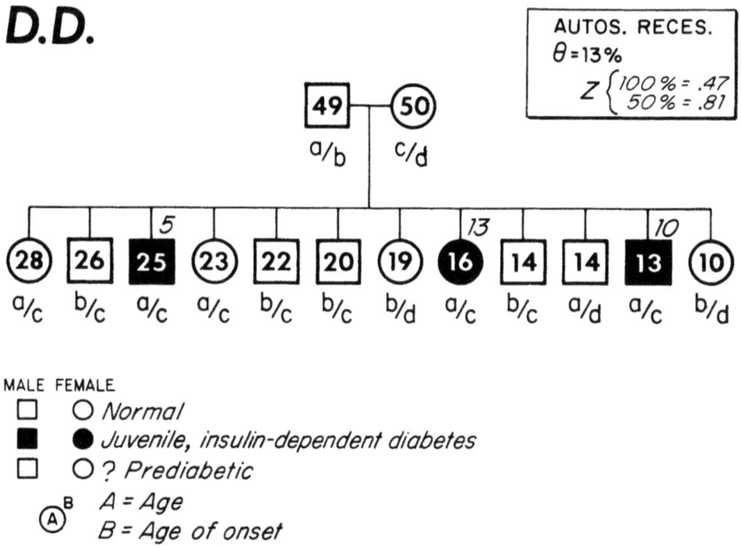

Fig. 1. Linkage analysis of diabetic family with multiple sibs affected (MS family). The lod score (Z) is 0.81 for a recombination fraction (θ) of 13% and assuming 50% penetrance. For 100% penetrance the lod score is only 0.47, reflecting the two HLA-JIDD discordant cases.

at onset of diabetes than the haploidentical sibs (one HLA haplotype identical) (2). The HLA identical sibs were also more concordant for seasonal incidence of disease in months (1.8 months difference), than were the haploidentical sibs (3.2 months difference). Moreover, the HLA identical siblings were more likely to develop diabetes in the winter months (78%), than the haploidentical sibs (21%). All these data are compatible with heterogeneity in this group of diabetics. It is noteworthy in this regard, that the diabetic concordant twins studied by Nelson et al. had onset of disease more frequently in January through March than the diabetics from the discordant pairs. The results from linkage analysis suggest the existence, at least in some of the families studied, of an autosomal recessive diabetic gene 13 map units away from the HLA region (Fig. 2). Whether its locus is on the A or D side of the HLA remains to be seen. Typing for the outside markers indicated in Fig. 2 may help to settle this issue. The fact that in these families no association could be seen between diabetes and particular HLA antigens, including B8, B18, and B7, whose frequencies in our population studies are abnormal, suggests to us that the HLA-JIDD associations, repeatedly described in population studies, underlie a mechanism different from that related to the presumed JIDD locus identified by the linkage analysis described above. The trait determined by the recessive JIDD gene located at 13 map units away from the HLA would express itself 50% of the time (penetrance), without necessarily showing an association with HLA antigens.

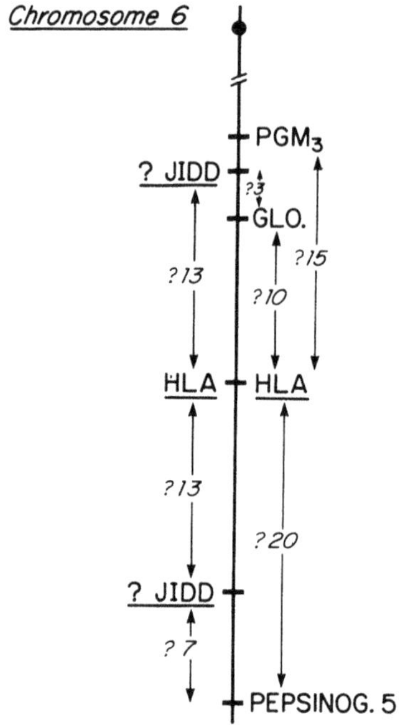

Fig. 2. The HLA region in the short arm of human chromosome #6. The JIDD autosomal recessive locus, suggested by studies of the MS families, is shown. Other loci known to exist in this are (outside markers) are also shown. All distrances from the HLA, given in map units, are tentative. Glo: glyoxalase; PGM3: phosphoglucomutase 3; JIDD: juvenile, insulin-dependent diabetes; Pepsinog. 5: pepsinogen 5.

Rubinstein et al. have published studies of HLA haplotype segregation in diabetic families apparently randomly ascertained. Most of these families included only one diabetic. On the basis of their results they concluded that JIDD is an autosomal recessive disease. We have re-analyzed their data by formal linkage analysis, assuming the autosomal recessive mode and 50% penetrance, as we did for our MS families (3). The kindreds with HLA recombinations were excluded since this finding has not been confirmed. When all the 22 families were analyzed, a total lod score of only 0.88 at a recombination fraction of 13% was found. This total lod score is not statistically significant and, therefore, does not support the authors' contention that these families have a homogenous form of autosomal recessive diabetes. When we restricted the linkage analysis to their six families (27% of the total sample) of MS type, the total lod score was 0.36 (41% of the total lod score) at a recombination fraction of 19%. For this small number of families the lod score was compatible with our results.

The segregation analysis reported above also strongly suggest that not all JIDD is autosomal recessive and there are probably many JIDD phenocopies.

We have proceeded with the study of 31 MG families. Although formal linkage analysis assuming on autosomal dominant type of JIDI is still in progress, it seems that heterogeneity will be more evident in these than in the diabetic MS families. There is, however, a group of MG families, like that shown in Fig. 3, with high lod scores when 50% penetrance is assumed for the gene. JIDD in these families is possibly due to an autosomal dominant gene in tight linkage with the HLA.

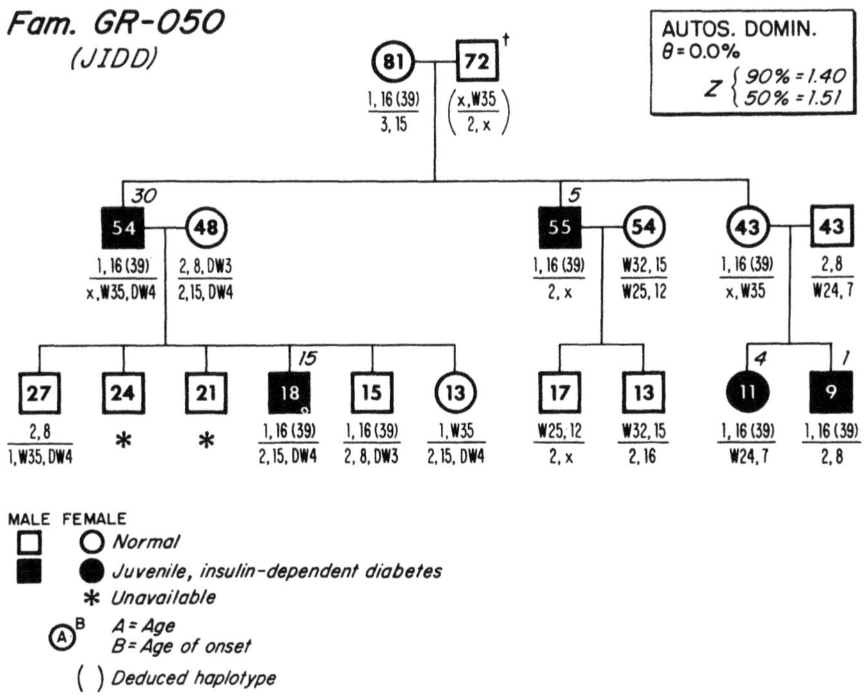

Fig. 3. Linkage analysis of family with individuals affected in several generations (MG family). The lod score (Z) was 1.51 for a recombination fraction (θ) of 0.0% assuming 50% penetrance. For higher penetrance the lod score is lower because three cases are discordant for HLA-JIDD.

MATURITY ONSET TYPE OF HYPERGLYCEMIA IN YOUNG PEOPLE (MOHY)

This type of hyperglycemia was first described by Fajans et al. (4) and later by Tattersall. It is not clear whether this is a homogeneous category of hyperglycemia different from maturity-onset, insulin-independent diabetes (IID), or simply the latter when recognized earlier. There is some evidence, however, that MOHY, at least in some of the families studied by us, may be a different disease. In two of these kindreds the hyperglycemia trait met all the criteria for the autosomal dominant model of inheritance, and the disease seemed clinically very mild as well as homogeneous (5). One of these families is shown in Fig. 4. More clinical heterogeneity seems to have been present in the clinical material reported by others. Plasma glucagon and growth hormone measured after oral glucose loads in four MOHY families, two of which have been reported before (5), also showed a pattern different from that frequently seen in IID. All MOHY patients had glucagon and growth hormone responses to glucose indistinguishable from normals, unlike most adult IID patients. Insulin deficiency, however, as determined by the ratio plasma insulin/plasma glucose, was present in most of our MOHY patients (5), not unlike many adult IID patients. We (6) and others (7) have found that, at least in some MOHY families, the hyperglycemic trait segregates with a HLA haplotype, as shown in Fig. 4 for one of our families. Formal linkage analysis between the HLA and MOHY trait in one family, assuming 50% penetrance, revealed the highest lod score of 1.2 for a recombination fraction of 5%. Although the lod score was not significant (lod scores are considered significant only above 3) it was appreciably high for only one family. More kindreds are being analyzed now. This finding, however, supports the concept of a monogenic autosomal dominant disease in MOHY. In view of the clinical, biochemical and immunogenetic evidence described above, we favor the opinion that in some families, such as the four we have been studying, MOHY is a distinct entity with apparent excellent prognosis. We are, therefore, opposed to labelling these patients as diabetics, a term with detrimental social and psychological connotations.

SUMMARY

We have briefly discussed immunogenetic studies of families with hyperglycemia which suggest the existence of at least four types of the disease: a) juvenile, insulin-dependent, ketosis prone diabetes determined by an autosomal recessive gene with 50% penetrance and in linkage with the HLA; b) juvenile, insulin-dependent, ketosis prone diabetes probably determined by an autosomal dominant gene; c) unidentified types of juvenile, insulin-dependent diabetes whose pathogenesis may be related to the HLA associations reported; and

d) maturity onset type of hyperglycemia in the young, probably determined by an autosomal dominant gene. There are probably other forms of juvenile hyperglycemia. Some may depend on genes unrelated to the HLA, others may be mostly or totally environmental, rather than genetic.

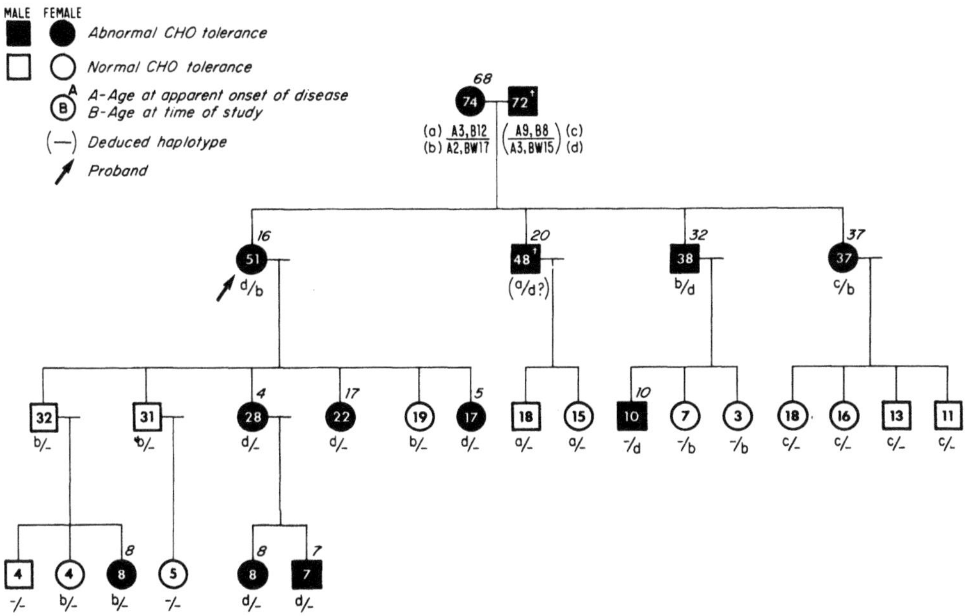

Fig. 4. Pedigree of family with maturity onset hyperglycemia of the young (MOHY). The haplotype A3-BW15 seems to segregate with the hyperglycemic trait. The lod score was 1.2 (recombination fraction 5% and penetrance 50%).

REFERENCES

1. *Barbosa, J., and Chern, M.M., (1978). Diabetes 27, 458.*
2. *Barbosa, J., et al., (1977). J. Clin. Invest. 60, 989.*
3. *Barbosa, J., et al., (1978). J. Clin. Invest. 62, 492.*
4. *Fajans, S.S. and Conn, J., (1960). Diabetes 9, 83.*
5. *Barbosa, J., et al., (1978). Annals of Intern. Med. 88, 595.*
6. *Barbosa, J., et al., (1978). Arch. Inter. Med. 138, 90.*
7. *Jaworski, M., et al., (1977). Clin. Res. 25, 701A.*

Supported by NIH Grants 1 R01 AM20729 GEN, 1 R01 EY02455, NIH Contract N01-HD-8-2846, and General Clinical Research Center Prog. (RR-400), The Division of Research Resources, NIH.

FAMILIAL PATTERNS OF INHERITANCE OF DIABETES MELLITUS. MATURITY-ONSET TYPE DIABETES OF YOUNG PEOPLE (MODY)

M. C. Cloutier and S. S. Fajans*

Since 1960, we have reported in prospective studies that non-progressive, maturity-onset type diabetes can be found in children, adolescents and young adults (1). We used the term maturity-onset type diabetes of the young in 1964, and reported that it occurred in a strong familial association. Since 1966, the occurence of maturity-onset type diabetes of the young has been amply confirmed by many investigators. In 1974, Tattersall reported three pedigrees with this type of diabetes and proposed that it was inherited in an autosomal dominant fashion and that it was distinct from JOD (2). In 1976, Tattersall and Fajans first used the abbreviation of MODY for maturity-onset diabetes of young people, gave data for 26 families with MODY, showed that there was a difference in the pattern of inheritence between classic juvenile-onset type diabetes and MODY, and provided further evidence for autosomal dominant inheritence of MODY (3). Barbosa et al. described data for two kindreds with MODY and suggested an association with HLA-A3 and BW15 in one of the two pedigrees (4), a finding not duplicated in pedigrees of other investigators, suggesting genetic heterogeneity in MODY.

It is the purpose of this presentation to present briefly six pedigrees of MODY to demonstrate that there is other evidence for heterogeneity within MODY.

We will indicate that 1) although some families are free of vascular complications, other MODY families contain members with typical macroangiopathic and microangiopathic complications of diabetes, indicating that this is a true diabetic syndrome and that MODY is not necessarily a benign disease, 2) some families with MODY members do not conform to the typical autosomal dominant pattern of inheritance, 3) there is heterogeneity of insulin responses between MODY pedigrees, to be discussed in greater detail later in this symposium, and 4) although many patients with MODY show little or no progression in severity over periods of more than 20 years, others do have progression to fasting hyperglycemia and to insulin requirement for the correcting of fasting hyperglycemia, but not for ketosis. We will also suggest that many patients first diagnosed as having conventional maturity-onset type diabetes of middle age (MOD) are members of MODY families, and that, conversely, MODY patients may represent the early stage of MOD diagnosed in later life.

The first pedigree is that of the R. W. family, an example of four generations of MODY diabetes (Fig. 1). Routine glucose tolerance tests were performed in 11 asymptomatic children of generation III, offspring of II-5. Seven of the 11 children in generation III were found to be diabetic in 1958. The three oldest siblings had fasting hyperglycemia while abnormal glucose tolerance tests were found in those aged 25, 21, 16 and 11 years. On followup, all have developed fasting hyperglycemia, except for the 21 year old. The fasting hyperglycemia has been normalized in all by diet plus sulfonylureas for the last 20 years. Seven members of generation IV have MODY, the youngest was nine years at diagnosis. Two have fasting hyperglycemia controlled by sulfonylyreas. One individual in this generation has classis JOD (age 13 years at diagnosis); she was islet cell antibody (ICA) positive at diagnosis as well as three years thereafter, while all MODYs are ICA negative. Background retinopathy is present in a member of generation III and IV, respectively. II-5 had diabetes diagnosed at the age of 41 and was controlled with chlorpropamide until his death at age 75. He was blind from diabetic retinopathy and had a leg amputated for peripheral vascular disease at ages 64 and 60, respectively. All members of generation III and IV have low insulin response to glucose.

In the diabetic siblings of generation II, myocardial infarctions, peripheral vascular disease with gangrene and leading to amputation have been associated with diabetes. Since asymptomatic members of generation III and IV have progressed from abnormal glucose tolerance to fasting hyperglycemia over a period of up to 20 years, it is possible that these five members of generation II may have had MODY which had been undectected.

Offspring of II-2 and II-3 (not shown in Fig. 1) have had MODY and MOD and some members have strongly abnormal cortisone-glucose tolerance tests. Patient III-10 was diagnosed at age 57 years and four years later was noted to have retinopathy which has progressed to visual impairment. II-4 was the only one of six brothers unaffected by diabetes (Fig. 1). There is no MOD or MODY in two generations of decendants. One grandaughter progressed from an abnormal glucose tolerance test to insulin-dependent diabetes over three years from age 18 to 21 years. Ketonuric during pregnancy, she had very strongly positive islet cell antibody levels measured in sera two years after diagnosis and one year before insulin therapy was instituted.

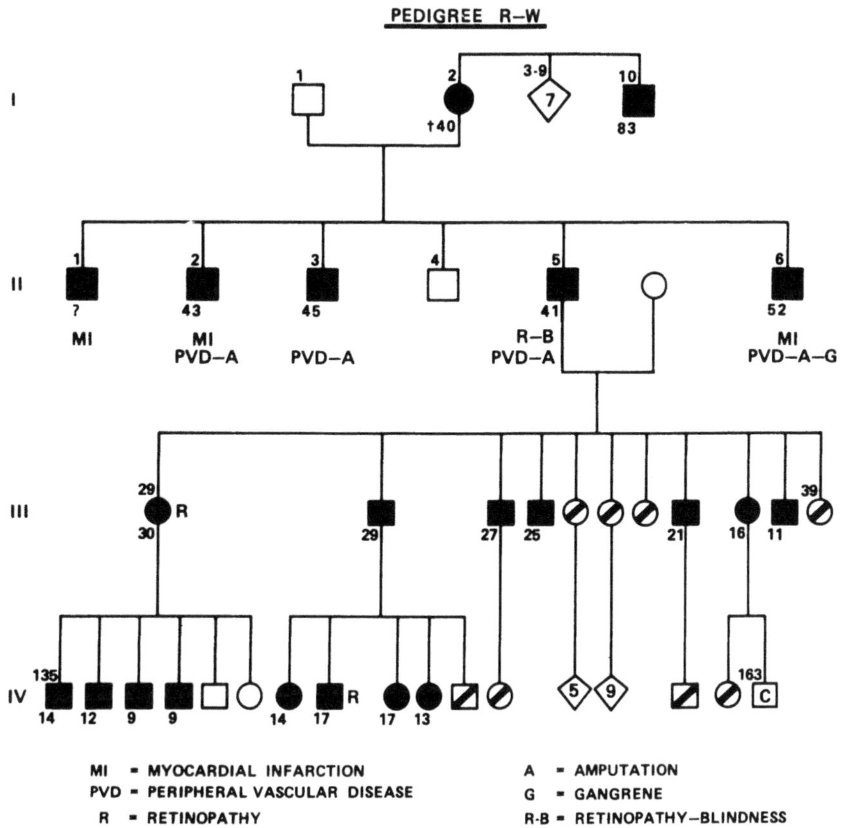

Fig. 1. Pedigree of R. W. family. Black squares (male) or circles (female) are diabetic members. All diabetics are MOD or MODY except for individual in generation IV and age 13 who has JOB diabetes. Circles or squares with heavy lines indicate subjects tested with normal glucose tolerance tests. Square containing C is a ten-year-old boy with borderline glucose tolerance test and strongly abnormal cortisone glucose tolerance test. Figures above squares and circles give number of member in generation, figures below give age at diagnosis of diabetes (Reproduced from DIABETES 27: 1112, 1978)

In pedigree VA there are four generations of maturity-onset type diabetes. In the propositus, generation III, a diagnosis was made with a fasting blood sugar level of 151 mg/dl in 1952. She was treated with insulin for one year, but has been controlled on diet since that time and has had normal fasting plasma glucose but diabetic glucose tolerance tests without progression of carbohydrate intolerance over 25 years (5). Abnormal glucose tolerance tests were found in both her sons at age 17 years and have been abnormal for 14 and 11 years, respectively. All three have displayed muscle capillary basement membrane thickening and plasma insulin response to glucose that are below the mean of control subjects. A diagnosis of diabetes was made in generation I, the paternal grandfather, at age 76 years. He was treated with insulin. Diabetes was diagnosed in the father (generation II) at age 76 with a FBS of 243 mg/dl. He had a myocardial infarction, and his diabetic brother had peripheral vascular disease and amputation. The propositus' mother and aunt had diabetes and retinopathy. A brother had diabetes and myocardial infarction.

In Pedigree HO, MODY and MOD was present in three generations. Myocardial infarction and background retinopathy have occurred in generation II. Both III-6. who is diabetic, and his brother, III-3, who has impaired glucose tolerance, neither of whom are obese, have sums of insulin responses to oral glucose which exceeded by 1 standard deviation the mean of control subjects. Incremental insulin response in III-5, the other nonobese diabetic, also exceeds the mean of controls. However, each of these three men had a 30-minute increment of insulin below the mean of the controls. To date, only one of the six, III-5, has progressed to fasting hyperglycemia. Capillary basement membrane thickening is present in III-2 and III-5.

In Pedigree TE, three siblings in generation IV have MODY diabetes. Incremental insulin responses to oral glucose also exceed the mean of control subjects or the mean +1 standard deviation of the mean.

Family PO has included four generations of MODY and MOD. Diabetes and severe vascular disease have coincided in three generations of this family. II-2 was diagnosed at age 26 years after discovery of glycosuria. She was never ketonuric. At age 37 years she developed diabetic gangrene leading to a metatarsal amputation. Over the next 18 years, before her death from breast cancer at age 63, she suffered a myocardial infarction at age 56 years and diabetic retinopathy with retinal detachment. Five of her six children are diabetic with ages of diagnosis ranging from 41 to 10 years. All except one are obese. The oldest, III-6, died from a myocardial infarction at age 42 years. The youngest, III-11, was diagnosed as diabetic at age 10 years. At age 28 years, she first developed fasting hyperglycemia. At age 33, she required insulin to control fasting hyperglycemia and had an EKG compatible with inferior wall ischemia. An abnormality of lipid metabolism has never been documented in this family.

Family HA does not conform to a typical MODY pedigree although it contains members with typical MODY. Three of four siblings in generation III presented with a similar picture of diabetes but have displayed varied clinical courses. III-3 and III-5 were discovered to have asymptomatic fasting hyperglycemia at ages 22 and 17 years respectively in 1961 and have required sulfonylureas for the last 17½ years to maintain fasting euglycemia. Each has an incremental insulin response to oral glucose less than 1 standard deviation below the mean of control subjects. Over 17½ years of observation, they have shown only mild progression of fasting hyperglycemia when off sulfonylureas for two weeks. To date both are free of complications of diabetes. Capillary basement membrane thickening has been found in both patients.

On the other hand, sibling III-4 had a normal fasting glucose but an abnormal glucose tolerance test at diagnosis in the Navy at age 22 years. He was treated with diet and oral antidiabetic agents for seven years before he developed ketotic diabetes. One year after initiation of insulin therapy he had hemorrhagic and neovascular retinopathy. In the intervening seven years, retinopathy has progressed to marked visual impairment in one eye and blindness in the other, and he suffered progressive nephropathy leading to renal failure requiring hemodialysis. Diabetes is present both on the maternal and paternal side of this sibship. A maternal grandmother was diagnosed at age 60 years and treated with oral agents. The paternal grandfather had ketotic diabetes diagnosed in his twenties with frequent episodes of ketoacidosis throughout the remainder of his life. He had progressive retinopathy leading to blindness. He died in his seventies of unspecified causes. Mild diabetes was diagnosed in the father, II-3, at age 25 years and managed with diet alone. He died at age 51 years of renal disease related to diabetes.

Susceptibility to the long-term vascular complications in MODY may be heterogenous. Reports to date have suggested that MODY is a relatively benign disease with a low incidence of vascular complications (2,4). The present data indicate that an optimistic prognosis cannot be assigned to members of MODY families with certainty any more than to other forms of idiopathic diabetes. In our six families, excluding four patients with JOD, 52% of patients followed for 15 years or more had evidence of macro-or microvascular complications (5). Since precise clinical details are missing in many instances, particularly among earlier generations, it is likely that this figure underestimates the actual incidence of vascular complications. In addition to our studies, Tattersall reported evidence of diabetic retinopathy in five of 12 patients from three families diagnosed under the age of 30 years, having a mean duration of diabetes of 37 years (2). Four of his patients had myocardial infarctions and one patient underwent amputation. Steele et al. have demonstrated rapid onset of proliferative retinopathy among five patients with apparently mild MODY type diabetes (6).

The prevalence of basement membrane thickening in our patients without clinical evidence of vascular disease was 61% of those tested after age of 19 years.

The precise incidence of MODY is unknown. Were it not for the application of glucose tolerance testing in successively younger patients in families with diabetes, this syndrome might be all together unrecognized. These affected persons are nearly always asymptomatic. Among the 86 diabetics in these six families, a diagnosis was made in 38 by testing asymptomatic relatives of diabetic patients. Of 31 patients diagnosed before the age of 31 years, a diagnosis was made by glucose tolerance testing only in 27.

Two of the families had many obese patients in each generation, but nonobese diabetics are found in these families and some obese members do not have diabetes. Increase in adiposity is a contributing factor in worsening carbohydrate tolerance in MODY as well as in MOD. In the six families in the present series. nothing distinguishes the older diabetics in these families from other patients with maturity-onset type diabetes.

Examination of these pedigrees suggests that MODY may be the same disease as MOD discovered at an earlier stage. Evidence has been gathered that MODY may be transmitted by autosomal dominant inheritance. Kobberling had suggested that autosomal dominant inheritance may occur in some classic MOD families as well. As many as 50% of patients with MOD manifest complications of the disease, such as retinopathy, at the time of diagnosis. This implies that the disease may have been long-standing prior to laboratory confirmation. Many of our MODY patients have had asymptomatic diabetes for more than 20 years. Without routine testing, it is likely that these patients would have been diagnosed in later life as classical MOD.

The occurence of two JODs with 27 MODYs or MODs in pedigree R.W. may be a chance occurrence of two different diseases in the same family. The presence of positive islet cell antibody titers in the two JODs and their absence in the rest of the MODY siblings may indicate distinct diseases. Since JOD is not an uncommon condition, it may be introduced and inherited in an independent fashion from the genotype for MODY.

Family HA presents greater problems of interpretation. JOD was expressed in generation I and III and MODY in generations I, II and III. From this family, one could conclude that JOD and MODY are merely spectrums of the same disease, a conclusion not in keeping with other data supporting heterogenity in genetic and environmental factors between JOD and MODY (5). Two JODs, one in R.W. and the other in the HA pedigree demonstrate that a JOD may masquerade as a MODY initially. These patients progressed to insulin-dependent diabetes, three and seven years respectively after recognition of carbohydrate intolerance. At the present, the only means of predicting the possible future course of an apparent MODY at a time of diagnosis is the ascertainment of presence or absence of islet cell antibody titers.

REFERENCES

1. *Fajans, S. S., et al., (1976). Arch. Int. Med. 136, 194.*
2. *Tattersall, R.B., (1974). Quart. J. Med. 43, 339.*
3. *Tattersall, R.B. and Fajans, S.S., (1975). Diabetes 24, 44.*
4. *Barbosa, J. et al., (1978). Arch. Int. Med. 138, 90.*
5. *Fajans, S.S., et al. (1978). Diabetes 27, 112.*
6. *Steel, J.M., et al. (1976). Brit. Med. J. 2, 846.*

Supported in part by U.S. Public Health Service Grants AM-0888 and AM-02244; NIH-5 M01 RR-42 General Clinical Research Centers; and Grants from the Upjohn Co., Kalamazoo, Michigan; and Pfizer, Inc., New York, New York.

DISCUSSION

P. RUBINSTEIN: *Dr. Barbosa, a clinical heterogeneity need not be synonymous with genetic heterogeneity, and in fact may not be the consequence of it. Now some questions: First, the liped program that was used here does not by itself compute gene frequencies. How did you put these frequencies into the program? Second, how can you explain the persistent linkage disequilibrium between juvenile diabetes and B8, B15, B18, DW3, DW4, if the distance has a theta of .13? That would lead to elimination of linkage disequilibrium in about 11-15 generations. The third question is: when you compute your dominant pedigrees, did you calculate them together with the rest of the patients, to account for the chance that these may be the few pedigrees where the homozygous parent may express the disease?*

J. BARBOSA: *About the second question, we have the impression that associations, in population studies between B8, B15 and diabetes identifies a type of diabetes which is different from those found when you do family studies. There are several reasons why we think so. One of them is that in our families we don't find any association between the JIDD trait and any of these particular antigens. In fact, we have quite a few families where JIDD is homozygous for B7, whereas in our study populations, we find that B7 seems to be associated with the protective factor. Probably these underlie different mechanisms. And we do not expect diabetic genes in linkage disequilibrium with HLA.*

P. RUBINSTEIN: *That would mean that your cases are totally different from Cudworth and ours. The other question is gene frequency computation into the liped program. How did you manage that?*

J. BARBOSA: *This was a slightly modified liped program where the gene frequencies were included.*

P. RUBINSTEIN: *How did you compute for gene frequency?*

J. BARBOSA: *I couldn't give you the details because that was done by our statistician.*

P. RUBINSTEIN: *The third question was for the dominant pedigrees. Did you put them as a part of the total body of the data, as well as separate, to see whether they could fit into your overall hypothesis by being those few cases where the homozygous parent expressed his--*

J. BARBOSA: *You mean putting together the MS families with MG families? No, because even the computer programs are different.*

You know, we use a liped program for the autosomal dominant and another liped program for autosomal recessive.

G.M. REAVEN: *Dr. Fajans, have you had a chance to figure the relationship in your patients between macroangiopathy, lipoprotein metabolism, and insulin response; those three variables?*

S. FAJANS: *In the families where there was the greatest incidence of micro-and macroangiopathy, there was no evidence of a hyperlipoproteinemia.*

T. PROUT: *Thank you. Now I would like to pose Dr. Camerini's question in a different way. If you find hyperglycemia as defined by the workshop, what is your diagnosis of record on these patients? I pose it in this way because I think that whether or not you feel that there is a condition called "pre-diabetes" as stated by Dr. Camerini, there should be some concern as to whether or not we place a label of diabetes on patients prematurely. The diagnosis of "hyperglycemia" is not penalized by insurance carriers, or by our society in general. Pedigrees that you have shown sharpen the need for an answer to that question, because you have a 50% chance of being wrong either way whether or not you label them as being diabetic.*

S. FAJANS: *I did not deny that there is a prediabetic state. But what I said is that we don't know, as of today, particularly in the MODY-MOD families, how to recognize pre-diabetes prospectively. I think it may be somewhat simpler if you have a sibling who shares the same HLA type as his diabetic sibling; then, I think the chances are greater. If you find islet cell antibodies at the time the glucose tolerance is normal, then you have a great likelihood that you're dealing with prediabetes with the definition of normal glucose tolerance. Now, coming back to the MODY, this is a very difficult problem, since we do not have a marker other than glucose intolerance. And, as you indicated, the chances are 50%, and our advice is frequent testing at periodic intervals.*

E. PFEIFFER: *A couple of years ago, we were influenced by the observation that early diabetes, which we call protodiabetes, is influenced by environmental factors. Obesity, diabetes and hyperlipidemia influence arterial sclerosis, and we see how everything gets together. But, I should like to challenge you in the following way: These families with so many children probably come from lower class which, within the last 40 years, became affluent and required less physical work. Now, haven't you been describing the development of the disadvantages of the industrial age instead of inheritance? What they inherited was their grandmothers' cooking.*

S. FAJANS: *Well, I think the majority of our MODY families are hard working, lean individuals, but as I tried to indicate earlier, small increases in body weight may bring out glucose intolerance. So certainly there is a superimposed environmental factor.*

PHOSPHATE TRANSLOCATIONS DURING SECRETORY STIMULATION OF PANCREATIC ISLETS

N. Freinkel*

In 1974, we described a new phenomenon: During a study of various aspects of phosphorus metabolism in isolated rat pancreatic islets, we noted that exposure of islets prelabeled with radiophosphate to nutrient secretagogues elicits a rapid transitory efflux of radioactivity (1). In much earlier experiments with thyroid, we had already reported that functional activation of tissues with appropriate stimuli (e.g. thyrotropin in the case of thyroid) may induce acute changes in tissue inorganic phosphate (P_i) (2,3). For our islet experiments, the protocol was as follows: Pancreatic islets isolated by collagenase were prelabeled by incubation with [^{32}P] -orthophosphate in modified Krebs-Ringer bicarbonate medium (KRB). After washing to remove adherent extracellular radioactivity, they were introduced into small chambers for perifusion with KRB and various secretagogues. The efflux was monitored for radioactivity and insulin.

With two different perifusion systems, having entirely different "dead space" characteristics (1,4), we noted that the release of radioactivity increases almost immediately when glucose in the perifusion medium is increased from 0.5 to 3.0 mg/ml (Fig. 1). The heightened release of radioactivity achieves peak values rapidly and then returns to basal levels despite continuing secretory stimulation with the 3.0 mg/ml glucose. Extensive biochemical characterization clearly established that virtually all the released radioactivity consists of [^{32}P] -orthophosphate. Accordingly, we called the phenomenon, the phosphate flush.

The temporal features of the phosphate flush exhibited certain intriguing correlations with activated insulin secretion. It should be recalled that the latter occurs in a biphasic pattern

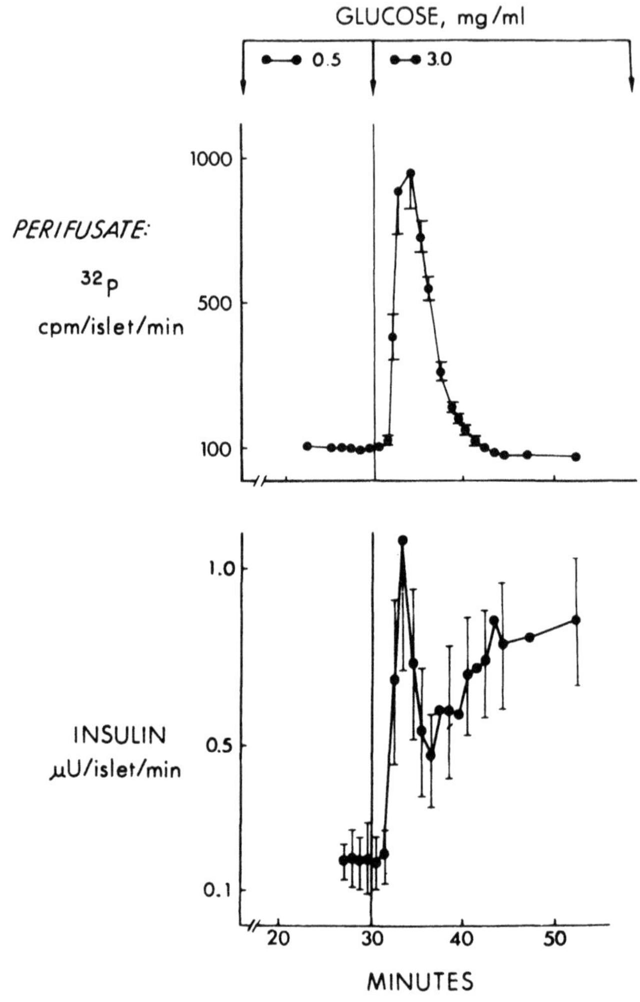

Fig. 1. Temporal correlations between the phosphate flush (upper panel) and stimulated insulin release (lower panel): Rat pancreatic islets were isolated with collagenase, and prelabeled with [^{32}P] -orthophosphate, before perifusion at the rate of 0.3 ml/min with media containing 0.5 mg/ml glucose for the first 30 min and 3.0 mg/ml glucose thereafter. Volume of the perifusion chamber was 40 µl and that of the total perifusion system with tubing was 230µl. The illustration depicts Mean ± SEM values for the rates of release of ^{32}P (cpm/islet/min) and insulin (µU/islet/min) into the perifusate. Adapted from Asplund and Freinkel(4).

(5, 6): there is a short-lived, transitory first phase of heightened insulin release which is then followed by a more prolonged second phase persisting throughout the period of islet exposure to ambient secretagogues. Concurrent examination for insulin and P_i indicated that the phosphate flush was initiated slightly before, or directly coincident with, the first phase of activated insulin release. The actual phosphate flush encompassed the entire first phase and was completed shortly after inception of the second phase of stimulated insulin release (1,4,7) (Fig. 1).

A number of other characterizations were soon secured: It was shown that the phosphate flush could be elicited with all nutrient secretagogues but with a high decree of specificity paralleling insulin-secretory potentialities. Thus, with respect to sugars, the phosphate flush is triggered by D-glucose but not L-glucose (1) and by alpha rather than the beta anomer of the D-glucose (8). It can also be elicited by D-mannose (1), and D-glyceraldehyde (Pierce, M. and Freinkel, N., unpublished observations) but not by D-galactose, D-fructose, or i-inositol (1). Mannoheptulose blocks glucose-mediated phosphate flush (7). Secretagogic amino acids also cause a phosphate flush. Thus, leucine elicits the phosphate flush -- an action that is not impaired by mannoheptulose (7). Moreover, the phenomenon does not require intracellular metabolism of the secretagogue because the appropriate stereosomers (9,10) of the non-metabolizable analogue of leucine, 2-aminobicyclo (2,2,1), heptane-2-carboxylic acid (BCH) appear to be equally effective (7). With amino acids, as with the stimulatory sugars, the same temporal correlations between phosphate flush and first phase of stimulated insulin release appear to obtain (7).

However, the phosphate flush is not a consequence of the exocytotic process. It can be readily dissociated from activated extrusion of insulin per se. Thus, the phosphate flush still occurs during islet exposure to nutrient secretagogues even when stimulated release of insulin is inhibited by omission of Ca^{++} from the suspending medium or inclusion of Ni^{++}(1, 11). The phosphate flush is also seen with nutrient secretagogues even when the vagaries of islet isolation have compromised the highly sensitive first phase but not the second phase of stimulated insulin release. In addition, the phosphate flush can be dissociated from intracellular processes involved in the propagation or amplification of stimuli. For example, we have been able to promote insulin secretion without increasing ongoing rates of phosphate efflux by supplementing perifusates with dibutyryl cyclic AMP (Freinkel, N. and Botos, C., unpublished observations) or by promoting acute transcellular Ca^{++} flux with the ionophore, A23187 (11).

The experimental ability to separate the phosphate flush from exocytosis and from intracellular processes involved in stimulus propagation and/or amplification has prompted our suggestion that the phosphate flush is linked to earlier components of stimulus-secretion coupling, i.e. to some aspect of the recognition of nutrient stimuli at the cell surface. Such a proposition implies that membrane perturbations are involved. Our early finding, that heightened efflux of [^{32}P] -orthophosphate from prelabeled islets can be abolished by local anesthetics, such as tetracaine (1, 11), is in concordance with that suggestion. The hypothesis is reinforced further by the demonstration that the phosphate flush can be inhibited reversibly by stabilizers of membrane organization, such as deuterium oxide (1,7).

All of these considerations heightened the desirability of identifying the intracellular origin of the release orthophosphate. Initial efforts were directed towards characterizing tissue radioactivity before and after the phosphate flush during our standard perifusion experiments with KRB (4,12). It was documented that [^{32}P]-orthophosphate accounts for approximately one-half of the total radioactivity that is present in rat pancreatic islets after prelabeling by batch incubation with [^{32}P] - orthophosphate for 90 minutes and then perifusing for 30 or 45 minutes with KRB containing 0.5 mg/ml glucose. Analyses of paired islets following an additional ten (4) to fourteen (12) minutes of perifusion with 3.0 mg/ml glucose, and elicitation of the phosphate flush, indicated that all the heightened efflux of radioactivity during the latter period could be accounted for by a reduction in tissue [^{32}P] -orthophosphate [$^{32}P_i$]. Approximately half of the tissue $^{32}P_i$ pool is released into the effluent during the phosphate flush (4,12). Contributions via net hydrolysis of high energy phosphates were excluded by our finding that the labeling of AT^{32}P and GT^{32}P actually increased during the same interval (4,12). Similar changes in tissue radioactivity were found during perifusions with KRB from which all phosphate had been omitted (i.e., "Phosphate-free media") (13,14). Thus, simple ionic exchange could be excluded as the basis for the phosphate flush. Nonetheless, the possibilities remained that: a) the phosphate flush merely represented an isotope anomaly due to incomplete equilibration of ^{32}P with exchangeable tissue P_i; or b) that the prolonged preparative manipulations for prelabeling of islets had caused artifactual "leakiness" for ions. It was therefore, deemed extremeley important to obtain direct chemical estimates of islet orthophosphate content, and to do so under conditions which would minimize preparative delay.

To meet these objectives, islets were perifused with "phosphate-free media" immediately following isolation. They were analyzed by the microchemical methods of Lowry before and 11 minutes after glucose in the perifusate was increased from 0.5 to 3.0 mg/ml. Such stimulation effected a brisk first phase and an early second phase of heightened insulin release. It also reduced total islet orthophosphate content an average of 47% -- that is, from 19.8 ± 3.1 to 10.4 ± 1.0 pmol per islet (Mean ± SEM) in 10 experiments ($p<0.05$) (13,14). Concurrent estimates of ATP content in the same islets failed to disclose any significant change (5.8 ± 0.8 vs. 7.3 ± 0.6 pmol per islet in the unstimulated vs. stimulated islets respectively). These first estimates of islet P_i provided direct chemical documentation that a pool of orthophosphate which is labilized during early secretory stimulation and available for release into the extracellular phase exists within pancreatic islets.

Some documentation of the participating cell types and the subcellular localization of the labile orthophosphate was clearly desirable. Accordingly, we sought to develop an appropriate electron microscopic histochemical technique for inorganic phosphate. A variant of the classical reaction with lead acetate, in which phosphate is precipitated as lead phosphate (15) was finally established (16). To enhance specificity, we instituted prior perifusion of the islets with saline media from which bicarbonate and phosphate had been omitted (so that precipitation of lead carbonate or phosphate of extracellular origin could be avoided). In practice (16), the following procedure was followed: isolated islets were perifused with "phosphate-free," bicarbonate-poor tris-HCl buffered saline media at pH 7.4. Immediately before and directly after elicitation of "phosphate-flush" (by increasing perifusate glucose from 0.5 to 3.0 mg/ml), islets were introduced into fixation fluid containing sodium cacodylate (0.1 M). glutaraldehyde and lead acetate (2%) at a pH of 7.0. Islets were then dehydrated and embedded according to standard electron microscopic procedures. Osmium tetroxide and uranyl acetate were not used since these removed all the lead precipitate present in the section. Microprobe analysis was performed to identify the composition of the precipitates (16).

In the B cells of the islets prior to stimulation, punctate precipitates were concentrated at or on the plasmalemma and over the nucleolus. There was no significant amount of precipitate on or near the plasmalemmas of the A and D cells or on the plasmalemma of any of the exocrine cells remaining at the edges of the islets. By contrast, in the glucose-stimulated islets, precipitate was not seen on the plasmalemma or nucleolus of the B cells. No precipitate was seen on any other type of cell present. Microprobe analysis shows that the precipitate on the nucleolus and at the plasmalemma of the B cell contained only lead and phosphate in significant amounts. The exact location of the precipitate on the plasmalemma was difficult to determine. However, with the resolution available, nearly all the particles of precipitate appeared to be on the internal surface of the plasmalemma (16). As far as we are aware, these findings represent the first demonstration by an electron microscope technique of a specific localization of phosphate at the plasmalemma.

Clearly these ongoing histochemical efforts may not have identified all the inorganic phosphate in islet tissue: formation of visible precipitates with lead must necessitate a critical concentration of reactive phosphate at any given site. By the same token, the reactivity with lead does not necessarily characterize the nature of the prior association of that phosphate. From the available data, we cannot say whether the phosphate found at or near the plasmalemma is directly bound to the membrane; or combined with cations; or complexed in some other combination. However, regardless of physicochemical characteristics, a labile intracellular component has been visualized and identified isotopically,chemically and histochemically as orthophosphate. If truly linked to stimulus-secretion coupling, the labilization should bear some stoicheometric relationship to the magnitude of stimulation and/or excitation. This has proved to be the case. Concentrations of nutrient secretagogue and magnitude of phosphate flush have displayed clear dose-response correlations in every circumstance examined to date (1,7,17).

Thus, the data strongly indicate that there is an intracellular pool of orthophosphate in the beta cell which is directly responsive to nutrient secretagogues and strategically placed to subserve a role in the events incident to stimulus recognition. The temporal correlations between heightened translocations of intracellular orthophosphate and the first phase of stimulated insulin release are consistent with the possibility that the phosphate flush may be an integral component of those metastable and disequilibrated intracellular events which determine the first phase of stimulated-insulin release. In a more practical sense, the phosphate flush is also providing us with a convenient biochemical probe to characterize the beta cell in physiological states in which insulin secretion is faulty but underlying determinants may be different, such as neonatal life (4) or starvation (18).

REFERENCES

1. *Freinkel, N., et al.(1974). J. Clin. Invest., 54, 1179*
2. *Freinkel, N. (1957). Endocrinology, 61, 448*
3. *Freinkel, N. (1963). Nature, 198, 889*
4. *Asplund, K.and Freinkel, N. (1978). Diabetes, 27,611*
5. *Curry, D.L., et al.(1968). Endocrinology, 83, 572*
6. *Porte, D. and Pupo, A.A. (1969). J. Clin. Invest., 48, 2309*
7. *Freinkel, N., et al.(1976). Proc. Natl. Acad. Sci. USA, 73,3403*
8. *Pierce, M. and Freinkel, N. (1975). Biochem. Biophys. Res. Commun., 63, 870*
9. *Tager, H.S. and Christensen, H. N. (1971) Biochem. Biophys. Res. Commun., 44, 185*

10. *Christensen, H. N., et al.(1971). Biochim. Biophys. Acta, 241, 341*
11. *Bukowiecki, L. and Freinkel, N. (1976). Biochim. Biophys. Acta, 436, 190*
12. *Pierce, M., et al.(1978). Endocrinology, 103, 971*
13. *Bukowiecki, L., et al.(1976). Diabetes, 25 (Suppl. 1), 346*
14. *Bukowiecki, L., et al.(1979). Biochim. Biophys. Acta, in press*
15. *Libanati, C.M. and Tandler, C.J. (1969). J. Cell Biol., 42, 754*
16. *Freinkel, N., et al.(1978). Science, 201, 1124*
17. *Pierce, M., et al.(1976). Horm. Metab. Res., 8, 358*
18. *Asplund, K. and Freinkel, N. (1978). Acta Endocrinol., 88, 545*

The author should like to express his gratitude to the following colleagues for stimulating collaborations in various aspects of this work: K. Asplund, M.D., Ph.D.; J. Bonnar, B.A.; C. Botos, M.A.; L. Bukowiecki, Ph.D.; R.M.C. Dawson, Ph.D., D.Sc.; F.M. Matschinsky, M.D.; K.C. Pedley, Ph.D.; M. Pierce, M.D., Ph.D.; M. Trus, Ph.D.; P. Wooding, Ph.D.; C. El Younsi. The studies have been supported in part by Research Grants AM-10699 and HD-11021 and Training Grants AM-05071 and AM-07169 from the NIH, Bethesda, Maryland, and by a Research Grant from The Kroc Foundation.

THE ROLE OF PHOSPHOENOLPYRUVATE AND LACTATE PRODUCTION IN INSULIN SECRETION

C. J. Hedeskov* and K. Capito

We have previously shown that inosine is an initiator or primary stimulus of insulin secretion (1). Inosine also stimulates insulin biosynthesis (2) and has further been shown to exert a protective effect on the β-cell glucoreceptor function during culture of pancreatic islets (3). The effect of inosine on insulin secretion is almost completely abolished after 48 hours starvation of the animals but normal secretion rates during starvation can be maintained in the presence of caffeine (1). This normalization of the insulin secretory response may be due to either a direct effect of caffeine on the intracellular distribution of calcium (4) or to an effect of caffeine on the islet cAMP content by inhibition of the phosphodiesterases, since the normal elevation of cAMP on stimulation by both glucose and inosine is curtailed by starvation (5,1).

In islets inosine is first split by a nucleoside phosphorylase to hypoxanthine and ribose-1-phosphate which is then further metabolized to glyceraldehyde-3-phosphate and lactate. The starvation-depressed insulin secretion during stimulation by inosine is accompanied by an augmented accumulation in the islets of fructose-1,6-diphosphate and triose-phosphates indicating a possible inhibition of the glyceraldehyde-3-phosphate dehydrogenase (1). Initiation of insulin secretion may therefore depend on the production of a metabolic signal below the triose-phosphate level (1,6). It has recently been suggested that phosphoenolpyruvate (PEP) may play such a role as intracellular trigger to insulin release (7) since the concentration of PEP was shown to be positively correlated to glycolytic flux after exposure of islets to glucose and D-glyceraldehyde both in the absence and presence of mannoheptulose.

In order to test this hypothesis we have examined the effect of some known potentiators of insulin release on the islet content of PEP, islet lactate output and insulin secretion, both in the fed state and during starvation. The potentiators used were fructose, N-acetylglucosamine (NAG) and pyruvate, all of which may circumvent the hexokinase-glucokinase system and enter the glycolytic pathway at or below the triose-phosphate level during their metabolism.

In the reported experiments we have used islets from normal mice isolated by a collagenase technique. Inosine was applied as primary insulin secretagogue. Insulin, lactate and cAMP were measured as previously described (5,8). PEP was measured after conversion to ATP by a luciferase technique. Endogenous ATP was first removed by the aid of hexokinase and glucose as described (7).

The results suggest that glycolytic flux is of overall importance for insulin secretion. On the other hand, an increased concentration of PEP does not seem to be a sufficient condition to elicit insulin release.

RESULTS AND DISCUSSION

The data of Table I show that inosine clearly stimulated insulin secretion in the fed state but not in islets from starved mice. None of the potentiators, fructose, NAG and pyruvate, stimulated insulin secretion by themselves. Fructose, NAG, pyruvate and caffeine, potentiated insulin secretion in the starved state. They also potentiated insulin secretion in islets from fed mice although with one obvious exception: fructose did not potentiate insulin secretion in the fed state.

Table II showns the results of measurements of islet PEP content. In the fed state inosine increased the concentration of PEP, as glucose and glyceraldehyde previously have been shown to do (7), but a similar increase of PEP content was seen with fructose and NAG although these agents do not stimulate insulin secretion. An increased PEP concentration may thus be a necessary but not a sufficient condition to elicit insulin secretion. It is noteworthy that pyruvate did not increase the content of PEP. It is not known whether islets contain the enzyme phosphoenolpyruvate carboxykinase. The potentiation of insulin secretion in the fed state by NAG and pyruvate was not associated with an additional increase in PEP content. Overall there was no statistical correlation between PEP content and insulin secretion rates.

In starved state (see Table II) inosine and NAG enhanced the PEP content without having any effect on insulin secretion. The potentiation of insulin secretion in the starved state by fructose, NAG and pyruvate was not accompanied by an additional increase in PEP content above that seen with inosine alone. It should be

TABLE 1. POTENTIATION OF INSULIN SECRETION

ADDITION	INSULIN SECRETION (μU/ml per 5 islets per 2 h) FED	48 h STARVED
NONE	382 ± 39 (59)	244 ± 24 (55)
FRUCTOSE (20 mM)	405 ± 54 (12)	137 ± 52 (12)
NAG (20 mM)	551 ± 76 (18)	264 ± 69 (13)
PYRUVATE (2 mM)	371 ± 69 (13)	348 ± 60 (24)
INOSINE (10 mM)	1198 ± 101 (69)	305 ± 31 (81)
INOSINE + FRUCTOSE	1166 ± 122 (24)	729 ± 89 (24)**
INOSINE + NAG	1673 ± 155 (18)*	527 ± 68 (13)**
INOSINE + PYRUVATE	1766 ± 242 (12)*	561 ± 49 (21)**
INOSINE + CAFFEINE	1717 ± 194 (15)*	1509 ± 118 (15)**

Batches of 5 islets were incubated for 2 hours in 0.6 ml of Krebs-bicarbonate buffer containing albumin. Insulin was measured by radioimmunoassay. Results are given as mean ± S.E.M.

* $p < 0.01$ vs Inosine

** $p < 0.005$ vs Inosine

emphasized that some caution has to be exercised in the interpretation of these results concerning islet PEP content. The really interesting concentration of PEP is the cytoplasmic concentration. What we have measured is the total content of PEP in the islets. It is known from other tissues, however, that PEP may be compartmentalized between cytoplasm and mitochondria.

We have also evaluated the relation between insulin secretion and glycolytic flux under these conditions. Lactate output (see Table III) was taken as an expression of glycolytic flux although we are aware that this assumption may not be completely valid. In the fed state, inosine increased the lactate output to a value of about 1000 pmol per 2 hours per ug DNA. Fructose and pyruvate

TABLE 2. PHOSPHOENOLPYRUVATE (PEP) CONTENT OF ISOLATED MOUSE ISLETS

	PEP CONTENT (% OF BASAL)	
ADDITION	FED	48 h STARVED
NONE	100	100
INOSINE (10 mM)	179 ± 16 (15)*	160 ± 22 (15)*
FRUCTOSE (20 mM)	167 ± 33 (8)*	138 ± 43 (9)
NAG (20 mM)	160 ± 12 (8)*	125 ± 9 (8)*
PYRUVATE (2 mM)	123 ± 17 (7)	134 ± 23 (7)
INOSINE + FRUCTOSE	217 ± 35 (8)*	182 ± 45 (9)*
INOSINE + NAG	145 ± 15 (8)*	141 ± 14 (8)*
INOSINE + PYRUVATE	176 ± 23 (8)*	185 ± 31 (7)*

Batches of 20 - 40 islets were incubated for 30 min. in Krebs-bicarbonate buffer and the PEP content determined as described. The basal value was 203 ± 34 fmol/islet (n = 15) in the fed state and 191 ± 34 fmol/islet (n = 15) in the starved state. Results are given as means ± S.E.M.

*$p < 0.05$ vs NONE

also enhanced lactate output but without increasing secretion. Perhaps there exists a threshold value for the lactate output of around 800 pmol/2 hours/ug DNA, which has to be surpassed in order to elicit insulin release. Assuming that approx. 15% of utilized glucose is converted to lactate (8) this value would correspond very well with the threshold value for glycolytic flux suggested by Zawalich et al. (9) of 50 pmol glucose equivalents perhour per islet. The NAG and pyruvate induced potentiation of insulin secretion in the fed state was clearly associated with an increased lactate output.

In the starved state, fructose and pyruvate also stimulated lactate output somewhat, but the potentiation of inosine-induced insulin secretion by fructose, NAG and pyruvate was not associated with any additional increase lactate production.

TABLE 3. LACTATE PRODUCTION OF ISOLATED PANCREATIC MOUSE ISLETS

	LACTATE PRODUCTION (pmoles / μg DNA / 2 hours)	
ADDITION	FED	48 h STARVED
NONE	318 ± 101 (7)	167 ± 41 (8)
FRUCTOSE (20 mM)	806 ± 121 (5)*	517 ± 75 (5)*
PYRUVATE (2 mM)	740 ± 79 (4)*	570 ± 51 (8)*
NAG (20 mM)	418 ± 109 (6)	286 ± 80 (7)
INOSINE (10 mM)	992 ± 75 (8)*	1051 ± 115 (8)*
INOSINE + FRUCTOSE	1282 ± 79 (5)**	1166 ± 108 (6)
INOSINE + NAG	1348 ± 121 (6)**	1024 ± 96 (8)
INOSINE + PYRUVATE	1286 ± 125 (7)**	1193 ± 118 (8)

Batches of 40 - 60 islets were incubated for 2 hours in Krebs-bicarbonate buffer. Lactate was determined fluorimetrically. Results are expressed as means ± S.E.M.

*p ± 0.05 vs NONE

**p ± 0.05 vs INOSINE

Statistical analysis of the data revealed a highly significant positive correlation between lactate output and insulin secretion in both the fed and starved state. The correlation coefficients were 0.89 ($p < 0.005$) and 0.77 ($p < 0.05$), respectively. However, the slope and the intercept of the two regression lines differed widely. Especially was the slope of the regression line for the data in the starved state much less steep than in the fed state. The highest values for lactate production were similar in the two states. This seems to indicate that starvation-depressed insulin secretion is not solely due to a decreased glycolytic flux. Additional factors may be involved in causing the defect. Changes in cAMP metabolism (8) and in intracellular Ca^{++} (10) distribution have been suggested.

Preliminary experiments have shown that potentiation of insulin release in the fed state could not be explained by an enhanced cAMP production. In contrast, the potentiation of insulin release by fructose, NAG and pyruvate in the starved state was accompanied by an augmented cAMP production.

IN SUMMARY

There is a positive correlation between lactate output and insulin secretion but there is no correlation between total islet PEP content and insulin secretion and no correlation between cAMP production and insulin release. Neither PEP or cAMP seem to be primary triggers to insulin release but may rather act as positive modulators of insulin secretion. Potentially, PEP can maintain an elevated cytoplasmic Ca^{++} concentration by inhibiting Ca^{++} uptake in the mitochondria, increase the concentration of cAMP in the β-cells by activating the adenylate cyclase (11) and change the phosphorylation state of the plasma membrane (12). The possible trigger effect of an increased glycolytic flux on insulin secretion may be mediated perhaps via changes in the $NADH/NAD^+$ ratio (13). As regards the mechanism of potentiation of insulin release: in the fed state potentiation may be related to an increased glycolytic flux whereas this is not the case during starvation. Here enhancement of cAMP may play a role.

The relevance of these studies to the problems of early diabetes is the assumption that changes in β-cell metabolism may be involved in the abnormal insulin secretion observed in human diabetes and that starvation diabetes in rodents may relate to human diabetes.

REFERENCES

1. *Capito, K., and Hedeskov, C.J., (1976). Biochem. J. 158, 335.*
2. *Ashcroft, S.J.H., et al., (1978). Biochem. J. 174, 517.*
3. *Gylfe, E., Biochem. J. in press.*
4. *Formby, B., et al., (1976). Am. J. Physiol. 230, 441.*
5. *Capito, K., and Hedeskov, C.J. (1974). Biochem. J. 142, 653.*
6. *Hellman, B., et al., (1974). Arch. Biochem. Biophys. 162, 448.*
7. *Sugden, M.C., and Ashcroft, S.J.H.(1977), Diabetologia 13, 481.*
8. *Hedeskov, C.J., and Capito, K. (1974). Biochem. J. 140, 423.*
9. *Zawalich, W.S., et al., (1977). J. Biol. Chem. 252, 8519.*
10. *Wolters, G.J.H., et al. (1978). Diabetologia 15, 282.*
11. *Capito, K., and Hedeskov, C.J. (1977). Biochem. J. 162, 569.*
12. *Davis, B., and Lazarus, N.R., (1975). J. Membrane Biol. 20, 301.*
13. *Sener, A., et al., (1978) Diabetologia 15, 269.*

The cost of these studies has been met in part by grants from the Danish Medical Research Council, Nordisk Insulinfond, Novo's Fond, Dr. med. Erik Garde og Elizabeth Gardes legat and the Danish Diabetic association. The expert technical assistance of Mrs. Anne-Marie Fabricius, Mrs. Anette Garval and Mrs. Ingrid Mikkelsen is gratefully acknowledged.

EFFECTS OF INSULINOTROPIC AGENTS ON CATIONIC FLUXES IN ISLET CELLS

W.J. Malaisse*, A. Sener and A. Herchuelz

In the stimulus-secretion coupling for insulin release, a remodelling of ionic fluxes in the pancreatic B-cell may represent the essential link between the site of identification of secretagogues and the site of release of secretory granules (1). This paper reviews the participation of several cations (K^+, Na^+, H^+, Mg^{2+}, Ba^{2+}, and Ca^{2+}) in the process of insulin release and in delineating the influence of insulinotropic agents, especially glucose, upon the handling of such cations.

1. K^+

Glucose causes a dose-related, rapid, sustained and rapidly reversible decrease in the fractional outflow of $^{42}K^+$ or $^{86}Rb^+$ from isolated islets (2-5). This is accompanied by a marked increase in the steady-state values for $^{86}Rb^+$ (or $^{42}K^+$) net uptake and $^{39}K^+$ content of the islets (3,4). Assuming that all K^+ is located in a single pool, no effect of glucose upon the steady-state values for K^+ inflow-outflow rate could be detected (Table 1).

The inflow of K^+ in the islet cells is mediated, in part at least, by an ouabain-sensitive ATPase (4). The outflow of K^+ apparently corresponds to a passive movement driven by the electrochemical gradient of K^+ across the plasma membrane, and mediated by a native ionophoretic system (6). Indeed, it is facilitated by valinomycin or cell depolarization, little affected by ouabain, and inhibited by verapamil or omission of extracellular K^+ (6). The effect of glucose upon $^{86}Rb^+$ efflux does not appear to be directly attributable to changes in either glucose transport, Na^+ influx, cyclic AMP concentration, insulin secretion or cytosolic Ca^{2+} concentration. The experimental data rather suggest that the glucose-induced modification of $^{86}Rb^+$ fractional outflow rate is directly linked, for its major part, to metabolic events such as the generation of reduced pyridine nucleotides and/or H^+ (6).

Table 1

EFFECT OF GLUCOSE UPON THE HANDLING OF MONOVALENT CATIONS BY RAT PANCREATIC ISLETS
The outflow of H^+ was measured using a bicarbonate-free incubation medium.

Ionic parameter	Glucose concentration NIL	Glucose concentration 16.7 mM	Reference (number)
Totak K^+ pool (pmol/islet)	161 ± 11	312 ± 38	(3, 4)
K^+ inflow-outflow rate (pmol/islet/min)	14.3 ± 1.6	13.8 ± 1.6	(3, 4)
K^+ fractional outflow rate (percent/min)	8.88 ± 0.34	4.23 ± 0.74	(3)
Total Na^+ pool (pmol/islet)	157 ± 7	119 ± 7	(14)
Na^+ inflow-outflow rate (pmol/islet/min)	28.4 ± 3.3	40.6 ± 5.0	(14)
Na^+ fractional outflow rate (percent/min)	18.3 ± 1.3	29.8 ± 2.0	(14)
H^+ net outflow rate (pmol/islet/min)	1.10 ± 0.18	2.35 ± 0.33	(16)

The glucose-induced accumulation of K^+ in islet cells may have several consequences. On one hand, it is thought that the glucose-induced change in K^+ conductance may lead to B-cell depolarization, as indeed observed in B-cells exposed to glucose (7-9) and, by doing so, cause the gating of voltage-dependent channels for the entry of Ca^{2+} in the islet cells (5). At concentrations close to 0.01 μM, valinomycin which fails to affect adversely the oxidation of glucose, concentration of NAD (P)H and adenylate charge in islets exposed to glucose (16.7 mM), increases the fractional outflow rate of $^{86}Rb^+$, decreases the glucose-stimulated net uptake of $^{45}Ca^{2+}$, and inhibits insulin release (10). However, even at higher concentrations of the drug, a modest effect of glucose on $^{45}Ca^{2+}$ handling (such as the induction of a secondary rise in $^{45}Ca^{2+}$ efflux) is still observed, despite complete suppression of the effect of glucose on $^{86}Rb^+$ handling by the islets. It appears, therefore, that the effect of glucose upon $^{45}Ca^{2+}$ handling can be dissociated, to a limited extent, from the effect of the sugar upon $^{86}Rb^+$ efflux (10).

On the other hand, the intracellular concentration of K^+ may affect the rate of glucose metabolism. Indeed, when extracellular K^+ is removed, the K^+ content of the islets is reduced by at least 80% and the rate of glucose oxidation concomitantly falls (11). This situation could be due to a change in the rate of glycolysis. Thus, in the islets, like in other tissues (12), the activity of pyruvate kinase is markedly influenced by the K^+ concentration, the latter effect being observed within the range of K^+ concentrations expected to be found in the cytosol of B-cells exposed to either a normal of K^+-depleted incubation medium (Figure 1, left panel). In the presence of K^+, Na^+ causes a dose-related inhibition of the enzyme activity (Figure 1, right panel). In considering these effects it should be kept in mind that the glucose-induced change in intracellular K^+ concentration is a relatively slow process. For instance, upon raising the glucose concentration from zero to 16.7 mM, the exponential increase in the K^+ content of the islets occurs with a half-life of about 16 min, and, hence, displays a time course which could account for delayed effects of glucose upon B-cell function, such as the priming action of the sugar upon subsequent stimulation by insulinotropic factors (13).

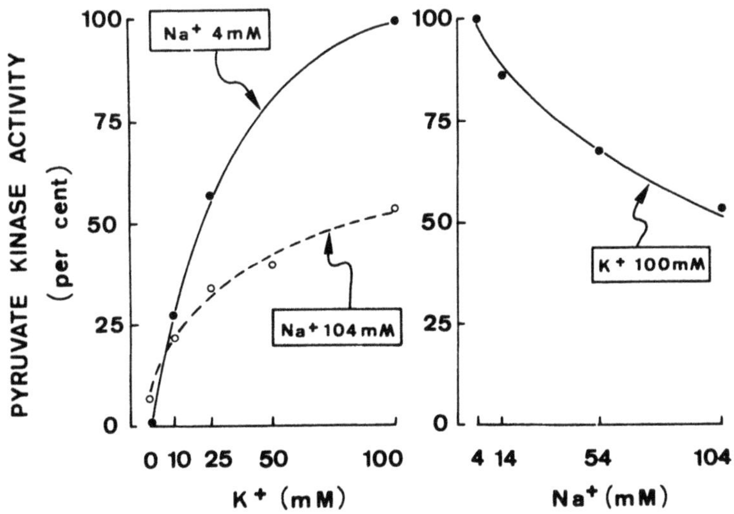

Fig. 1. Influence of Na^+ and K^+ upon the activity of pyruvate kinase in rat islets homogenates. The reference value (100 percent) observed in the presence of K^+ 100 mM and Na^+ 4 mM averaged 2.43 $\pm$ 0.43 nmol/min per islet (n = 3). Each point is the mean of 3-6 individual determinations. All measurements were made at 37°C in the presence of PEP 2.0 mM and ADP 2.5 mM.

2. Na^+

The study of Na^+ handling by isolated islets meets with severe methodological difficulties. First, the fractional outflow rate of Na^+ is so rapid that the efflux of $^{22}Na^+$ must be investigated immediately after prelabelling, without prior removal of extracellular $^{22}Na^+$ by a washing procedure. Second, the intracellular/extracellular ratio of Na^+ concentration in islet cells amounts to 0.3-0.5, so that the correct estimation of $^{22}Na^+$ net uptake is critically dependent on the adequate behaviour of the tracer molecule used as the extracellular marker. Third, Na^+ is apparently distributed in the islet cells in two compartments (14). Despite these difficulties, 3 significant effects of glucose upon $^{22}Na^+$ handling could be documented (Table 1); namely an apparent increase in the inflow rate of Na^+, an immediate and sustained increase in Na^+ fractional outflow rate, and a modest decrease in the steady-state concentration of Na^+ inside the islet cells (14). The outflow rate of Na^+ exceeds the value expected from the inflow rate of K^+, on the assumption of a 3/2 stoichiometry for Na^+/K^+ active transport by a (Na^+ + K^+)-activated ATPase. Thus a significant amount of Na^+ may be extruded from the islet cells by an ionophoretic modality different from the ouabain-sensitive ATPase. Our findings do not support the speculation according to which glucose affects Ca^{2+} handling and insulin release by increasing the intracellular concentration of Na^+ in islet cells (15).

3. H^+

We were unable to detect a significant effect of glucose upon the intracellular pH of islet cells, as judged by the ^{14}C-DMO method (16). However, glucose clearly augments H^+ output from the islets (Table 1). The dose-response curve for H^+ output at increasing glucose concentrations displays a hyperbolic pattern, with a half-maximal value being reached at a glucose concentration close to 2.9 mM. Such a dose-response curve is closely similar to that characterizing the magnitude of the glucose-induced initial fall in $^{45}Ca^{2+}$ fractional outflow rate (16). It also resembles the dose-response curve for the glucose-induced changes in $^{86}Rb^+$ or $^{42}K^+$ fractional outflow rate (17). Thus, it could be speculated that a nutrient-induced increase in H^+ generation somehow participates in the reduction of K^+ and Ca^{2+} fractional outflow rates. In an artificial system for the study of ionophoresis, an increase of pH in the chamber simulating the intracellular compartment indeed results in a decreased outflow of Ca^{2+} from such a chamber (17).

4. Mg^{2+}

High concentrations of Mg^{2+} (5-10 mM) are known to inhibit glucose-induced insulin release, and this was attributed to a decrease rate of Ca^{2+} entry into the islet cells (18). At physiological concentration (ca. 1 mM), Mg^{2+} also influences B-cell function. Thus, the glucose-induced electrical activity of the B-cell is suppressed in the absence of extracellular Ca^{2+}, but not when both Ca^{2+} and Mg^{2+} are removed (19). And indeed, in media deprived of both Ca^{2+} and Mg^{2+}, glucose is able to stimulate insulin release above basal value (Figure 2). Under the latter experimental condition, the secretory response to glucose is enhanced by theophylline and abolished by verapamil (Figure 3). In the simultaneous presence of glucose and theophylline, no stimulation of release occurs when EGTA (0.15 mM) is added to the Ca^{2+}- and Mg^{2+}-depleted media. Thus, in physiological concentration, Mg^{2+} exerts an inhibitory effect upon the process of glucose-induced insulin release. However, even in the absence of extracellular Mg^{2+}, the secretory process remains apparently dependent on the availability of minute amounts of extracellular Ca^{2+} (20). The effect of glucose upon Mg^{2+} handling remains to be evaluated. In isolated rat islets, the total concentration of Mg averages 50 ± 9 pmol/islet (3).

5. Ba^{2+}

Exposure of the isolated perfused rat pancreas or isolated islets to Ba^{2+} (1.0-2.0 mM) represents one of the sole experimental conditions in which an active process of insulin release is seen in the absence of extracellular Ca^{2+}, with or without EGTA (21). The insulinotropic action of Ba^{2+} is enhanced by theophylline. In isolated islets, the secretory response to the combination of Ba^{2+} and theophylline is abolished by epinephrine, verapamil, antimycin A and dinitrophenol. It is associated with an increased oxidation of endogenous nutrients. It is enhanced by glucose (3.3 or 16.7 mM), the enhancing action of the sugar correlating with the rate of glucose oxidation (Figure 4). The aptitude of 3.3 mM glucose to augment Ba^{2+}-induced insulin release contrasts with the fact that, under normal conditions, 3.3 mM glucose fails to stimulate insulin output. However, in the Ca^{2+}-depleted media containing Ba^{2+} and theophylline, 3.3 mM glucose is also sufficient to augment the concentration of reduced pyridine nucleotides from 145 ± 14 to 228 ± 17 fmol/islet. These findings (Sener & Malaisse, unpublished data) suggest that, even when insulin release is stimulated by a direct interference with divalent cations' availability to the B-cell, a modulatory role of reducing equivalents upon the handling of such cations could still be operative. Under suitable experimental conditions, glucose exerts a modest stimulatory effect upon $^{133}Ba^{2+}$ net uptake (21).

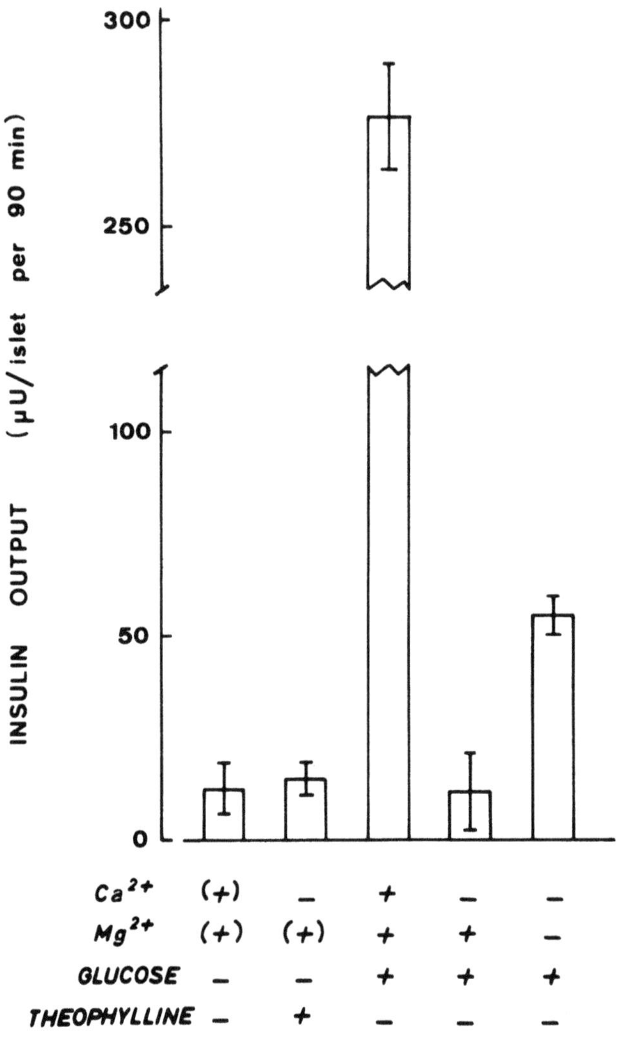

Fig. 2. Absolute values (± SEM) for insulin release in the presence (+) or absence (–) of glucose (16.7 mM), theophylline (1.4 mM), Ca^{2+} (1.0 mM) and Mg^{2+} (1.0 mM).

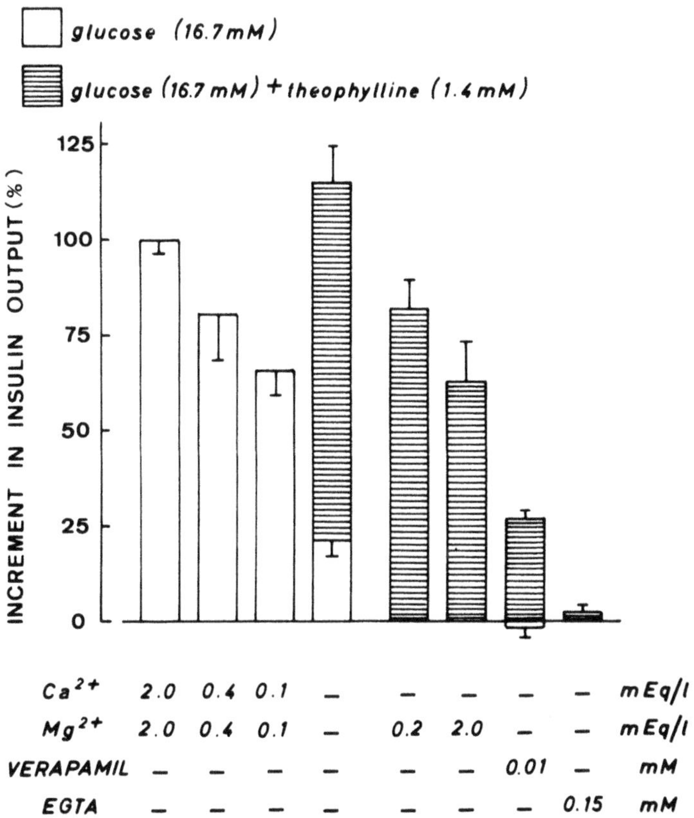

Fig. 3. Increments in insulin release attributable to either glucose alone or theophylline (in the presence of glucose) in rat isolated islets incubated for 90 min under different experimental conditions.

6. Ca^{2+}

Two distinct movements of Ca^{2+} were recently characterized in prelabelled perifused islets suddenly exposed to an increase in extracellular glucose concentration. Each of these movements may participate in the rapid regulation of Ca^{2+} availability at the site involved in controlling insulin release (16, 22,23). The first movement consists in a reduction of $^{45}Ca^{2+}$ efflux. As already mentioned, its relationship to increasing glucose concentrations displays a hyperbolic pattern. Its time course is analogous to that characterizing the change in K^+ conductance. The second movement consists in a secondary rise in $^{45}Ca^{2+}$ efflux. Its dose-response curve is sigmoidal and, as such, closely resembles the pattern of changes in either NAD(P)H

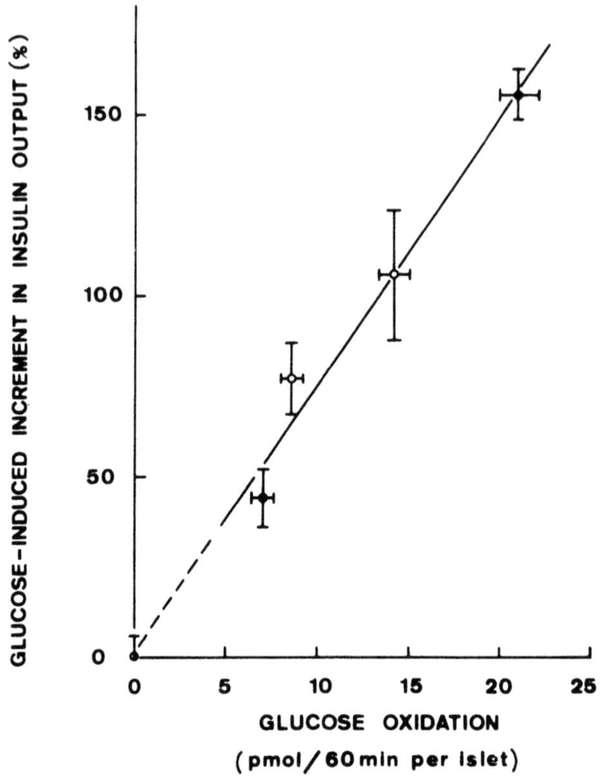

Fig. 4. Correlation between the increment in insulin output evoked by glucose 3.3 or 16.7 mM (relative to the control value for insulin release found in the absence of glucose) and the rate of oxidation of the sugar in islets incubated in the absence of Ca^{2+} but presence of Ba^{2+} (2.0 mM) and theophylline (1.4 mM), with (open circles) or without (closed circles) EGTA 0.5 mM.

concentrations or insulin release (16). Its time course is almost identical to that of insulin release. Its magnitude is thought to be proportional to the rate of Ca^{2+} influx in islet cells; and, it may thus represent a Ca^{2+}- Ca^{2+} exchange process (23). It could coincide with the increase in Ca^{2+} inflow held responsible for the depolarization of the B-cell,from a silent polarised level to a spiking depolarised plateau potential(24).

We have exposed elsewhere our reasons to believe that, in the process of nutrient induced insulin release, an increased generation of H^+ and NAD(P)H, which occurs in concert with an increased generation of high-energy phosphate intermediates, represents an essential coupling system between metabolic and cationic

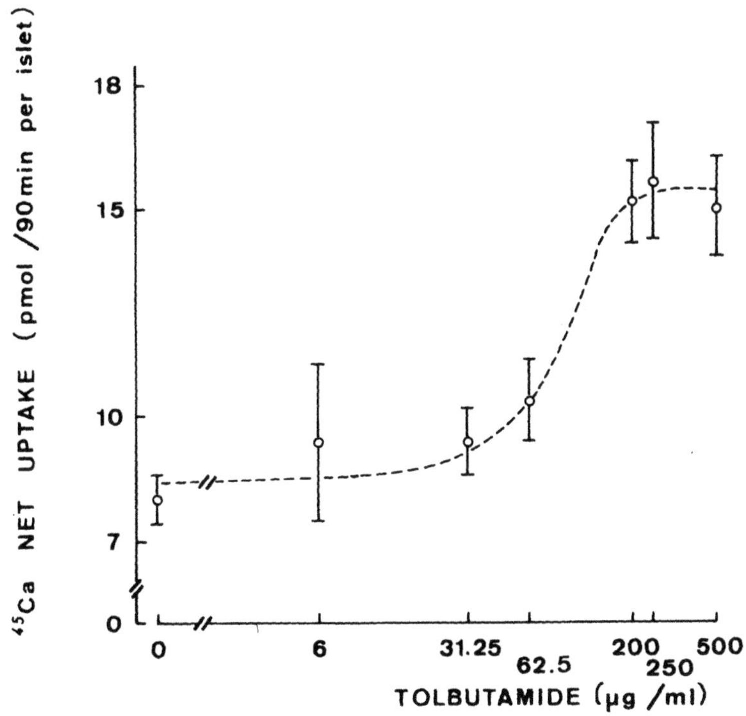

Fig. 5. Dose-related effect of tolbutamide upon 45 calcium net uptake by isolated islets incubated in the absence of glucose.

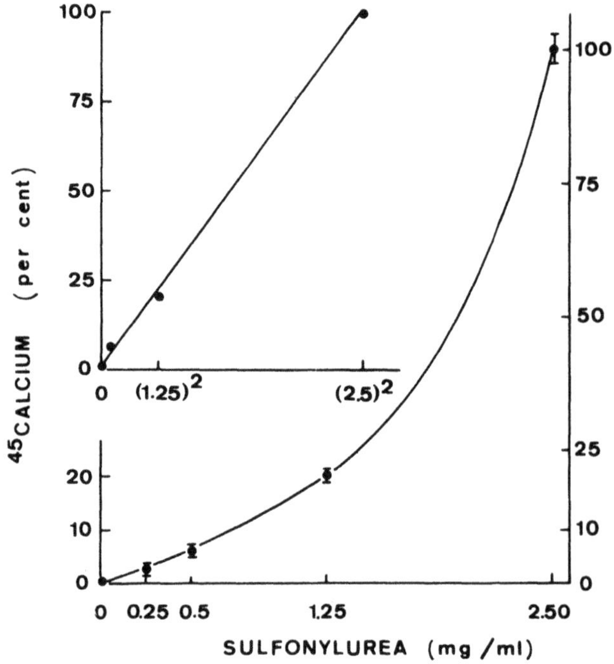

Fig. 6. Dose-related effect of sulfonylurea upon ^{45} calcium translocation in an artificial system (27). The data are expressed in percent of the mean value found at the highest concentration of the drug.

events (16,17). We are presently exploring to which extent the situation encountered in the intact B-cell can be reproduced in an artificial system for the study of ionophoresis.

We were led to the latter experimental approach by the following considerations. First, the movements of Ca^{2+}, at least those occurring at the level of the plasma membrane, may be mediated by native ionophoretic systems. The rate of Ca^{2+} entry into islet cells at increasing extracellular Ca^{2+} concentration is compatible with the existence of a finite number of transport units (1). The native system, like the antibiotic ionophore A23187, is sensitive to organic calcium-antagonists, the inhibitory effect of which is overcome at high concentrations of extracellular Ca^{2+} (25-27). Second, the artificial system allows for the reproduction of such phenomena as Na^{+}/Ca^{2+}, H^{+}/Ca^{2+} and Ca^{2+}/Ca^{2+} counter transport, each of which may contribute to the dynamics of Ca^{2+} inflow-outflow in the pancreatic B-cell (28). And last, the artificial system may help to elucidate the intimate mode of action of insulinotropic agents. For instance, hypoglycemic sulfonylureas, which cause a dose-related stimulation of ^{45} Ca net uptake by isolated islets (Figure 5), are able to translocate ^{45}Ca into an organic immiscible phase (29,30). The translocation phenomenon represents a power fuction of the sulfonylurea concentration (Figure 6), a behaviour reminiscent of that seen with A23187. Non-hypoglycemic derivatives of the sulfonylureado not cause ^{45}Ca translocation in our system, so that the ionophoretic capacity of the drug may indeed be relevant to its insulinotropic action.

In summary, the present observations confirm that the movements of cations across membrane systems in the islet cells represent an essential aspect of B-cell physiology. The experimental findings also suggest that our understanding of such movements may gain from a comparison with the situation found in artificial systems for the study of ionophoretic processes.

REFERENCES

1. *Malaisse, W.J., et al.(1978). Ann. N.Y. Acad. Sci., 307, 562*
2. *Sehlin, J. and Täljedal, I.-B. (1974). J. Physiol. (Lond.), 242, 505*
3. *Boschero, A.C., et al.(1977), FEBS Lett., 83, 151*
4. *Malaisse, W.J., et al.(1978). Pflügers Arch. 373, 237*
5. *Henquin, J.C. (1978). Nature, 271, 271*
6. *Boschero, A.C. and Malaisse, W.J. (1979). Amer. J. Physiol (In press)*
7. *Dean, P.M. and Matthews, E.K. (1968). Nature, 219, 389*

8. *Pace, C.S. and Price, S. (1972). Biochem. Biophys. Res. Commun., 46, 1557.*
9. *Meissner, H.P. and Atwater, I.J. (1976). Horm. Metab. Res., 8, 11.*
10. *Boschero, A.C., et al. (1978). Diabetologia, 15, 221 (Abstract)*
11. *Sener, A., et al. (1979). Excerpta Medica I.C.S. (In press) (abstract)*
12. *Seubert, W. and Schoner, W. (1971) in Current topics in cellular regulation, Horecker, B.L. and Stadtman, E.R.,eds., Academic Press, New York, vol. 3, pp. 237.*
13. *Grill, V., et al. (1978). J. Clin. Invest. 61, 1034.*
14. *Kawazu, S., et al. (1978). Pflugers Arch., 375, 197.*
15. *Donatsch, P., et al. (1977). J. Physiol. (Lond.), 267, 357.*
16. *Malaisse, W.J., et al. (1979). Diabetologia (In Press)*
17. *Malaisse, W.J., et al., (1979). Metabolism (In Press).*
18. *Malaisse, W.J., et al. (1976). Diab. Metab. 2, 1*
19. *Atwater, I.J. and Beigelman, P.M. (1976). J. Physiol. (Paris) 72, 769.*
20. *Somers, G., et al. (1979). Acta Diabetol Lat. (In Press).*
21. *Somers, G., et al. (1976). Pflugers Arch. 365, 21.*
22. *Malaisse, W.J., et al. (1973). Amer. J. Physiol, 224, 389.*
23. *Herchuelz, A. and Malaisse, W.J. (1979). J. Physiol. (Lond.) (In Press).*
24. *Preissler, M. and Meissner, H.P. (1978). Diabetologia, 15, 262 (Abstract).*
25. *Devis, G., et al. (1975). Diabetes, 24, 547.*
26. *Somers, G., et al. (1976). Endocrinology, 99, 114.*
27. *Malaisse, W.J., et al. (1977). Experientia, 33, 1035.*
28. *Malaisse, W.J. and Couturier, E. Nature (1979).*
29. *Malaisse, W.J., et al. (1977). Excerpta Medica I.C.S., 413, 95.*
30. *Malaisse, W.J., et al. (1977). Diabetes, 26 (suppl. 1) 216 (Abstract)*

The experimental work mentioned in this account was supported by grants from the Fonds de la Recherche Scientifique Medicale (Brussels, Belgium).

GLUCOSE-INDUCED CHANGES OF THE MEMBRANE POTENTIAL OF PANCREATIC B-CELLS: THEIR SIGNIFICANCE FOR THE REGULATION OF INSULIN RELEASE

H. P. Meissner* and M. Preissler

The D-glucose molecule is recognized by the pancreatic B-cell as the major physiological stimulus for insulin release, and it is generally accepted that calcium ions are an essential prerequisite for the insulin releasing process. However, the precise mechanism of the regulation of insulin release by D-glucose and calcium is not yet clear. Electrophysiological experiments in B-cells have shown that D-glucose and other insulin secretagogues induce membrane depolarization and electrical activity (1,2) which seem to be directly connected with insulin release. By these studies it has been suggested that the glucose-inducted potential changes play an important role in the regulatory process of insulin secretion. Hence, the investigation of the membrane potential of B-cells seems to be appropriate to obtain a further insight into the stimulus-secretion coupling process.

MATERIALS AND METHODS

The methods of recording the membrane potential in single B-cells have been previously described in detail (3). Briefly, B-cells of partially microdissected islets of fed NMRI mice were impaled with ultra-fine microelectrodes filled with 2 M K-citrate and having a tip resistance greater than 200 Megohms. The membrane potential was continuously recorded on tape and monitored on ink writer and oscilloscope. The figures shown were usually obtained by play-back of the tape to a fast ink recorder (Brush 220). The preparation was continuously perfused at a rate of 3-5 ml/min in a small Plexiglas chamber (volume 1 ml) with a modified Krebs-Henseleit-buffer (NaCl 103 mM, KCl 4.7 mM, $CaCl_2$ 2.56 mM, $MgCl_2$ 1.13 mM, $NaHCO_3$ 25 mM, NaH_2PO_4 1.15 mM, D-glucose 2.8 mM, Na-pyruvate 4.9 mM, di-Na-fumarate 2.7 mM, Na-glutamate 4.9mM) equilibrated with O_2:CO_2 (95:5) and maintained at 37°C.

When the glucose concentration was changed, isotonicity was maintained by altering the NaCl concentration correspondingly. In experiments with elevated Ca concentrations or addition of cobalt a Hepes buffer (Hepes 10 mM, NaCl 115.5 mM, KCl 4.7 mM, $CaCl_2$ 2.56 mM, $MgCl_2$ 1.13 mM, Na-pyruvate 4.9 mM, di-Na-fumarate 2.7 mM, Na-glutamate 4.9 mM, glucose 11.1 mM; pH adjusted with NaOH to 7.4 mM) was used to avoid precipitations. When the $CaCl_2$ concentration was increased NaCl was reduced to maintain isotonicity.

RESULTS AND DISCUSSION

Glucose Dependence of the Electrical Activity of B-Cells

Glucose-induced electrical activity occurs only with glucose concentrations which also stimulate insulin release (1-2).

As shown in Figure 1 this electrical activity is characterized by a regular burst pattern. It consists of rhythmic oscillations of the membrane potential (slow waves) between the maximum repolarization potential V_r and the plateau potential V_p; superimposed on these slow waves is a fast spike activity which starts at V_p. Each burst is preceded by a slow depolarization to the threshold potential V_t which marks the beginning of the slow waves.

As shown previously (2,3) the spikes vary considerably in amplitude, duration, and shape, and there is no clear dependence of these parameters on the external glucose concentration.

In contrast, the time course of the slow waves is strongly glucose dependent in the individual B-cell (Figure 1) (3). Thus, with increasing glucose concentrations the duration of the slow waves increases and consequently the spike periods are markedly prolonged. In "unphysiologically" high glucose concentrations (above 16.6 mM) the burst pattern usually disappears, and the spike activity is continuous (Figure 1 C). As furthermore shown in Figure 1 D the membrane hyperpolarizes, and the electrical activity ceases when the glucose concentration is reduced to values which also stop insulin release.

Based on this marked dependence of the electrical activity of the individual B-cell on the external glucose concentration, it has been suggested that electrical activity and insulin release are directly related, and that insulin is released from the single cell only during the plateau phase. This suggestion is strongly supported by the observation that the electrical activity (defined as relative duration of the plateau phase) exhibits a sigmoid relation to the external glucose concentration (Figure 2); this curve is almost identical to the dose-response curve of insulin release (e.g. 4).

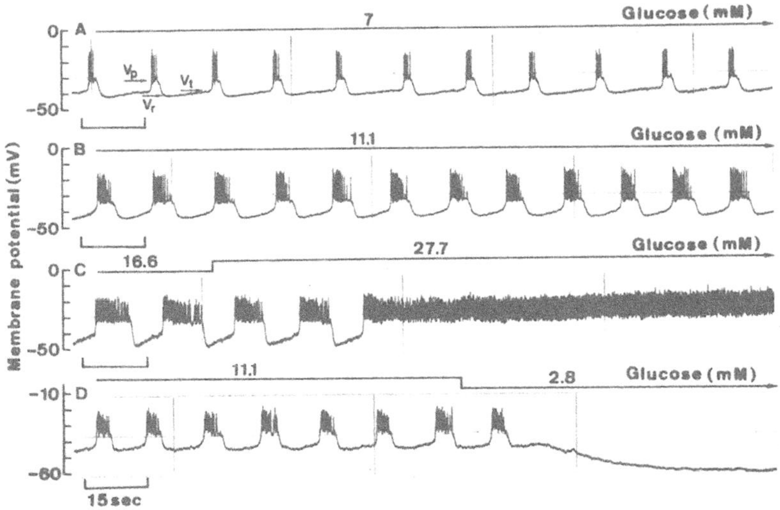

Fig. 1. Effect of external glucose concentration on the electrical activity of single B-cells. A and B were obtained from the same cell, C and D are records from two other cells. The arrows in A mark the threshold potential V_t, the plateau potential V_p, and the maximum repolarization potential V_r. Note, that there is no difference of V_t, V_p and V_r in A and B despite the variation of the glucose concentration. In C and D the glucose concentration was altered at the step of the trace on top of each record. The time scale is the same for all records.

A sigmoid relationship also between incidence of electrical activity and glucose concentration was described (3). This observation was explained by assuming a widespread glucose sensitivity among B-cells. However, in our experiments (2) there was only a narrow range of glucose concentrations, namely about 5 to 8 mM, in which electrically silent as well as active cells were detected. At glucose concentrations below 5 mM all cells were silent, while above 8mM glucose all cells exhibited electrical activity. This observation was also confirmed by others (5).

Another discrepancy between our results and those of Dean and Matthews (6) refers to the relationship between membrane potential and glucose concentration. While Dean and Matthews (6) reported a progressive depolarization with increasing glucose concentrations, we found a discontinuous relationship between the two parameters (Fig. 3). At low glucose concentrations (<3 mM) B-cells have a high membrane potential (about - 62 mV), and there is no significant difference between a glucose-free medium and 2.8 mM glucose. According to our recent studies (7) this high "resting" potential seems to be determined mainly by the potassium permeability of the B-cell membrane. When the glucose concentration is raised beyond<3 mM the membrane depolarizes, and at a critical potential of about - 48 mV it starts to oscillate between V_r, V_p and V_s; these oscillations are quite independent of the glucose concentration. Finally, at concentrations above 16.6 mM the membrane remains depolarized at V_p and continuous spike activity is observed.

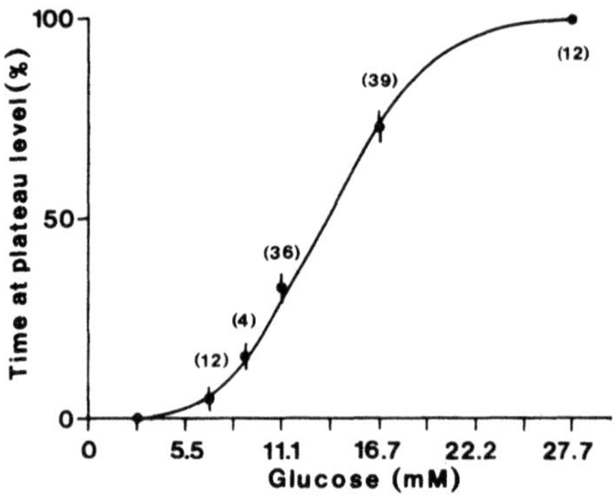

Fig. 2. Relationship between glucose concentration (abscissa) and relative duration of plateau phase (ordinate). The latter was obtained from perifusion periods of several minutes by measuring the total time during which the membrane potential was at V_p. 100% time at plateau level means continuous activity. Results are given as mean ± SEM; number of cells in parentheses.

Dynamics of Electrical Activity

By examination of the dynamics of the electrical response to a sudden rise of external glucose from a non-stimulating to a stimulating concentration we could show that individual B-cells exhibit a biphasic pattern of electrical activity (5-7) analogous to the well known biphasic insulin release.

A typical example is shown in Figure 4. After raising the glucose concentration from 2.8 to 16.6 mM there is first a slow depolarization of the membrane from - 62 to - 50 mV; then a rapid depolarization to the plateau potential ensues, and a fast spike activity occurs which lasts for about 1 minute (Fig. 4A and B). Thereafter, the burst pattern reappears. At first the duration of the spike periods is short but their duration

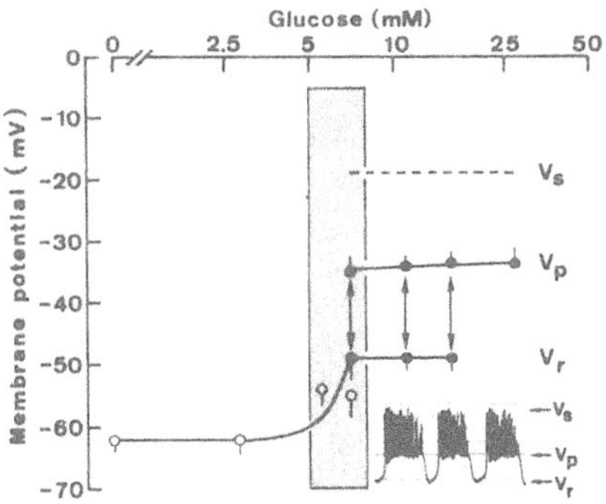

Fig. 3. Relationship between membrane potential and glucose concentration. Values are given as mean ± SEM, and were obtained from 4 (5.5 mM glucose) up to 29 (2.8 mM glucose) cells. The unfilled circles correspond to membrane potential values at which no electrical activity was observed. The hatched column indicates the range of glucose concentrations at which cells in an electrically active or silent state could be found. The inset with the 3 bursts clarifies the potential levels used in the plot. V_s means the reversal potential of spikes.

increases progressively with time (Fig. 4 B and C).

In order to quantify these results we determined, from successive 30 sec periods, the total time during which the membrane potential was at its plateau level; results obtained from 7 cells are plotted in Figure 5 against the time of perifusion. Comparison of Figure 5 with the biphasic insulin release reveals that the dynamics of the electrical activity in single B-cells and insulin release closely follow the same time course. A similar conformity could also be found under the influence of sulphonylureas (5).

These findings corroborate further the direct relationship between insulin release and electrical activity. Moreover, these results suggest that the multiphasic, glucose or sulphonylurea-induced changes of the membrane potential may play an important role in the control or even in the occurence of the biphasic insulin release (1).

As further shown in Figure 4 D, there is also a multiphasic response of the membrane potential, when the glucose is reduced from a higher to a lower stimulating concentration. Initially, the duration of the bursts is shortened; then the membrane hyperpolarizes slightly, and the electrical activity is transiently blocked completely. After a while the membrane depolarizes again slightly, and the activity reappears, first as abortive slow waves without spikes, thereafter as normal bursts with shortened duration according to the reduced glucose concentration. Similar observations were also made by others (11). In accordance with this transient "overshooting" inhibition of electrical activity a short "refractory period or negative spike" of insulin release has been found under similar experimental conditions.

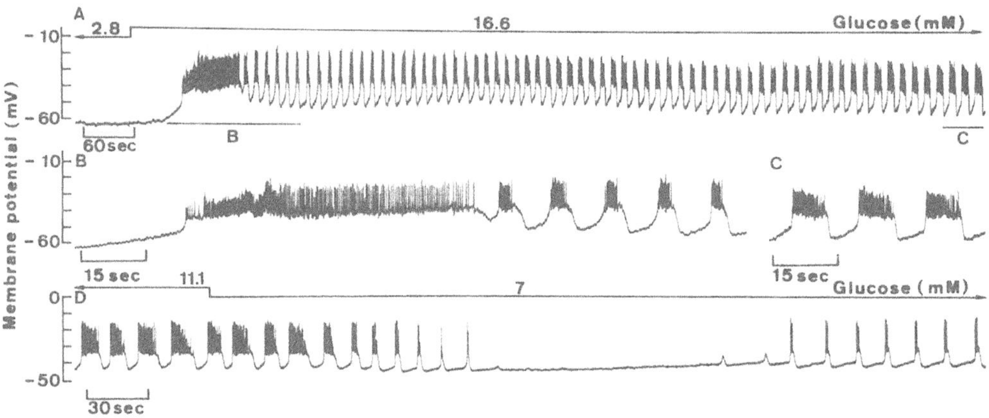

Fig. 4. Dynamics of changes of the membrane potential in response to variation of the external glucose concentration. A, continuous recording of the membrane potential of a single B-cell; glucose concentration raised from 2.8 to 16.6 mM as indicated. Sections labeled by bars are shown in B and C with faster time resolution. D, continuous recording of another cell during reduction of the external glucose concentration from 11.1 to 7mM. Note that V_t, V_p, V_s and V_r are identical in 11.1 and 7 mM glucose.

Ionic Mechanism of Glucose-Induced Potential Changes

As mentioned above the "resting" membrane potential of normal B-cells at glucose concentrations below 3 mM seems to be determined mainly by the potassium permeability (7). At stimulating glucose concentrations (>5 mM) the membrane depolarizes from the resting state to the level from which the slow waves start. Since it has been shown that calcium-uptake increases with increasing glucose concentrations (8), it would be conceivable that this depolarization is caused by an increase of the calcium permeability. However, as

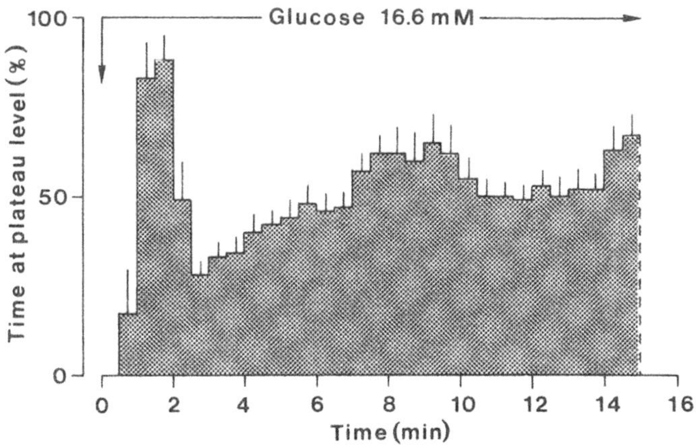

Fig. 5. Relationship between time at plateau level with spike activity and perifusion time in response to a stimulation with glucose. After stimulation with glucose (time zero) the total time at plateau was determined and expressed as a percentage of successive 30 sec periods. The histogram summarizes the results from 7 different experiments as shown in Figure 4A. Values are given as mean ± SEM.

demonstrated in Figure 6, this explanation is unlikely because the depolarizing effect of a stimulating glucose concentration is unchanged in the presence of 5 mM cobalt which has been shown to inhibit calcium uptake and insulin release (9), probably by blocking calcium channels. Similarly, removal of external sodium has no effect on the depolarization induced by glucose in the presence of cobalt. In contrast, the depolarization is prevented by addition of the potassium ionophore valinomycin. Hence, these findings suggest that the glucose-induced depolarization is due to a decrease of the potassium permeability. This conclusion is strongly supported by observations showing that increasing glucose concentrations decrease the ^{86}Rb or ^{42}K efflux from isolated islets. In particular, it could be demonstrated that the effect of glucose on the potassium efflux was most pronounced in the concentration range between 0 and 6 mM glucose (10).

As further shown in Figure 6 cobalt prevents the appearance of the electrical activity, although the membrane is depolarized beyond the threshold from which the slow waves usually start (compare potential values in Figure 6 A and B). The activity only reappears when cobalt is removed from the external medium (Figure 6 C and D). Since cobalt is assumed to inhibit the calcium influx, this observation indicates that electrical activity is somehow linked with calcium entry.

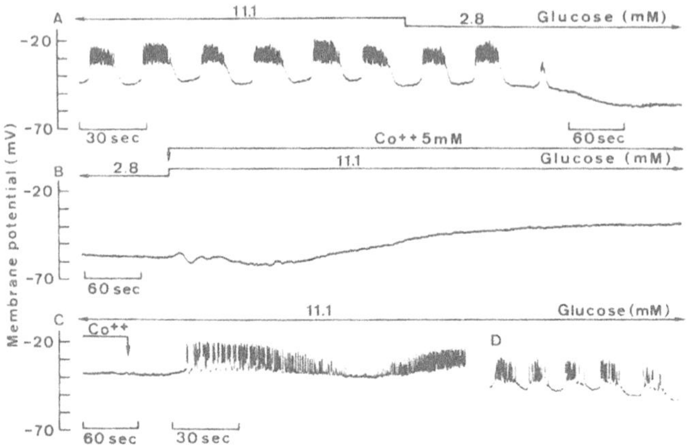

Fig. 6. Depolarizing effect of glucose on the membrane potential in the presence of cobalt. All records from the same cell. A to C, continuous recording; interval of 6 min between C and D. A: control burst activity in 11.1 mM glucose and change to 2.8 mM glucose. B: glucose increased from 2.8 to 11.1 mM; at the same time addition of 5 mM $CoCl_2$. C and D: perifusion with 11.1 mM glucose and removal of $CoCl_2$ at the arrow. Note the change of time scales in the different records.

Matthews and coworkers (11) concluded that the spikes arising from the plateau potential are mainly due to a voltage dependent calcium influx which triggers the exocytotic insulin release. The results shown in Figure 7 are incompatible with this hypothesis. From this figure it becomes clear that 1) the amplitude and the velocity of depolarization of the slow waves increase markedly with the external calcium concentration while the spikes disappear (Figure 7 E),and 2)addition of cobalt immediately abolishes the electrical activity by preventing the depolarization phase of the slow waves (Figure 7 A); the membrane remains polarized at a level between V_r and V_t. The effect of cobalt is completely reversible; however, after removal of cobalt a remarkable "off response" can be observed before the normal burst pattern is restored (Fig. 7 A, C and D).

Both, the effect of cobalt and calcium ions suggest that the depolarization phase of the slow waves is initiated by an increase of the calcium permeability. The marked threshold phenomenon suggests a voltage dependence of this permeability. This increased calcium permeability leads to an influx of calcium ions eliciting the exocytotic process. The spikes, however, may be considered as the consequence rather than the cause of exocytosis. For that

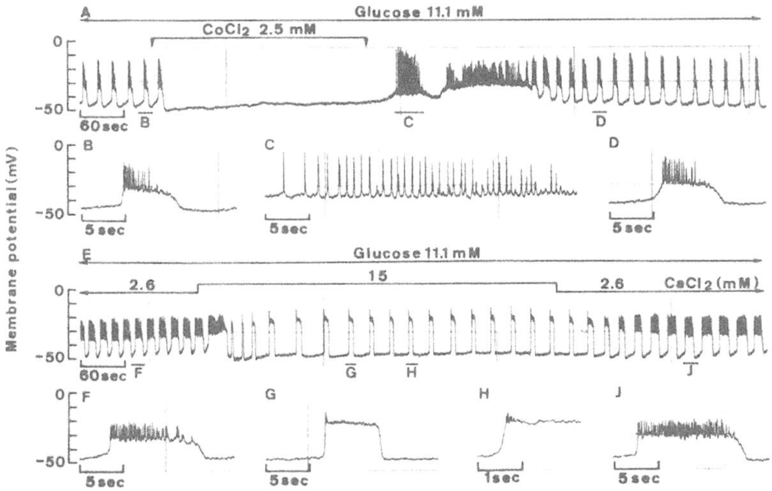

Fig. 7. *Effect of cobalt and high external calcium on the glucose induced burst activity. A and E continuous recordings from two different cells. B,C,D,F,G,H,I show the sections marked by bars in A and E at higher time resolution. In both experiments the preparations were perifused with a Hepes-buffer, containing 11.1 mM glucose. Note, that there is no difference in the burst pattern compared with that in the Krebs-Henseleit buffer.*

reason we regard the slow waves as the main electrical event which regulates insulin release.

Concerning the repolarization phase of the slow waves it seems to be brought about partially by the activity of an electrogenic Na/K-pump (12). Recent results (8), however, point also to an important contribution of the potassium permeability, because addition of TEA or 9-aminoacridine, both substances known to block potassium channels inhibits the repolarization phase (Figure 8); consequently the slow waves are prolonged or the spike activity becomes continuous under these conditions. On the contrary, in high calcium concentrations the duration of the slow waves is shortened by acceleration of the repolarizing phase (Figure 7 E). This shortening may be explained by a calcium-induced activation of the potassium permeability, a mechanism which presumably exists in many other tissues (for ref. see 9).

From Figure 7 E it is furthermore obvious that the slope of the depolarization preceding the slow wave is considerably reduced, and that the duration of the periods between the slow waves is increased in the high calcium concentration. This effect could also be the consequence of this calcium-induced activation of the potassium permeability, particularly because it has been suggested that the slow depolarization may be due to changes of the potassium conductance (13).

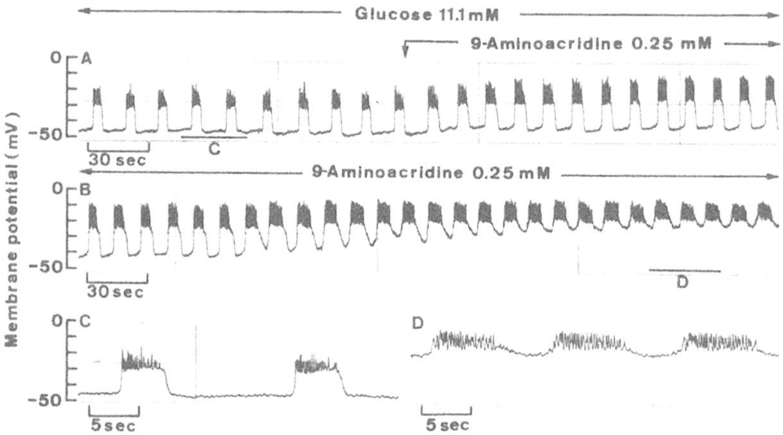

Fig. 8. Effect of 9-aminoacridine on glucose-induced electrical activity of a single B-cell. A and B are continuous recordings from the same cell. Preparation perifused throughout with 11.1 mM glucose. 9-aminoacridine was added in A as indicated. Sections marked by bars in A and B are shown in C and D with faster time resolution. Note the progressive decrease of the repolarization phase and the prolongation of the slow waves.

CONCLUSIONS

The experimental data reviewed in the present paper emphasize that the glucose-induced electrical activity of the individual B-cell, characterized by the regular burst pattern, is directly related to the insulin release. The findings therefore suggest that the glucose-induced changes of the membrane potential are essentially involved in the regulation of insulin release. Concerning the ionic mechanisms underlying the potential changes it seems that glucose in a first step induces a decrease of the potassium permeability; this leads to the depolarization from the resting state to the threshold level at which the burst activity, composed of slow waves and spikes, originates. The slow waves are considered as the main electrical event regulating the output of insulin. It is suggested that the depolarization phase of the slow waves is due to a voltage dependent calcium influx which is responsible for the exocytosis. The repolarization phase of the slow waves is assumed to be caused by the interaction of the activity of an electrogenic Na/K-pump, and by an increase of the potassium permeability which also may be activated by the entering calcium.

REFERENCES

1. *Meissner,H.P. and Atwater, I.J. (1976) Horm. Metab. Res. 8, 11*
2. *Meissner, H.P. (1976). J. Physiol., Paris, 72, 757*
3. *Meissner, H.P. and Schmelz, H. (1974). Pflugers Arch. 351, 195*
4. *Malaisse, W., et al.(1967). Endocrinology, 80, 99*
5. *Beigelman, P.M., et al.(1977). J. Physiol., Paris, 73, 201*
6. *Dean, P.M. and Matthews, E.K. (1968). Nature, 219, 389*
7. *Meissner, H.P., et al.(1978). FEBS Lett., 94, 87*
8. *Meissner, H.P. and Henquin, J.C. (1978). Diabetes, 27, Suppl.2, 457*
9. *Meech, R.W. (1976) in Symp. Soc Exp. Biol. No. XXX, Calcium in Biological Systems, Duncan, C.J. ed., Cambridge University Press, Cambridge, 161*
10. *Henquin, J.C. (1978). Nature, 271, 271*
11. *Matthews, E.K. and Sakamoto Y. (1975). J. Physiol., Lond., 246, 421*
12. *Atwater, I. and Meissner, H.P. (1975). J. Physiol., Lond., 247, 56*
13. *Atwater, I., et al.(1978). J. Physiol., Lond., 278, 117*

This work was supported by the Deutsche Forschungsgemeinschaft, SFB 38, Bonn-Bad Godesberg. We thank Prof. H. Schmidt for critical reading of the manuscript. We are grateful to Mrs. T. Neumuller for secretarial help and Mr. W. Schmeer for skilled technical assistance.

DISCUSSION

E. TUTWILER: *Dr. Malaisse, is the sulfonylurea calcium ionophoric effect accompanied by a change of the redox state?*

W. MALAISSE: *Yes, but in the sense opposite to glucose. In all, it's exposed to the sulfonylurea; the NADH over NED, and NEDPH over NED ratio decreases. And this goes along with impairment of other certain metabolic parameters.*

C. HELLERSTROM: *Dr. Freinkel, is the phosphate flush specific property of the B cell, or is it the more general phenomenon which can be observed in other cell types? And, if so, would the pattern you observe in your system be superimposition of B cell phosphate fluxes and fluxes from other cell types in the rat fibers?*

N. FREINKEL: *With regard to the specificity in the islets, one can never be absolutely certain, but there are certain lines of evidence which would make us feel that the Beta cell is chiefly implicated. One was the histochemical evidence I tried to demonstrate. The second is that the phosphate flush has been observed in micro-dissected islets from the obese mouse, where there are more than 90% beta cells. The third line of evidence is in streptozotocin rats. We were unable to elicit a flush presumably following ablation of the beta cell. A fourth line of evidence is that Metzger and I and others, in islet cell tumors of pure beta cell progenitor composition, have been able to get phosphate flushes directly concording with the secretogogic potency of what's tested. For example, islet cell tumors poorly responsive to glucose elicit no phosphate flush, whereas the same tumors were well responsive to leucine. Is it confined to islets? In 1956 and 1963, I demonstrated changes in tissue inorganic phosphate content acutely responsive to stimulation, using the exciting system there, thyroid and thyrotropin. We made a considerable effort in the laboratory to use lymphocytes, stimulated with a variety of mitogens, to see whether we elicited the phosphate flush with secretogogues. Quite suggestive evidence accrued there. It may indeed be a component; in other words, an acute translocation of phosphate attending the initiation of the stimulated state by a membrane perturbation. Whether it is seen quite as markedly in any other tissue than the beta cell, I'm not quite prepared to say at this time.*

G. HOET: *Dr. Freinkel, is this phosphate flush present only in the adult or in a special situation like the fetus? And the second question is: would certain situations like starvation change the phosphate flush?*

N. FREINKEL: *For us, one of the most intriguing aspects of the phosphate flush has been that we feel it is a potential tool for characterizing responsiveness to nutrient secretogogue. We feel it is a recognition rather than an amplification mechanism, recognition mechanisms in situations where poor insulin secretion may be differentially mediated. I'll give an example of that in a moment. Two of the situations we were interested in applying it to were the fetal islets and secondly, starvation, both of which are situations where there is impoverished insulin release in response to glucose. Collaborative studies done with Asplundh and with Hellerstrom have been strongly addressed to the fetus, and here it would appear that, in association with the blunted insulin release, there is a markedly obtunded to absent phosphate flush. The fetal phosphate flush which does occur, seems to exhibit the same dose response characteristic as adult islets. In other words, their recognition systems are relatively well preserved and the limiting factor is in the capacity for phosphorus sequestration. The second event is starvation. Here, the impoverished insulin response seen in starvation is associated now with a reasonably well preserved phosphate flush, but the dose response characteristics are displaced to the right. Thus, the initiation of the response occurs at a higher glucose concentration as if there is a relative insensitivity of the recognition system. One of the most fascinating aspects of the phenomenon is that it does give a biochemical tool for characterizing recognition systems. There may very well be an anionic net throughout the B cell. I'm not sure that the phosphate flush is necessarily an expression of that anionic net. What the major determinant will be is something that no one knows yet. In other words, does it participate in the determination of electrical neutrality within the cell? That won't be established until we define what the bonding, the linkage, or the association is of what showed histochemically.*

T. PROUT: *One of the interesting things that keeps us from going into ketoacidosis is the continuous release of insulin, the so-called "slow" release that goes on in the fasting state which keeps from immobilizing fat. I wonder if any of the speakers have any idea of what that mechanism is?*

H. MEISSNER: *The interesting point is that the phosphate flush is not inhibited in the presence of nickel. Nickel is known to block the calcium channel.*

N. FREINKEL: *What we're really discussing is a labile intracellular pool. And intracellular determinants really delimit the magnitude of the efflux and the magnitude of that flush.*

R. CAMERINI-DAVALOS: *Dr. Meissner, is it true that when the blood sugar concentration goes up one reaches a stage where there is no cell response, apparently unrelated to the concentration of the glucose?*

H. MEISSNER: *No. In very high glucose concentration, the burst pattern disappears and the membrane remains depolarized at a level which is the same as in the lower glucose concentration. But there is a continuous spike activity. Regulation of the membrane potential or regulation of insulin by the slow waves seems not to exist at this high glucose concentration.*

R. CAMERINI-DAVALOS: *What would be the difference with a very low and a very high concentration in that case?*

H. MEISSNER: *In lower glucose concentration, the duration of the slow waves is very short and the spike periods are very short. The intervals are longer between the periods and in very high glucose concentration, you have indefinite slow waves without any interruption.*

J. TOBIN: *Dr. Freinkel, have you had the opportunity to look at the other end of the age spectrum, at islets from elderly animals?*

N. FREINKEL: *Not yet.*

S. FAJANS: *I wonder whether any of the speakers are going to address themselves to Dr. Prout's question, particularly to the circumstances of nutrient deprivation in starvation?*

W. MALAISSE: *I think, first of all, it is debatable whether there is such a thing as basal insulin release in isolated islets not exposed to nutrients. There is no doubt there is a basal insulin release occurring in vivo at concentrations of glucose which are not supposed to stimulate insulin release. Yet, under those conditions, there are a number of other insulinotropic nutrients present in the fasting state and these may be responsible for a minimal level of secretory activity and, by doing so, prevents the development of fatal ketoacidosis. I would assume that, in addition to the presence of glucose, which is admittedly below the threshold concentration for stimulating release, there are a number of other exogeneous nutrients present; this may account for the basal rate of insulin release.*

M. VRANIK: *Dr. Malaisse, can this be reproduced in isolated systems? If you have a medium containing the concentration of nutrients, which are seen in the fasting state, will this low glucose stimulate insulin release?*

W. MALAISSE: *As far as I know, nobody has really tried to see whether the plasma with its normal constituency is able to maintain a high rate of insulin release.*

E. PFEIFFER: *By putting isolated islets in a medium containing some of these glucocidases like neuroaminadase, it's possible to separate clearly the mechanism of secretion of insulin from the mechanism of production of insulin. That means that biosynthesis goes on undisturbed and glucose is not capable anymore of stimulating insulin secretion. Sulfonylureas are active on the others too. Now, my question goes to all of the five speakers. Are there any data existing in the literature concerning the effect of nickel cobalt on the other drugs or removal of calcium from the medium, and what is the action of these measures in insulin biosynthesis? Perhaps it's related to the basal secretion of insulin in the islets.*

N. FREINKEL: *May I answer one phase of that. I think that one has certain physiological models that partly answer this. I think Hellstrom, a long time ago, demonstrated that cells in late fetal life had the capacity of responding to glucose in terms of the biosynthetic mechanism of acute insulin secretory response. That's why we were so gratified to find that, in this system, at least the capcity to affect a retention of phosphate, and appropriately then to respond to recognition, in terms of secretory events not yet present despite the fact that recognition, with regard to biosynthetic events, was well operative. It's perhaps the perfect physiological model of that type of dissociation.*

J. HOET: *Drs. Fajans and Savage, can a comparison be made between the obstetrical histories of these mothers with the MODY type to those with no diabetes? Not only heavy birthweight history, but also perinatal pathology and congenital malformations?*

S. FAJANS: *I'm afraid I have no detailed information, Joe, but I can tell you that some female members of these pedigreees certainly gave birth to large babies and some of them had some perinatal events which one associates with typical diabetes.*

G.M. REAVEN: *I want to pick up on what Fajans said about those patients with atherosclerosis and normal lipoprotein levels. I think heterogeneity is becoming more and more an important word in discussing these patients.*

K.G.M.M. ALBERTI: *I'd like to press Dr. Fajans a little bit further on the particular point where you said there was no tie-up with the triglycerides and cholesterol, in view of a study suggesting an association between low insulin and a development of microangiopathy, and high insulin and macroangiopathy. I wonder if you've got any differences there between your low and high insulin families and the two types of complications?*

S. FAJANS: *We've seen both macroangiopathic and microangiopathic complications in the families in which generations 3 and 4 have lower insulin responses. Now, we don't have the insulin responses in generations 2 and 1, where the greatest incidence of macro-angiopathic and microangiopathic complications are. As I pointed out, we do have some background retinopathy in generations 3 and 4, and those were exclusively families with low insulin responses. As far as macroangiopathy is concerned, if you examine it in the literature, I think it will bear out that there have been reports of an association with both low insulin response such as from the Hammersmith group, as well as those with high insulin responses. So, I think this is still a rather confused field.*

W.J. IRVINE: *Drs. Barbosa and Fajans, could you give a brief statement of the present state of knowledge of HLA and diabetic complications in Type 1? Is there any new knowledge on that?*

J. BARBOSA: *About MODY, I have not studied as many families as Dr. Fajans. We have studied in detail two families and we have done now some vitreous fluometry, which presumably would be the most sensitive way of looking at any leakage of fluorescein into the vitreous. We have not seen any signs of leakage.In the JIDD, we are preparing a report, where we have an association between B-15 and severe proliferative retinopathy.*

S. FAJANS: *I don't think it should be surprising that there is heterogeneity in vascular disease in MODY because there's heterogeneity of vascular disease in JOD. Now, even among Dr. Knowles' long term study of juvenile onset type diabetes, there are 20% who after 30 years of diabetes, have no detectable clinical evidence of retinopathy, nephropathy or neuropathy. Now there are six studies from five different countries of insulin-requiring diabetics, who've been followed for 20 to 40 years, having no evidence of clinically recognizable vascular disease. So, if we have individuals with a prototype of insulin-dependent diabetes without vascular disease, I don't think we should be surprised that there are MODY families who have no vascular disease, while others do. I think it's simply another manifestation of the heterogeneity. We have heterogeneity in genetics. We have heterogeneity in environmental factors. We have heterogeneity in insulin responses to glucose. And I also think we have heterogeneity in the finding of vascular disease in both JOD and MOD diabetes.*

R. CAMERINI-DAVALOS: *We are in a more comfortable situation because we proved that there is microangiopathy even before hyperglycemia. (J. Clin. End. & Med. in press). When we compare our prediabetics with normals and controls, we found no differences in blood glucose or insulin levels. But, when we compare those prediabetics with thickening of the muscle capillary basement* *membrane to those without, we found that those with the thickening basement membrane have increased immunoreactive insulin levels at 180 minutes ($p < .05$).*

EFFECT OF MATERNAL CARBOHYDRATE INTOLERANCE ON THE DEVELOPMENT OF THE AUTONOMIC INNERVATION OF THE FETAL RAT PANCREAS

M. de Gasparo*, P. de Herdt, and J. J. Hoet

In vitro experiments with cultured fetal pancreas have indicated that amino-acid enrichment of the culture medium stimulated the cellular growth of the fetal pancreatic rudiment (1). This was associated with a higher concentration of insulin per B cell, a larger diameter of insulin granules and a greater release of insulin after a glucose stimulus. However, while it is generally accepted that hormones and nutrients control β-cell function in the fetus, the role of the autonomic nervous system should also be emphasized. The preservation of parasympathetic innervation and the absence of orthosympathetic innervation in the cultured rat pancreatic rudiment might partially explain the high sensitivity of the tissue to the stimulatory effect of glucose on insulin release (2).

Infants born to diabetic mothers also have major morphological and functional modifications of the islets of Langerhans (3). The histological signs of hyperactivity of the B cells are associated with an insulin content and insulin secretion which are dependent upon the severity of the maternal diabetes. It was therefore interesting to analyse the effect of varying degrees of maternal carbohydrate intolerance on the pancreatic autonomic nervous development of their pups.

MATERIALS AND METHODS

Female rats (Tif:RAIf, SPF, from Tierfarm Sisseln AG) were mated overnight and pregnancy was timed from the detection of sperm in a vaginal plug the next morning (day 0). Streptozotocin was freshly dissolved in a 5 mM citrate buffer (pH 4.5) and injected (30, 40, or 50 mg/kg body weight) into the tail vein on day 2 of gestation. An oral glucose tolerance test with 350 mg/100 g body weight was performed in normal and streptozotocinized (30 mg/kg body weight) rats on day 20. The animals were sacrificed on day 22. Blood was collected from the mother on the day of sacrifice for enzymatic glucose determination (glucose oxidase/peroxidase method = glucose GOD perid[R], Boehringer). The pancreas of the mothers and their fetuses were dissected as quickly as possible and frozen on dry ice. Noradrenaline content was determined by a fluorimetric method based on the formation of trihydroxyindole derivatives (4). The limit of sensitivity of this method is approximately 1 ng noradrenaline/ml extract, which is equivalent to an apparent minimum assay sensitivity of 35 pg noradrenaline/mg wet tissue. The heart of some fetuses was also extracted for determination of noradrenaline content.

Fetal blood from the same litter was pooled for the determination of serum insulin concentration by a radioimmunoassay technique using rat insulin as standard (gift from Dr. Schlichtkrull, Novo, Copenhagen) and charcoal for separation (5). Statistical analysis was made using Wilcoxon's test.

RESULTS

Effect of streptozotocin on the maternal carbohydrate metabolism

The result of the oral glucose tolerance test is shown in Table I. While there was no signifcant difference in the fasting blood sugar between normal and treated rats, whether pregnant or not, the 60 min. value was significantly higher after treatment with streptozotocin. The glucose intolerance was further impaired during the gestation period. A normal fasting blood sugar with an abnormal glucose tolerance test is suggestive of chemical diabetes.

The blood sugar of the pregnant rats treated with 40 and 50 mg/kg streptozotocin was measured on day 22 when the animals were sacrificed. As seen in Table II, the animals from these groups developed a severe diabetes with a morning blood sugar above 300 mg/100 ml.

Effect of streptozotocin on the noradrenaline content

The low and moderate doses of streptozotocin did not modify the noradrenaline content of the maternal pancreas (Table II), while the dose eliciting a very severe diabetes with acetonuria significantly reduced it by 20%. The fetal pancreas was similarly affected. In the very mild or chemical diabetes the noradrenaline content of the fetal pancreas was almost double that of the control, in contrast with the value measured in the more severe diabetes where the content was decreased by about 50%. It was not

TABLE 1

Oral glucose tolerance test (350 mg/100 g b.w.) in normal and streptozotocin-treated (30 mg/kg b.w.) rats

	Body weight (g)	Blood sugar (mg/dl)	
		0	60 min.
non-pregnant controls (n = 9)	234.0 ± 6.7	72.8 ± 3.5	116.0 ± 2.1**
non-pregnant + strepto 30 (n = 10)	242.0 ± 3.6	68.1 ± 3.7	239.0 ± 11.6**
pregnant controls (n = 9)	265.5 ± 10.5	70.1 ± 4.2	90.7 ± 3.2**
pregnant + strepto 30 (n = 9)	230.0 ± 6.2	79.7 ± 4.3	389.3 ± 17.0**

(mean ± SEM)
Significance of the difference between the experimental and the corresponding control groups: ** $p < 0.01$

possible to make any correlation between the noradrenaline content in the fetus with that of the mother or with the maternal blood sugar levels.

The effect of maternal diabetes on the noradrenaline content of the fetal pancreas appears to be specific, since the noradrenaline content of the fetal heart was not affected by the diabetic condition of the mother (Table III) and amounted to about 50 ng/g wet tissue. Therefore the increase or decrease of the fetal pancreatic content did not seem to be a generalized toxic effect of streptozotocin on the adrenergically innervated tissue of the fetus.

Further, the effect of streptozotocin on the fetal noradrenaline content of the pancreas was not related to a significant change of the pancreatic weight (Table II).

Effect of streptozotocin on the serum insulin level

At 22 days, there was a significant increase of the fetal insulin level in the group treated with a low dose of streptozotocin

TABLE II

Effect of streptozotocin on maternal and fetal parameters

Treatment	MOTHER Blood sugar mg/dl	MOTHER Noradrenaline content (ng/g pancreas w.w.)	FETUS Insulin plasma levels (ng/ml)	FETUS Noradrenaline content (ng/g pancreas w.w.)	FETUS Pancreatic wet weight (mg)
Controls	66 ± 2.8 (15)	319 ± 13 (25)	6.28 ± 0.17 (15)	110 ± 7 (25)	23.7 ± 0.7 (25)
strepto 30	86 ± 4.4* (13)	319 ± 12 (13)	8.57 ± 0.37** (10)	180 ± 8** (13)	23.1 ± 0.9 (13)
strepto 40	351 ± 32.0** (13)	351 ± 13 (13)	4.01 ± 0.30** (6)	57 ± 6** (13)	22.3 ± 1.3 (13)
strepto 50	486 ± 19.0** (11)	259 ± 14* (11)	5.57 ± 0.22* (6)	75 ± 5* (11)	22.8 ± 1.1 (11)

mean ± SEM. Number of observations in parentheses.
Significance of the difference between the experimental and control groups: * $p < 0.05$; ** $p < 0.01$

(Table II). A larger dose of the beta-cytotoxic drug produced a low but statistically significant decrease in fetal insulin. A relationship between the insulin level in the fetal serum and the fetal pancreatic noradrenaline content was observed (r = 0.98).

TABLE III

Noradrenaline content of the rat fetal heart (ng/g w.w.)

Controls	(n = 10)	57.4 ± 5.6
strepto 30	(n = 16)	46.7 ± 2.1
strepto 40	(n = 10)	45.2 ± 3.2

mean ± SEM

DISCUSSION

The noradrenaline content of an organ reflects the extent of its sympathetic innervation. However, the content of an organ is of limited value since it is the consequence of a double phenomenon, i.e. synthesis and release. It is nevertheless indicative of the maturation of the tissue and interesting as a primary approach. The measurement of noradrenaline in the pancreas or in islets was reported in 1964 by Loubatieres (6), and more recently by Christensen and Neubauer (7) and Snyder and Feldman (8). In the human, non-pregnant diabetic adult, the noradrenaline content of the pancreas was unaffected, although a significant reduction was observed in the cardiovascular system (9). No change was detected in the pancreatic noradrenaline content of ob/ob mice (10).

These results have been confirmed in the present study. The noradrenaline content of the maternal pancreas remained unaffected by streptozotocin except at a dose which induces severe carbohydrate intolerance with ketosis. The net changes in noradrenaline content of the adult pancreas may be dependent upon the severity of diabetes or the sensitivity of the tissues in relation to their metabolic state as, for example, during pregnancy.

The measurement of plasma catecholamine levels has produced conflicting results (11). However, abnormalities of autonomic nerve function may be observed at diagnosis, i.e., at an early stage, much before the occurrence of diabetic autonomic neuropathy (12). Goldberg et al (1977) (13) speculated that the low plasma cAMP levels in juvenile onset diabetic subjects were due to decreased sympathetic activity. Also, Sacca et al (1977) clearly showed that the integrity of the sympathetic nervous system was essential for an efficient homeostatic response to insulin-induced hypoglycemia (14).

Reports on the effect of abnormalities in gestational metabolism on the noradrenaline content of fetal organs are scarce, but a reduction of the adrenergic neurotransmitters has been recognized in infants of diabetic mothers. Persson (1976) has described the small left colon syndrome in relation to a functional disturbance due to the immaturity of ganglionic cells in the intermyenteric plexus (15). Further, adrenaline release is impaired in hypoglycemic infants of diabetic mothers. The immaturity and/or the impairment of the adrenaline release mechanism was cited as a contributing cause to the often stormy changes in their blood sugar levels during the neonatal period (Light et al., 1965 (16); Stern et al., 1968 (17); Bloom and Johnston, 1972 (18)). Our findings concerning the alteration in fetal catecholamine levels in pancreas confirm the clinical observations mentioned and suggest the following comments.

Streptozotocin itself is not responsible for the variation in the fetal pancreatic noradrenaline content, since other noradrenergic organs such as the fetal heart remain unaffected. Therefore, the noradrenaline content of the fetal rat pancreas is dependent upon changes in the carbohydrate metabolism of the mother. In the normal adult, the tissue noradrenaline levels usually remain constant despite wide changes in turnover. This is attributed to the reuptake of noradrenaline at the sympathetic nerve ending (19). The variations in noradrenaline levels found in the fetal pancreas could be due to several mechanisms: increased synthesis without appropriate release; immaturity in synthesis and/or release mechanism; or ineffectiveness of active reuptake at the presynaptic level. These possible mechanisms may be related to the severity of the maternal diabetes.

Insulin as well as nerve growth factor (NGF) was reported to increase significantly. directly or indirectly, the cellular volume and activity of neurons in sympathetic ganglia (20). Further, sucrose overfeeding increased the sympathetic activity in the adult rat with an acceleration of noradrenaline turnover (19). The specific effect of sucrose upon the fetal noradrenergic activity has not been studied. Amino acids could also possibly be involved. In pups from mothers with mild glucose intolerance, we found high plasma insulin levels and an elevated pancreatic noradrenaline content. The histology of the fetal B cells shows a marked hyperplasia and hypertrophy as well as a high insulin content (3). The high insulin level in the plasma could be a consequence of increased glucose and amino acids acting upon the B cells. This insulin would act as a trophic substance and stimulates noradrenaline synthesis without affecting noradrenaline release.

An inhibition of insulin release by catecholamine has been demonstrated in the adult (21). Stress in the mother, such as that induced by anesthesia, will markedly reduce the blood insulin levels in the rat fetus for more than 24 hours. The inhibition is not complete, however (Reusen and Hoet, 1978, unpublished observation). Consequently, a reduction of insulin levels in the fetal pancreas as well as in fetal blood of pups born to severely affected diabetic mothers could be the result of chronic increased noradrenaline release. Further, continuous stimulation of the fetal pancreas by the increasing load of nutrients may lead to exhaustion of the stored hormones in both endocrine pancreas and sympathetic nerve endings. The observations of Aerts and van Assche (3), Guillaume and Kervran(22) and Eriksson et al. (23) concerning the effect of the severity of the maternal diabetes upon the morphological and functional changes in the fetal endocrine pancreas are consistent with this interpretation. Indeed, degranulation, low insulin levels in the endocrine pancreas and in the fetal blood, as well as reduction in insulin biosynthetic rate are observed with severe maternal diabetes.

Our data shed more light on the complexities of the adaptation of fetal endocrine activity in relation with gestational metabolism. They indicate that fetal sympathetic activities may also be challenged in these circumstances and react in a diversified way related with the severity of the metabolic disturbances. This adrenergic activity may modulate further the hormonal changes in endocrine organs sensitive to adrenergic activity.

REFERENCES

1. *de Gasparo, M., et al(1978). J. Endocr., 77, 241*
2. *de Gasparo, M., et al (1978). J. Endocr., 79, 49*
3. *Aerts, L. and Van Assche, F.A. (1977). J. Endocr. 73, 339*
4. *Waldmeier, P., et al (1974). Clin. Chem., 20, 81*
5. *Herbert, V., et al (1965). J. Clin. Endocr. Metab., 25, 1375*
6. *Loubatieres, A., et al (1964). C.R. Soc. Biol., 158, 607*
7. *Christensen, N.J. and Neubauer, B. (1976). Acta Endocr., 82,753*
8. *Snyder, J.H. and Feldman, J.M. (1977). Diabetes, 26, 418*
9. *Neubauer, B. and Christensen, N.J. (1976). Diabetes, 25, 6*
10. *Feldman, J.M. and Henderson, J.H. (1978) Diabetes, 27, 389*
11. *Cryer, P.E. (1976). Diabetes, 25, 1071*
12. *Fraser, D.M., et al (1977). Diabetes, 26, 546*
13. *Goldberg, M.L., et al (1977). Diabetes, 26, 936*

14. *Sacca, L., et al (1977). Endocrinology, 101, 1016*
15. *Persson, B. (1976) in Perinatal Management in 5th European Congress of Perinatal Medicine, Rooth, G. and Bratteby, L.E., eds., Almquist and Wiksell International, Stockholm, p. 103*
16. *Light, I.J., et al (1967). New Engl. J. Med., 277, 394*
17. *Stern, L., et al (1968). Pediatrics, 42, 598*
18. *Bloom, S.R. and Johnston, D.I. (1972). Br. Med. J., 4, 453*
19. *Young, J.B. and Landsberg, L. (1977). Nature, 269, 615*
20. *Angeletti, P.U., et al. (1966). Ann. 1st. Super. Sanita, 2, 420*
21. *Woods, S.C. and Porte, D. (1974). Physiol. Rev., 54, 596*
22. *Guillaume, M. and Kervran, A. (1977). Diabetologia, 13, 397*
23. *Eriksson, U., et al (1977). Acta Endocr., suppl. 209, 22*

The very skilled technical assistance of Mrs. G. Hostetter is gratefully acknowledged. Also we are most grateful to Drs. K. Hauser and L. Maitre for critical reading of the manuscript.

DISCUSSION

W. MALAISSE: *In your measurement of the noradrenaline content of the pancreas, what fraction represents noradrenaline in the islets?*

M. de GASPARO: *We have no direct measurement of the noradrenaline content in the islets.*

H. LEBOVITZ: *Did you have histochemical measurements of where the norepinephrine was located?*

M. de GASPARO: *It was not possible with our technique to determine if the immunofluorescence corresponds to alpha, beta, delta, or SNI cells. But, we know from the literature that all cell types in the pancreas are involved. If we were using a more sensitive technique, for example, electromicroscopy, we would have the answer to your question.*

H. LEBOVITZ: *Does your method differentiate norepinephrine from dopamine?*

M. de GASPARO: *Yes, there is no dopamine measureable in the embryo pancreas. In vitro or in utero, nothing.*

W.J. IRVINE: *In regard to the immunofluorescent technique, it should be quite possible to answer that point using a double staining technique with rodamine for antibodies against the A, B, C, or D cells for precise identification.*

M. de GASPARO: *Thank you very much for the suggestion.*

A. NOTKINS: *In diseases of the autonomic nervous system, do you find any abnormalities of the beta cell function with glucose intolerance or diabetes?*

M. de GASPARO: *I don't know.*

SUPPRESSION OF INSULIN SECRETION BY PROTEIN DEPRIVATION IN OBESITY

D. E. Schteingart*, A. K. McKenzie,
R. S. Victoria, and H. S. Tsao

Hyperinsulinemia, decreased sensitivity of peripheral tissues to both exogenous and endogenous insulin and abnormalities of glucose tolerance are frequent findings in obesity (1). These abnormalities are frequently reversed by dietary deprivation and weight reduction (2) and induced in normal subjects made obese by overfeeding. The role played by specific nutrients in the hyperinsulinemia of obese people has not been clearly defined. Studies by Grey and Kipnis (3) suggest that diets high in carbohydrate are associated with hyperinsulinemia while isocaloric diets low in carbohydrate decrease circulating insulin levels. In contrast to these observations, Brunzell, et al, (4) reported that high carbohydrate diets given to normal subjects or mildly diabetic patients decrease basal and glucose stimulated insulin levels and improve glucose tolerance.

The present study investigates the effect of low protein diets on insulin levels in obesity. The results to be reported suggest that protein deprivation even in the presence of high calorie and carbohydrate intake suppresses basal insulin levels.

MATERIALS AND METHODS

Seventeen obese, non-diabetic, hyperinsulinemic subjects were studied. Twelve were male and five were female; their mean age was 30.9 $\pm$ SE 2.1 years; their mean weight was 271% (range 73) of ideal weight. On a weight-maintaining mixed diet, mean basal glucose levels were normal, 96.6 ($\pm$ SE 3.8) mg/dl; but mean basal glucose levels, 47.8 ($\pm$ SE 5.3) uu/dl, and mean insulin/glucose ratio, .59 $\pm$ SE .05, were high. These levels were in contrast to those obtained in 235 non-obese, non-diabetic patients whose values were 93.7 ($\pm$ 0.96), 8.15 ($\pm$ SE 0.58), and 0.086 ($\pm$ .005) respectively. The insulin/glucose ratio is being used as an expression of peripheral insulin sensitivity. The high values suggested insulin resistance.

The obese subjects were fed a control weight-maintaining diet. This diet was followed by either a low protein diet or a total fast.

Plasma insulin, glucose, glucagon and cortisol, urinary 17-hydroxycorticoids and free cortisol and plasma amino acid levels were measured at the end of each diet or on the last day of the total fast. Plasma insulin, glucagon and cortisol and urinary free cortisol were measured by radioimmunoassay; plasma glucose by autoanalyzer; urinary 17-hydroxycorticoids by the method of Silber and Porter and plasma amino acid levels by a Beckman amino acid analyzer. Values are expressed as mean $\pm$ SE of the mean. The data was analyzed for statistical significance by a student t test.

RESULTS

The well known decrease in plasma insulin levels observed in obese people during total fast is illustrated in Figure 1. Seven obese subjects were studied on a weight-maintaining, 3300 calorie, mixed diet for 14 days; they were subsequently fasted for four days. There was a significant fall in plasma insulin and glucose and the insulin/glucose ratio at the end of the fast.

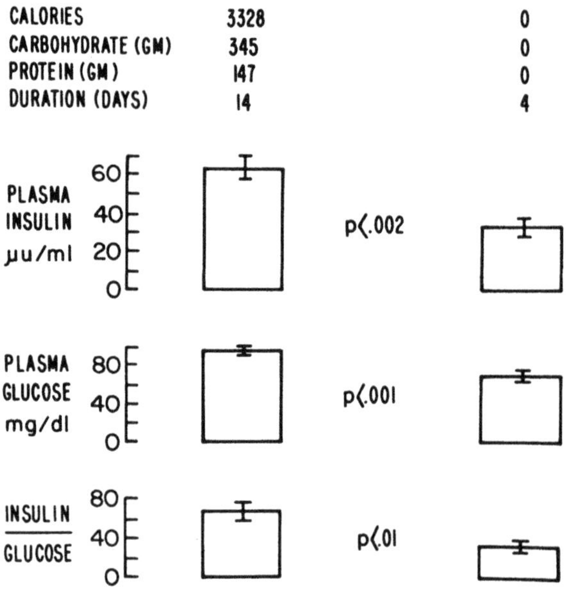

Fig. 1. Suppression of basal plasma insulin, glucose and I/G ratio by total fast in seven obese, non-diabetic patients.

As shown in Figure 2, a suppressive effect qualitatively similar to that produced by a total fast was also observed with diets deficient in protein, but adequate in calories to maintain weight. Nine obese patients were fed a weight-maintaining, 3700 calorie diet for 14 days. This diet contained 398 gm of carbohydrate and 170 gm of protein. The patients were then fed an isocaloric diet containing only 6 gm of protein for 14 more days. This diet contained 587 gm of carbohydrate.

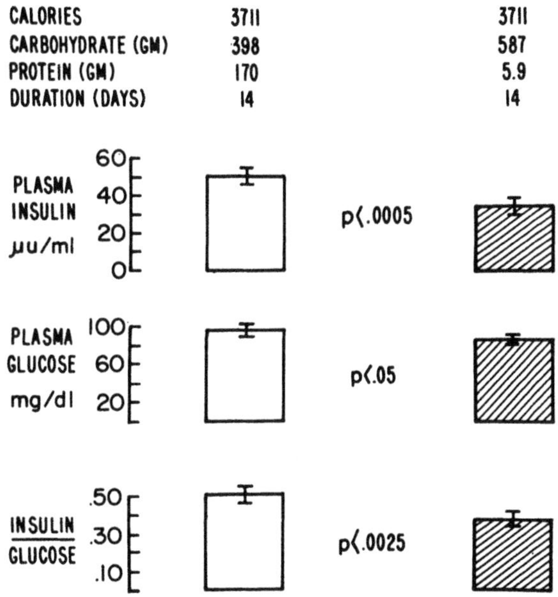

Fig. 2. Suppression of basal plasma insulin, glucose and I/G ratio by low protein diets in nine obese, non-diabetic patients.

Protein restriction caused a significant decrease in mean basal insulin levels from 50.4 to 34.7 uu/ml. This decrease was accompanied by a modest, but significant decrease in the mean plasma glucose level from 96 to 87 mg/dl and in the mean IRI/G ratio from 0.51 to 0.39.

To rule out the possibility that the decrease in insulin levels observed with protein restriction was due to the concommitant increase in carbohydrate intake, four obese subjects were fed a weight-maintaining, 3500 calorie diet for 28 days. This diet contained 130 gm of protein. For the first 14 days, the carbohydrate content was 375 gm; for the last 14 days, 612 gm. As shown in Figure 3, there was lack of suppression of plasma insulin, glucose and I/G ratio when the high carbohydrate diet was fed without restriction of protein.

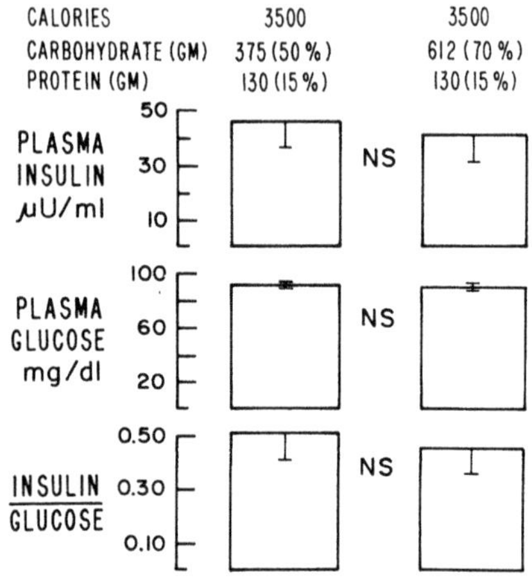

Fig. 3. Lack of suppression of plasma insulin, glucose and I/G ratio with high carbohydrate diets without protein restriction.

As shown in Figure 4, protein restriction can also prevent the post-refeeding recovery of plasma insulin levels previously suppressed by total fast. Seven patients were fed a weight-maintaining, 3300 calorie diet for 14 days. This diet contained 345 gm of carbohydrate and 147 gm of protein. They then fasted for four days. The fast was followed by a 3300 calorie diet containing only 6 gm of protein for 14 days. There was a significant decrease in values during fasting, but no significant recovery occurred during the low protein diet, despite the fact that the carbohydrate content of this diet, 582 gm, was higher than the control diet.

These findings are in contrast to the apparent recovery of basal insulin levels observed when the control, rather than a low protein diet, is refed following a fast. As depicted in Figure 5, a study in two obese patients showed that basal insulin and glucose levels and the IRI/G ratios decreased on a total fast but rose towards the control level at the end of two weeks of refeeding the control diet.

Although protein restriction in obesity decreases basal insulin levels, it does not affect the insulin response to the intravenous infusion of arginine, a potent insulin secretagogue. This lack of effect is shown in Figure 6. Eight obese subjects received intravenous infusions containing 30 gm of arginine while on a control diet and at the end of an isocaloric, 6 gm protein diet, fed for 14 days. On isocaloric low protein diets, basal insulin levels decreased to 63% of control. In contrast, arginine stimulated values did not change significantly. Similarly, no significant change was observed in either phase 1 or phase 2 insulin release. These findings differ from those observed in patients with protein calorie malnutrition who exhibit a decrease in phase 1 insulin release, but not in basal levels (5,6).

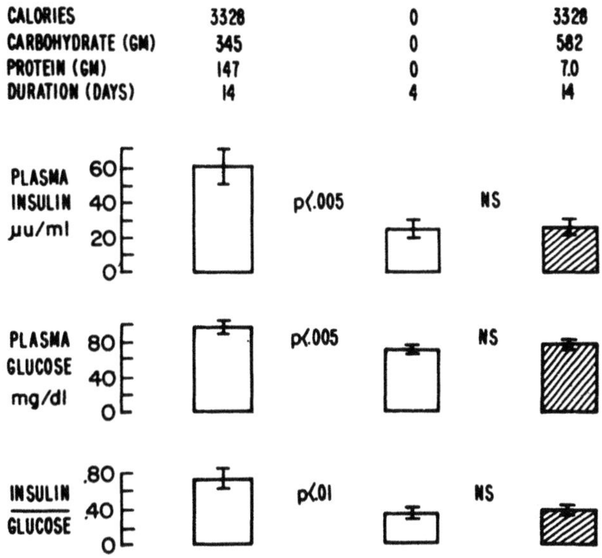

Fig. 4. Suppression of plasma insulin, glucose and I/G ratio by fasting in seven obese, non-diabetic subjects. Lack of recovery with low protein diets.

The mechanism by which protein restriction suppresses basal insulin levels in obesity is unknown. Several possibilities exist. Protein restriction may have directly suppressed β-cell function. Like and Chick (7) have reported decreased β-cell mitotic activity of diabetic mice fed diets low in protein and high in carbohydrate. Alternatively, factors known to influence insulin secretion and which are abnormal in obesity might have been affected by protein restriction and secondarily lowered basal insulin levels. Changes in plasma glucose, glucagon, cortisol, amino acids and body weight were measured among these factors. There was lack of correlation between changes in basal plasma insulin levels and changes in plasma glucose, glucagon, urinary 17-hydroxycorticoids (17-OHCS) and body weight during protein deprivation.

As shown in Figure 7, urinary 17-OHCS and free cortisol decreased significantly on protein restricted diets. However, as shown in Figure 8, the administration of cortisol in doses equivalent to basal cortisol secretion rates during isocaloric, low protein diets, did not prevent the decrease in basal insulin and glucose levels and in the insulin/glucose ratio induced by this diet.

The levels of branch-chain amino acids, valine, leucine and isoleucine, decreased in parallel to insulin levels on the

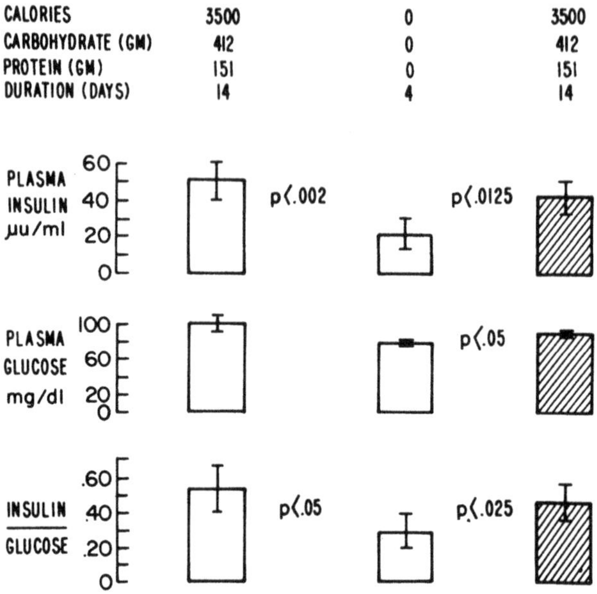

Fig. 5. Suppression of plasma insulin, glucose and I/G ratio by total fasting in two obese, non-diabetic patients. Recovery with control diet.

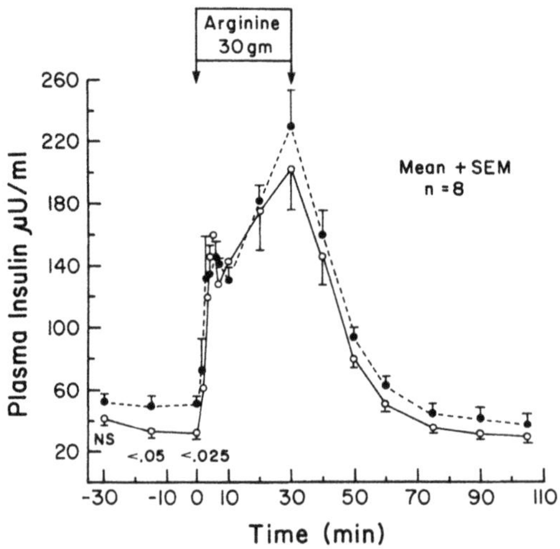

Fig. 6. Lack of effect of low protein diets on the insulin response to the intravenous infusion of arginine. The solid line depicts the response to a low protein diet.

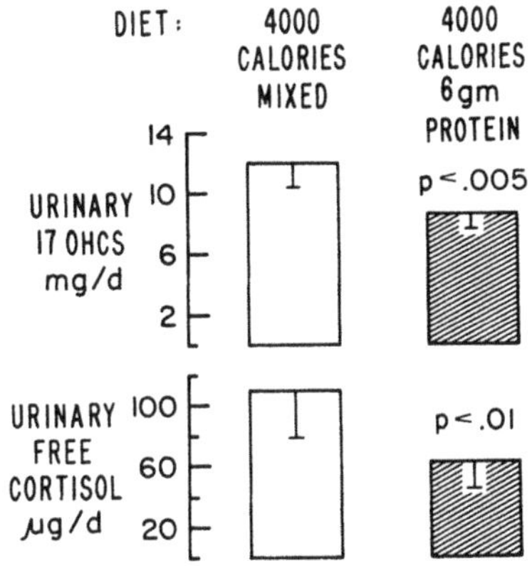

Fig. 7. Suppression of urinary 17 OHCS and free cortisol on low protein diets.

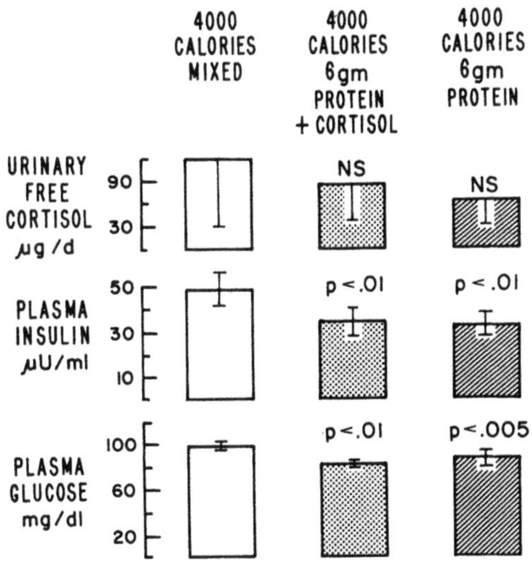

Fig. 8. Failure of cortisol treatment to prevent the suppression of plasma insulin by low protein diets in five obese patients.

isocaloric low protein diet. Levels returned back to control values when the control diet was refed. More definitive studies in which patients are fed branch chain amino acids to restore plasma levels to those of the control period during protein deprivation have not been carried out.

The role of gastrointestinal hormones in the suppression of insulin levels during protein restriction has not been studied.

The results reported here on protein deprivation do not necessarily imply that a high protein intake is responsible for hyperinsulinemia in obesity. However because of its well known ability to stimulate insulin secretion (8) protein may indeed play a role in the pathogenesis of the hyperinsulinemia and insulin resistance found in obesity.

SUMMARY AND CONCLUSIONS

1) Protein restricted diets decrease basal plasma insulin levels in obesity.
2) This effect occurs even in the presence of sufficient calories to maintain body weight and while the diet is high in carbohydrate.
3) The decrease in insulin is accompanied by a fall in plasma glucose and in the I/G ratio, suggesting an increase in insulin sensitivity.
4) Excessive protein intake, in addition to carbohydrate, may play a role in the pathogenesis of the hyperinsulinemia and insulin resistance found in obesity.

REFERENCES

1. *Rabinowitz, D. (1970). Annual Rev. Med. 21, 241.*
2. *Jackson, I.M.D., et al., (1969). The Lancet 1, 285.*
3. *Grey, N. and Kipnis, D.M. (1971). N. Engl. J. Med. 285, 827.*
4. *Brunzell, J.D., et al., (1971). N. Engl. J. Med. 284, 521.*
5. *Smith, S.R., et al., (1975). Metabolism 24, 1073.*
6. *Becher, D.J., et al., (1975). Diabetologia 11, 237.*
7. *Chick, W.L. and Like, A.A. (1971). Am. J. of Physiol. 221, 202.*
8. *Floyd, J.C., et al., (1966). J. Clin. Invest. 45, 1487.*

Supported in part by USPHS Grants AM 02244, 5 MO1 RR-4216 and T1-AM-05001.

DISCUSSION

J. ANDERSON: *Dr. Schteingart, the natural inclination is to assume that chronic high carbohydrate diets would stimulate insulin secretion. Our own work suggests that, in lean individuals, chronically feeding high carbohydrate diets enhance insulin sensitivity and decrease basal insulin secretion, as measured peripherally. In obesity, it's a different situation, as Kipnis showed that feeding high carbohydrate diets enhances insulin secretion and Stern and others have shown in animals that high carbohydrate diets in obese animals increase insulin secretion. The question is: is there evidence that protein deprivation decreases insulin secretion?*

D. E. SCHTEINGART: *You're absolutely right that there might be a difference between non-obese and obese individuals, humans or animals, in terms of response to either carbohydrate or protein. There is evidence that protein deprivation also seemed to inhibit insulin production. I might add that, in the studies where we increased the carbohydrate intake alone without changing the protein content of the diet, there was no significant change in insulin or glucose or insulin sensitivity. And the level of carbohydrate intake in these diets were certainly quite high, up to 650 grams.*

M. VRANIC: *Dr. Schteingart, how can you use the insulin-glucose ratio as an index of peripheral insulin sensitivity, since insulin affects glucose uptake in the periphery, glucose uptake in the liver, and in addition has an effect on glucose production in the liver? This is one-half of the feedback mechanism; the other half is the effect of glucose on insulin release.*

D. E. SCHTEINGART: *I'm well aware that expressing the insulin sensitivity as I/G ratio is not the most detailed way but, in a rough manner, it indicates the responsiveness of target tissues.*

P. L. POFFENBARGER: *A question for both Dr. Tobin and Dr. Pfeiffer-I'd like to know what arguments they can marshal that their data might be explained just by decrease in the total number of beta cell responsive mass in the pancreas.*

J. TOBIN: *The analysis of our data on isolated perfused pancreas is just at the beginning and wouldn't answer that question; in any event in terms of absolute number.*

E. PFEIFFER: *In our studies in humans, the number of the beta cells are different in the various groups. Since we used the same patients, I don't think there is much difference between the groups. This cannot answer for the different action of the sulfonylurea compounds and for the action on the surface of the beta cell.*

G. M. REAVEN: *I would like to make several comments about the effect of age on insulin secretion. We have used the electron microscope to quantify the number of beta cells per islet in rats. As rats age from 2 to 18 months their islets increase in volume. Since the proportion of beta cells remains the same, the number of beta cells per islet increases with age. This age-related increase in number of beta cells is associated with a concomitant increase in insulin content per islet. However, there is a progressive decrease in glucose-stimulated insulin release from isolated islets as rats age, and this decline is particularly dramatic when expressed per beta cell. However, the fact that insulin secretion per beta cell decreases with age does not mean that the total pancreatic insulin secretion will decrease with age. For example, if there are more beta cells, the intact animal may well maintain net insulin secretion. In this regard, I think it is necessary to question Jordan's interpretation of the hyperglycemic clamp studies. As pointed out, older subjects have worse glucose tolerance. Therefore, in order to carry out the hyperglycemic clamp, it is necessary to give significantly more glucose to young individuals than to old individuals. Since an increase in administered glucose load will give rise to a greater insulin output, it is possible that the decreased insulin secretion in older patients is simply a function of the fact that they received less glucose. I think it possible that Jordan's results are a function of this additional variable, and not indicative of an age-related defect in total pancreatic secretion.*

J. TOBIN: *Basically, if we go back to the glucose clamp, I agree that the third variable is the amount of glucose that you have to infuse into the body to maintain identical levels of plasma glucose. If we desire to bring someone 125 milligrams deciliter above basal, it's going to take a certain amount of glucose. If they're very tolerant to glucose, we must put in a lot more glucose to keep that level. If they're very intolerant, then we're going to need very little glucose to maintain that level. And that's what we mean by glucose load being the third variable, which we called M, glucose metabolized, which we haven't discussed today. What we are really aiming at is what the pancreas is seeing. We have to think of this as an isolated perfused pancreas. We want the pancreas to be presented with the identical stimulus, and the stimulus to the pancreas to release insulin in the absence of gut factor, or something else, is the glucose level.*

S. FAJANS: *I'd like to enlarge on Dr. Reaven's point. In a simpler model, if you take a normal subject and do a glucose tolerance of 75, 100 and 125 grams, respectively, you get identical glucose curves, but you get successively higher insulin response curves. So, I think that's another way of saying what Dr. Reaven just said, that glucose is a variable indeed, and in the model I just gave, you have identical glucose levels but different insulin responses.*

VIRUS-INDUCED DIABETES MELLITUS: INFECTION OF MICE WITH VARIANTS OF ENCEPHALOMYOCARDITIS VIRUS, COXSACKIEVIRUS B4, AND REOVIRUS TYPE 3

A. L. Notkins*, J. Yoon, T. Onodera and
A. B. Jenson

For many years, it has been suggested that an infectious agent, possibly a virus, might be involved in the etiology of some cases of the juvenile-onset type of diabetes (1). Numerous case reports have shown a temporal relationship between the onset of certain viral infections and the subsequent development of diabetes. The viruses most often implicated have been mumps and members of the Coxsackievirus B group. Despite these case reports, most of the evidence is circumstantial and proof that viruses actually produce diabetes in humans is still lacking.

The best evidence that viruses might be involved in the etiology of diabetes comes from experiments in mice. This brief review will be divided into two parts. First, we will summarize what is known about the diabetogenic capacity of the M-variant of encephalomyocarditis (EMC) virus and second, we will discuss recent data on variants of two viruses of human origin which can produce a diabetes-like syndrome in mice.

When inoculated into mice, the M-variant of EMC virus infects and destroys pancreatic beta cells (1,2). This results in hypoinsulinemia and the subsequent development of a diabetes-like syndrome which is characterized by hyperglycemia, glycosuria, polydipsia and polyphagia. Examination of over two dozen inbred strains of mice revealed that only certain strains develop diabetes when infected with EMC firus (3). Based on this information, it was possible to choose and mate the appropriate susceptible and resistant strains and study the susceptibility of the F1, F2 and backcross animals (4,5). Some of the more important findings are illustrated in Fig. 1. Each animal was bled four times.

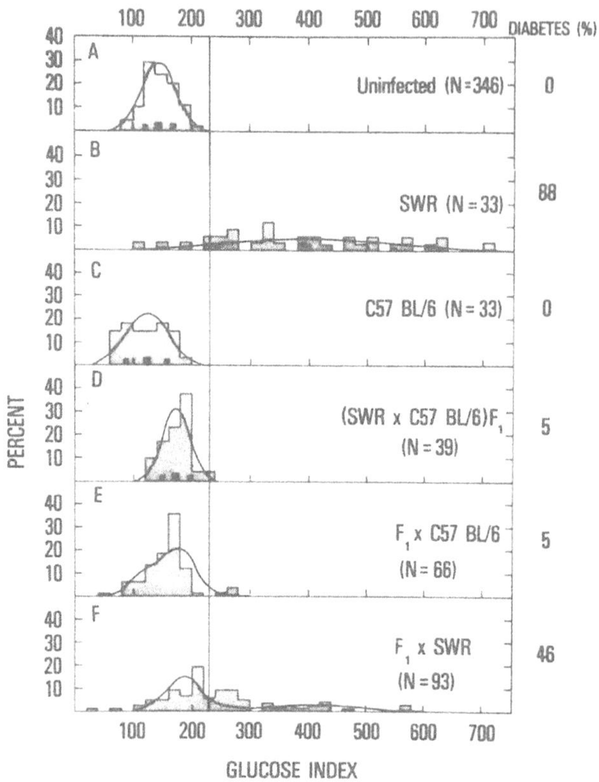

Fig. 1. Glucose index of male mice infected with EMC virus and uninfected controls (5). Glucose indexes were determined and the percentage of animals falling within each 20-unit interval was plotted (shaded areas). The small bars represent the mean ± SD. The curves represent the expected distribution of the data based on the assumption that each population is normally distributed. An animal was scored as diabetic if its glucose index was 3 SD above the mean of the uninfected animals (vertical line). N represents number of mice.

Non-fasting (NF) blood glucose levels were measured 7 and 14 days after infection and single point 60 minute glucose tolerance tests (GTT) were performed 10 and 17 days after infection. The data from these four determinations was used to calculate the glucose index (4) for each mouse: glucose index = (4 x NF day 14) + (3 x NF day 7) + (2 x GTT day 17) + (1 x GTT day 10) ÷ 10. Any animal with a glucose index greater than 220 (three standard deviations above the mean of uninfected animals) was considered diabetic. When

SWR mice were infected with EMC virus (Fig. 1B), the majority of the animals, 88%, developed diabetes. C57BL/6 mice, however, failed to develop diabetes when infected with EMC virus (Fig. 1C). Similarly, the F1 offspring of susceptible SWR x resistant C57BL/6 were essentially resistant to the development of EMC-induced diabetes (Fig. 1D). In contrast, a significant percentage of the F2 offspring developed diabetes (data not shown). From these and other studies, it was concluded that susceptibility to EMC-induced diabetes is inherited as an autosomal recessive trait.

Information on the number of loci involved comes from backcross data. F1 mice were mated with resistant C57BL/6 mice and the backcross animals infected. If a single locus were involved, half the animals would be expected to have glucose indexes similar to the F1 and the other half similar to the C57BL/6. As seen in Fig. 1E, the actual data fit quite closely the expected data (i.e. only 5% of the animals developed diabetes). F1 mice then were mated with susceptible SWR mice and the backcross animals infected. If a single locus were involved, half the animals would be expected to have glucose indexes similar to the F1 and the other half similar to the SWR. Fig. 1F shows a bimodal distribution with approximately half of the animals having glucose indexes similar to the resistant F1 and the other half having indexes similar to the susceptible SWR. Although there may be other interpretations, the data are consistent with a single locus being a major determinant in controlling susceptibility to EMC-induced diabetes (5).

Why do SWR mice develop diabetes while C57BL/6 mice do not? Certainly this could be explained if beta cells from SWR mice were more susceptible to infection than beta cells from C57BL/6. This problem was approached in several ways (6). First, at different times after infection, the pancreas was removed from strains of mice that developed diabetes and from strains of mice that did not develop diabetes. The amount of infectious virus in the islets then was determined. Approximately 10 times more virus was recovered from strains of mice that developed diabetes than from the strains of mice that did not develop diabetes. By immunofluorescence, using fluorescein-labeled antibody to EMC virus, many more infected cells were found in SWR than C57BL/6 islets.

To be certain that this difference in susceptibility resided at the level of the beta cell and was not secondary to the host's immunological defense mechanisms, the susceptibility of beta cells in culture was investigated (6,7). In these experiments, beta cells in cultures were prepared from strains of mice that developed diabetes (e.g., SJL) and from strains of mice that did not develop diabetes (C57BL/6). The cultures then were infected with EMC virus. By use of fluorescein-labeled antibody to EMC virus, approximately 10 times more infected cells were found in beta cell cultures from

SJL than from C57BL/6 mice (7). We conclude from both the animal and cell culture experiments that the difference in susceptibility resides at the level of the beta cell.

At the present time, we are trying to determine why beta cells from SJL mice are more susceptible to infection than beta cells from C57BL/6 mice. It is known that there are receptors on the surface of cells for at least certain of the picornaviruses. We have been studying the binding of infectious EMC virus to cultured beta cells from susceptible and resistant strains. More virus seems to bind to beta cells from SJL than from C57BL/6 mice (7). This suggests that there may be more receptors for EMC virus on the surface of SJL beta cells. However, these studies are difficult to perform because it is hard to get large numbers of beta cells and the cultures are not pure beta cells. If these binding studies can be confirmed, then it is possible that the locus controlling susceptibility might actually operate by controlling the expression of viral receptors.

From these and other studies, a picture is beginning to emerge concerning the pathogenesis of EMC-induced diabetes mellitus. First, the virus infects and destroys pancreatic beta cells, producing an insulin-dependent hyperglycemia. Second, only certain inbred strains of mice develop virus-induced diabetes. Third, susceptibility is inherited as an autosomal recessive trait. Fourth, the data is consistent with a single locus. Fifth, the genetic factors appear to operate at the level of the beta cell where they control susceptibility. And sixth, preliminary data suggest (but have not proven) that the gene product might be a receptor for the virus.

With the information gained from the EMC model, we begin to look for other viruses, especially of human origin, that might produce a diabetes-like syndrome in mice. Previous studies from our laboratory showed that Coxsackievirus B4 did not produce diabetes when inoculated into mice (8). However, as seen in Fig. 2, by passaging Coxsackievirus B4 in cultures enriched in mouse beta cells, it has been possible to enhance the diabetogenic capacity of this virus (9). Inoculation of mice with Coxsackievirus B4 that had been passaged 14 times in beta cell cultures resulted in destruction of pancreatic beta cells and a decrease in the immunoreactive insulin content of the pancreas (Fig. 3). The reduction in immunoreactive insulin correlated inversely with the elevation of glucose in the blood. Over 80% of the infected animals developed hyperglycemia within 14 days after infection (9). The percentage of animals with hyperglycemia decreased with time and at the end of 60 days, less than five percent of the animals were still hyperglycemic. Many of the normoglycemic mice, however, were metabolically abnormal when evaluated by glucose tolerance tests. During the acute phase of the infection, viral antigens were found in the islets of Langerhans (Fig. 4A). As in the case of EMC virus, only certain inbred strains of mice were susceptible to the development of

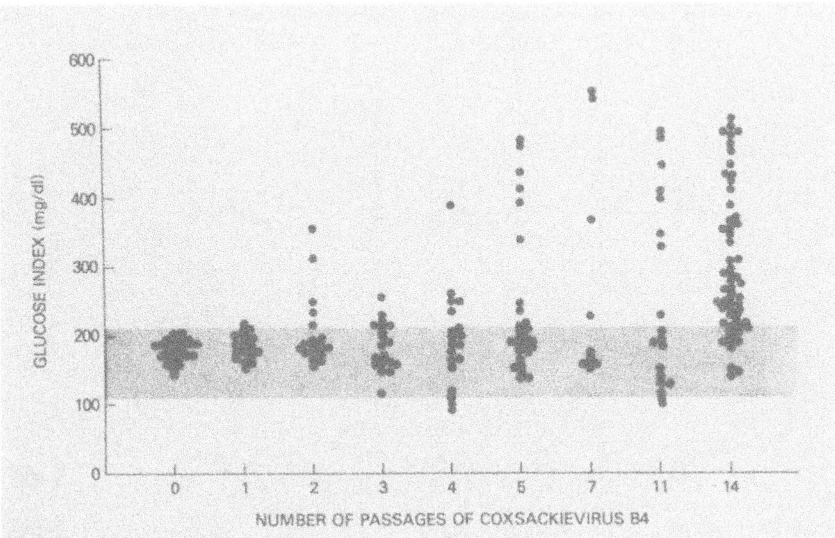

Fig. 2. *Effect of passage of Coxsackievirus B4 in beta cell cultures on the diabetogenic capacity of the virus (9). Virus harvested after each passage was titrated on secondary mouse embryo cells and $10^{5.0}$ plaque-forming units were inoculated intraperitoneally into mice. Shaded horizontal area represents the mean glucose index of 80 uninfected mice $\pm$ 3 SD. Each point represents the glucose index of an infected animal.*

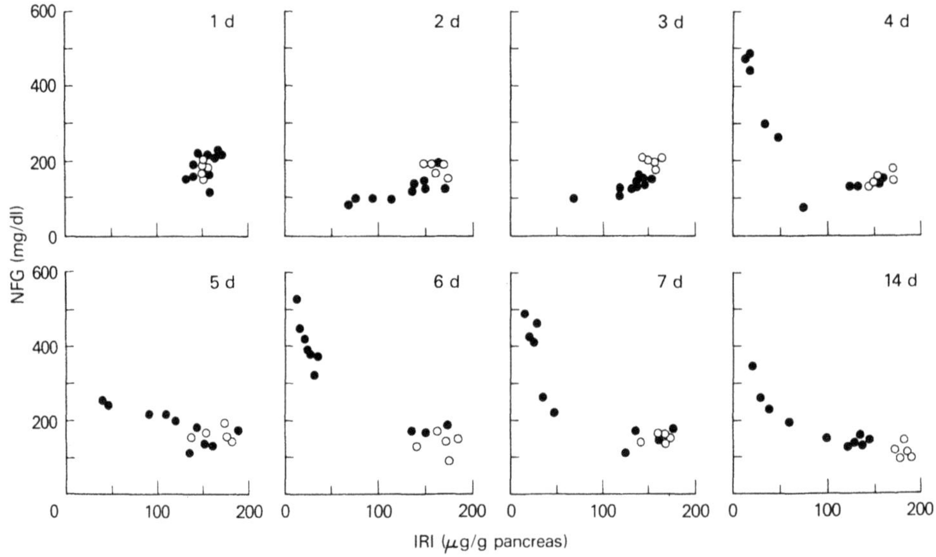

Fig. 3. Relationship of concentration of non-fasting glucose (NFG) in the plasma to the concentration of immunoreactive insulin (IRI) in pancreas at different times after infection with the 14th passage of Coxsackievirus B4 (9). Each point represents an individual mouse. (O) uninfected mice; (●) infected mice.

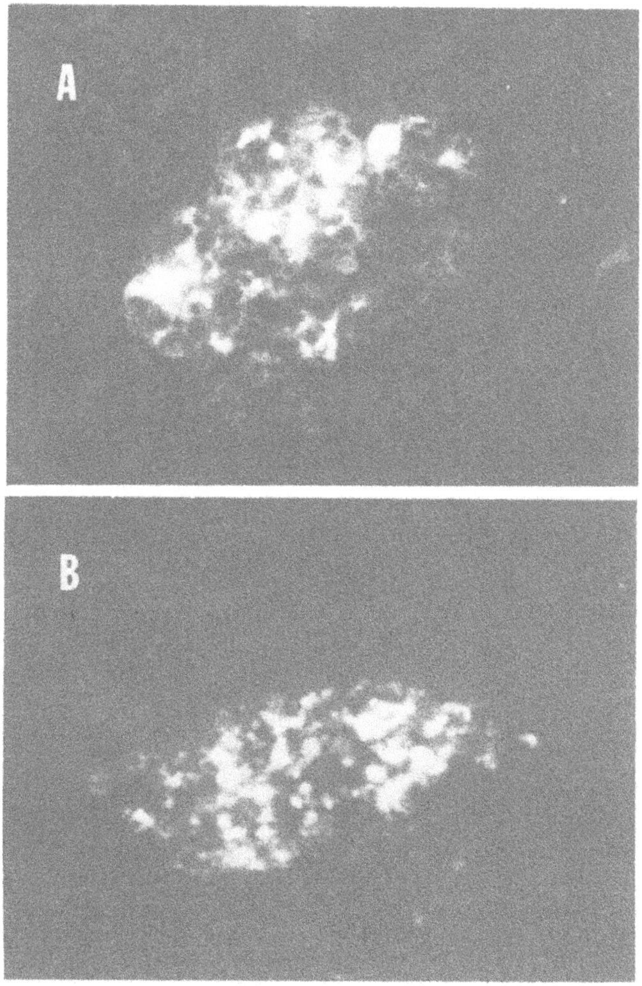

Fig. 4. *(A) Coxsackievirus B4 antigens in islet of Langerhans. Frozen sections from pancreas taken 4 days after infection and stained with fluorescein-labeled antibody to the variant of Coxsackievirus B4 (x 340). (B) Reovirus antigens in islet of Langerhans. Frozen sections from pancreas taken 7 days after infection and stained with fluorescein-labeled antibody to reovirus (x 340).*

Coxsackievirus B4-induced diabetes (Table 1). Many, but not all strains of mice which were susceptible to EMC-induced diabetes also were susceptible to Coxsackievirus B4-induced diabetes. It is concluded from these studies that both the passage history of the virus and the strain of the host influence the development of diabetes.

Table 1. Induction of Diabetes by Coxsackievirus B4 in Different Inbred Strains of Mice.

Strain of mouse	Sex	Glucose index	Diabetic
		Mean ± SD	%
SJL/J	M	253 ± 83	72
SWR/J	M	270 ± 91	75
NIH Swiss	M	325 ± 119	80
C57BL/6J	M	129 ± 27	0
CBA/J	M	157 ± 15	0
AKR	M	113 ± 32	0
BALB/C	M	92 ± 40	0
C3H/J	M	87 ± 33	0
DBA/1J	M	159 ± 25	0
DBA/2J	M	140 ± 25	0
SJL/J	F	216 ± 87	33
SWR/J	F	233 ± 25	50
NIH Swiss	F	174 ± 33	10
CBA/J	F	153 ± 17	0
AKR	F	125 ± 14	0
DBA/1J	F	100 ± 30	0
DBA/2J	F	158 ± 10	0

Mice, 5-to-6-week old, were infected intraperitoneally with the 14th passage of Coxsackievirus B4. Glucose indexes were determined and the percentage of diabetic animals calculated. Each group contained 30-40 mice. (See Ref. (9).

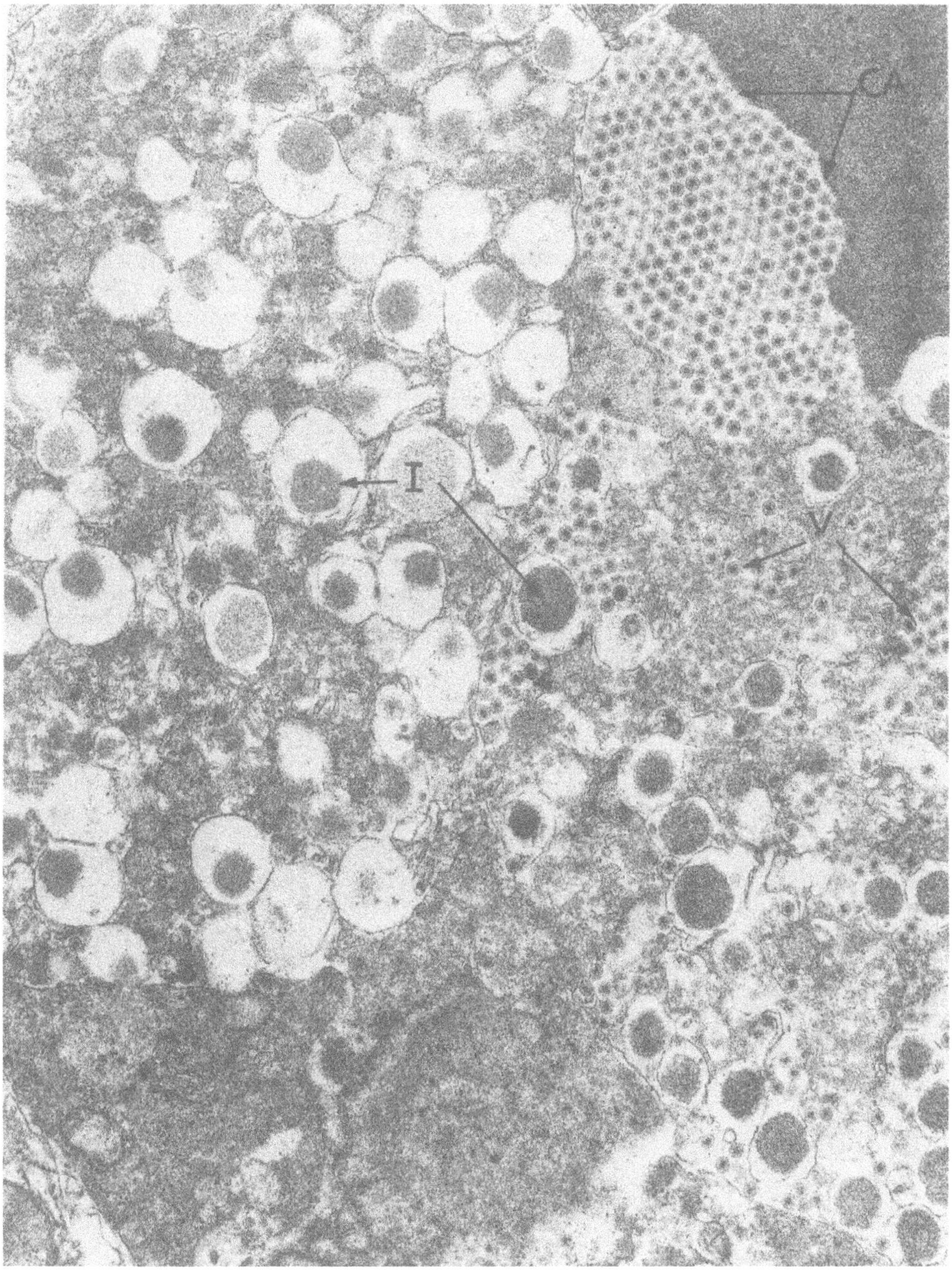

Fig. 5. Electron micrograph of damaged pancreatic beta cells from mouse infected with reovirus. Reovirus particles (V), sometimes in crystalline array (CA), are seen interspersed among typical insulin (I) granules (x 38,000).

Reovirus type 3 also was found to be capable of infecting beta cells (10). The diabetogenic capacity of this virus was enhanced by passage in mouse beta cell cultures. When reovirus was inoculated into 1-to-2 week old mice, insulitis and beta cell damage followed. By a double-label antibody technique, using fluorescein-labeled antibody to reovirus (Fig. 4B) and rhodamine-labeled antibody to insulin, reovirus antigens were found in beta cells. By electron microscopy, viral particles were observed in insulin-containing beta cells (Fig. 5). The damage to beta cells resulted in a decrease in the insulin content of the pancreas and altered the host's capacity to respond normally to a glucose load. The metabolic alterations in reovirus-infected animals were less severe than in animals infected with EMC virus or Coxsackievirus B4.

In conclusion, (1) animal models for virus-induced diabetes have been developed and these models are similar in many respects to juvenile-onset type of diabetes; (2) genetic factors, at least in the case of EMC virus and Coxsackievirus B4, control susceptibility; (3) beta cells from both animals and humans can be grown in culture and the interaction of viruses with these cells can be studied; (4) variants of two viruses that are present in the human population can produce a diabetes-like syndrome in mice. What role these and other viruses play in the etiology of juvenile-onset diabetes still remains to be determined.

REFERENCES

1. *Notkins, A.L. (1977). Arch. Virol. 54, 1.*
2. *Craighead, J.E. (1975). Prog. Med. Virol. 19, 161.*
3. *Boucher, D.W., et al. (1975). J. Infect. Dis. 131, 462.*
4. *Ross, M.E., et al. (1976). Diabetes. 25, 190.*
5. *Onodera, T., et al. (1978). Nature (Lond.) 274, 693.*
6. *Yoon, J.W., and Notkins, A.L. (1976). J. Exp. Med. 143, 1170.*
7. *Chairez, R., et al. (1978). Virology 85, 606.*
8. *Ross, M.E., et al. (1974). J. Infect. Dis. 129, 669.*
9. *Yoon, J.W., et al. (1978). J. Exp. Med. 148, 1068.*
10. *Onedera, T., et al. (1978). Science 201, 529.*

IMMUNOLOGICAL ASPECTS OF DIABETES MELLITUS

*W.J. Irvine

Clinical observation established that ketosis-prone, insulin-dependent diabetes, but not diabetes that can be controlled by diet or oral hypoglycemic agents, is associated with the organ-specific group of autoimmune disorders (1). There is a markedly increased prevalence of thyroid cytoplasmic and of gastric parietal cell cytoplasmic antibodies especially in young female diabetics compared to age and sex-matched controls, even when all patients are excluded who had any clinical features or past history of thyroid disease, atrophic gastritis or anemia. When insulin-dependent diabetics were compared with those who were non-insulin-dependent, it was found that the increased prevalence of these cytoplasmic antibodies (which was highly significant statistically) was solely confined to the insulin-dependent group (2).

CELL-MEDIATED IMMUNITY TO ISLET CELL ANTIGENS

Evidence for cell-mediated immunity to porcine, bovine (3) and to human (4) pancreatic antigen was obtained by the migration inhibition test using leucocytes from the peripheral blood of diabetics, although there is some uncertainty as to how specific this test is for type IV immune reactions (5).

Statistically significant positive findings were again confined to insulin-dependent diabetics. That the pancreatic antigen in question was in the islets was shown by using an antigen of very high islet-cell content derived from calf pancreas in which atrophy of the exocrine tissue had been induced by surgical ligation of the pancreatic duct 8 weeks before the organ was removed (3) and by using appropriate fresh human insulinoma tissue (6).

CYTOPLASMIC ISLET CELL ANTIBODIES (ICAb) IN DIABETICS

It was in the sera of patients with insulin-dependent diabetes plus autoimmune polyendocrine disease that ICAb was first independently described in late 1974 (7, 8), using the indirect immunofluorescence technique and unfixed cryostat sections of fresh group O human pancreas. The antibody or antibodies react with the cytoplasm of all the cells of the pancreatic islets. Rarely, a serum may only react with A cells or D cells, but this does not seem to be characteristic of diabetes in any of its forms (9).

ICAb occurs in about 60-70% of newly diagnoses Caucasian insulin-dependent (ketosis prone) diabetics, irrespective of age. Some diabetics only have ICAb detectable in the serum for a few weeks or less (ICAb transients) while others retain ICAb in the serum for many years (ICAb persisters) (10). The short duration of ICAb in most insulin-dependent diabetics is in contrast to the long duration of other organ-specific antibodies such as gastric parietal cell, thyroid and adrenocortical antibodies that characterize pernicious anemia, primary atrophic hypothyroidism and idiopathic (autoimmune) Addison's disease, respectively (11).

In contrast to insulin-dependent (ketosis prone) diabetes, the prevalance of ICAb in what used to be referred to as 'maturity onset' diabetics (who are insulin-independent and can be controlled by diet or by oral hypoglycemic agents) is very much less. In those controlled by diet alone, the prevalance is very similar to that in a control Caucasian population at about 0.5%. However, a significant minority of diabetics controlled on OHA have ICAb in the serum (10). Such patients have a very high tendency towards becoming insulin-dependent in subsequent years, indicating that they are at an earlier stage of the same disease process that culminates in insulin-dependent ketosis prone (type 1) diabetes (12) (Fig. 1).

ICAb AS A MARKER FOR POTENTIAL TYPE 1 DIABETES

Some 6% of patients with organ specific autoimmune disease, some 3% of first degree relatives (without clinical diabetes) of ICAb-positive diabetics and 0.5% of the normal Caucasian population have ICAb in the serum (10). A substantial number of these subjects go on to develop diabetes, sometimes acutely as ketosis-prone, insulin-dependent diabetics but sometimes only reaching this stage by going more slowly through milder stages of what would appear to be the same disease process that culminates in insulin-dependent diabetes (13). These findings therefore point to the value of ICAb as a marker for type I diabetes, especially in its less severe forms, and suggest that not all diabetics controlled by diet or oral

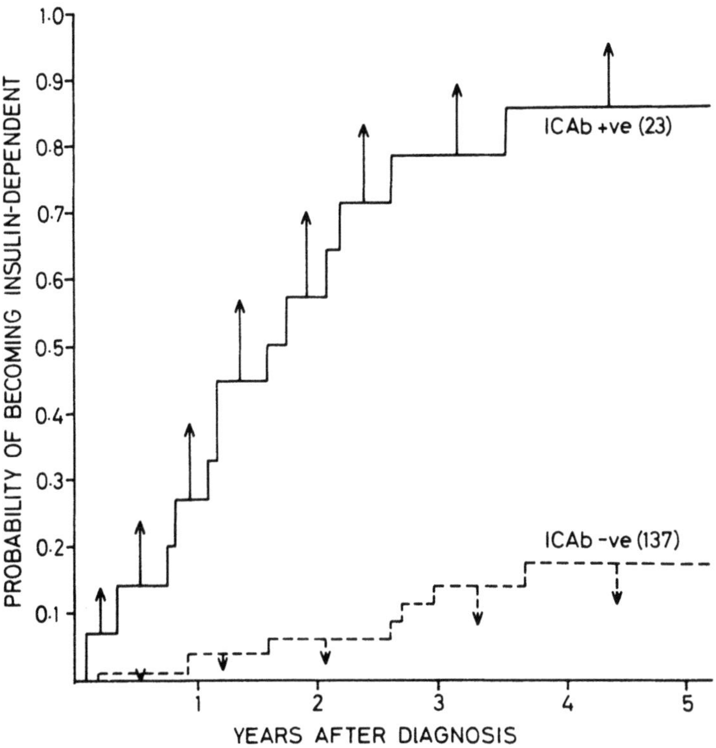

Fig. 1. The value of cytoplasmic islet cell antibody (ICAb) in predicting secondary failure of oral hypoglycemic agent (OHA) therapy in diabetes. From Irvine (12), by permission of the editor of J. Clin. Lab. Immunol.

hypoglycemic agents have the 'maturity onset' type of the disease (type II). At the present time, ICAb is the only in vitro marker for potential type I diabetes.

OTHER AUTOANTIBODIES

Antibodies in the sera of type I diabetics reactive with the cell surface of rat islet cells in culture have been described using the indirect immunofluorescence technique (13). Their relatively poor correlation with type I as opposed to type II diabetes and their higher prevalance in healthy controls (14), together with the fact that rat instead of human islet cells are used as antigen, raises some concern as to what in fact these 'antibodies' are reacting.

Auto-antibodies to insulin receptors have been described in the rare clinical situation of insulin resistance associated with acanthosis nigricans, but they are not characteristic of the common type I or type II diabetes (15).

CLASSIFICATION OF DIABETES

As inferred above, it would now appear to be established that the syndrome referred to as primary diabetes consists of two principal and distinct diseases which may be referred to as type I and type II (16). In addition, there is a multiplicity of rare disease processes that also may produce primary diabetes (17). The separation of primary diabetes into two main distinct types is also supported by the HLA studies described below.

Type I diabetes is characterized by the state of insulin dependency (i.e. proneness to ketosis). Although this condition commonly develops in young people, it is by no means confined to them, so that the term 'juvenile-onset' diabetes is not appropriate. Likewise, type II diabetes, while occurring predominantly in older persons, is not confined to them. As mentioned above, it is important to realize that a significant minority of diabetics controlled by diet or especially by oral hypoglycemic agents belong not to type II but to type I, and that such patients are indicated by the presence of cytoplasmic ICAb in the serum. Therefore, patients on oral hypoglycemic agents should only be called type II diabetics if their serum is negative for cytoplasmic ICAb at the time of diagnosis. Type II diabetics may be obese or non-obese, and may be treated by their physicians with insulin without being insulin-dependent. They are not prone to ketosis.

GENETICS OF DIABETES

The use of the age at discovery of diabetes as a basis for classifying primary diabetes into the two main types ('juvenile onset' and 'maturity onset') led to much confusion in the analysis of its familial and therefore of its genetic aspects (18). However, when the criterion of insulin dependency compared to non-insulin dependency was used and the age at discovery of diabetes ignored in relation to classification, results were obtained that strongly suggest that the two main types of primary diabetes as so defined breed true (19).

The three series of HLA alleles which appear to be in linkage disequilibrium with three immune response (Ir) genes and which are associated with type I diabetes in Caucasians are shown in figure 2. It is probably that the Ir genes are located near to the D locus or to the DR locus (20). The series A1, B8, DW3 and DRW3 and the series A2, CW3, B15, DW4 and DRW4 have a positive and additive risk factor for type I diabetes while the series

A3, B7, DW2 and DRW2 has a protective effect associated with a resistance to type I diabetes (21). Type II diabetes is not associated with any known HLA type.

HLA in TYPE I DIABETES

					RISK FACTOR
Ir 1 ←	DRW3/DW3 ←	B8 ←		A1	POS
Ir 2 ←	DRW4/DW4 ←	B15 ←	CW3 ←	A2	POS
Ir 3 ←	DRW2/DW2 ←	B7 ←		A3	NEG

Fig. 2. The three series of HLA antigens, each probably in linkage disequilibrium with an immune response (Ir) gene associated with type I diabetes; two with a positive and one with a negative risk factor. From Irvine (5), by permission of the editor of Medical Immunology, Teviot Scientific Publications, Edinburgh.

The series which includes B8 is associated with persistence of ICAb and with the occurrence of other clinical autoimmune disorders (22) (Fig. 3). In turn, the persistence of ICAb (even in the absence of other clinical immunological disorders) is associated with an increased prevalance of thyroid and of gastric autoantibodies (Fig. 3), indicating that persistence of ICAb is associated with an increased diathesis towards organ-specific autoimmunity in general (22).

The series which includes B15 is associated with an increased titre of antibodies to cocksackie B viruses (23) and to heterologous conventional insulin given as regular therapy (Figure 4) (24). Allergic reactions (type I and type III) to conventional therapeutic insulin have been reported to be associated with B7 (25).

IMMUNE COMPLEXES

The occurrence of immune complexes in the serum, detected by the solid phase C1q binding assay (C1q-SP), at diagnosis shows a significant correlation with the occurrence of ICAb (26). This suggests that some, if not most, of these complexes consist of islet cell antigen and antibody to it, in the presence of antibody excess. This could be important in the pathogenesis of type I diabetes through the immune mechanism of antibody-dependent cell-mediated cytotoxicity (ADCC). In preliminary studies, there was no significant correlation with viral antibody titres, including those to the cocksackie B group (27).

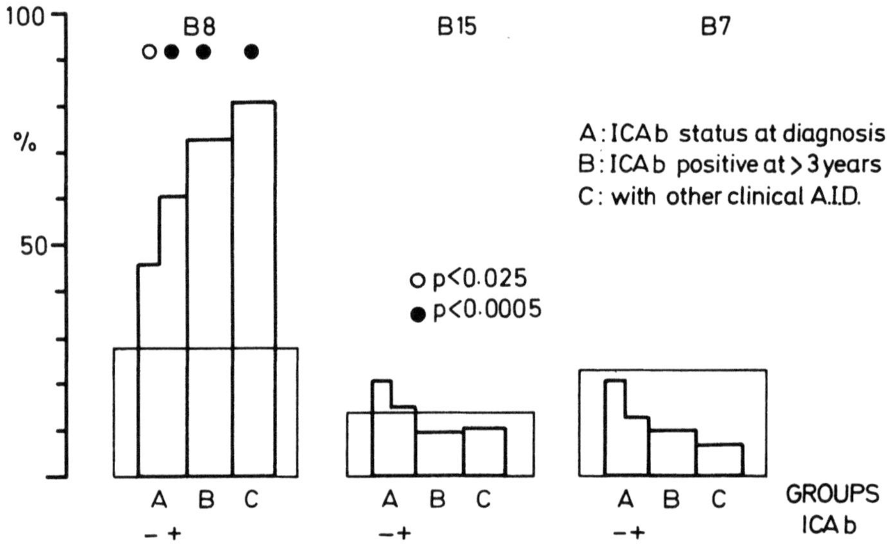

Fig. 3. The positive association of the autoimmune aspects of type I diabetes with HLA-B8 and the lack of it with B15 and with B7. From Irvine et al. (22), by kind permission of the editor of J. Clin. Lab. Immunol.

When type I diabetics have been treated with conventional heterologous insulin for some months, they generally form antibodies to insulin (28). A correlation has been reported between high titres of insulin antibodies in the serum and microvascular disease (28). However, it appears unlikely that the majority of complexes detected in diabetics by Clq-SP or Raji assays are related to insulin (29). This is probably due to the low valency of insulin and consequently its poor lattice formation in the presence of antibody (13). Except when ICAb, immune complexes developing many years after diagnosis are probably not related to islet cell antigens either. There is a correlation between the development of microangiopathy and immune complexes in insulin-dependent diabetes. However, type II diabetics show a similar correlation between the presence of immune complexes and microangiopathy, although the prevalance of both immune complexes and microangiopathy is less than in type I diabetes (13). It is possible that impaired clearing mechanisms which would normally remove such complexes may be responsible for their presence (13). In this way, immune complexes may aggravate the development of vascular complications (26). The efficiency of mechanisms for clearing the circulation of immune complexes may be impaired by poor metabolic control (e.g. hyperglycemia) or by the presence of an excess amount of immune complexes which in itself blocks the clearing mechanisms. Thus, the suspected relationship between poor metabolic control and microvascular disease could be at least partially accounted for in terms of immune complexes.

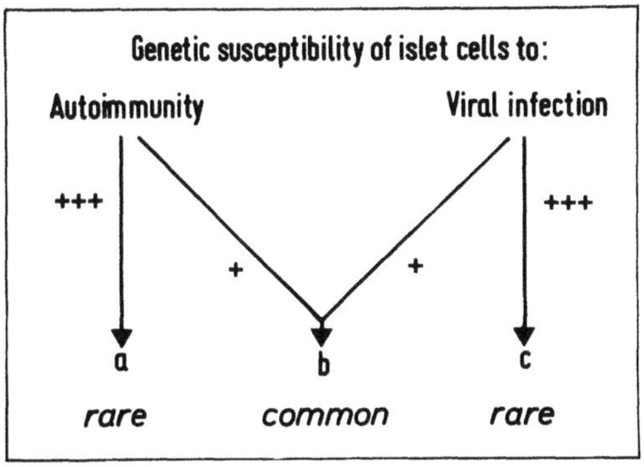

Fig. 4. The concept of an interaction between islet cell autoimmunity and viral infection in the pathogenesis of type I diabetes. Uncommonly one or the other may play the predominant role (i.e. types Ia and types Ic) but in most type I diabetics some genetic susceptibility to both probably exists (type Ib). From Irvine (16), by permission of the editor of The Lancet.

THE POSSIBLE ROLE OF AUTOIMMUNITY IN THE PATHOGENESIS OF TYPE I DIABETES

Cytoplasmic ICAb is unlikely on its own to be a main pathogenic agent (30). Experiments whereby glucose intolerance was induced in nu/nu mice by the transfer of washed leucocytes from the peripheral blood of insulin-dependent diabetics are suggestive that immunological mechanisms that are cell-dependent may be important (31). Exactly what immune mechanisms may be operative will have to await improved islet cell culture techniques so that such mechanisms can be analyzed more precisely in vitro.

In type I diabetes autoimmunity may uncommonly be the only pathogenic mechanism (type Ia) in which case the patient is likely to have polyendocrine autoimmune disease(16) (Fig. 4). In other cases (type Ic), other genetically determined factors, such as susceptibility to viral infection of the islets, may be the main factor without there being any significant autoimmune reaction to the islet cells. However, it is tempting to speculate that more commonly (type Ib) there is both a greater susceptibility to a pancreatotrophic viral infection and to islet cell autoimmunity which augments the damage done by the virus (16). This would fit the observations described above that there are two HLA-related positive risk factors for type I diabetes that are additive in their effects and that only one of these is associated with autoimmunity. It would also fit the transient nature of islet cell antibodies in the majority of type I diabetics. It is to be stressed, however, that type Ia, b and c are stages in the continuing spectrum of interaction between autoimmunity and some other agent such as viral infection.

REFERENCES

1. *Irvine, W.J., (1974). Proc. R. Soc. Med. 67: 548.*
2. *Irvine, W.J., et al., (1978). Lancet i: 163.*
3. *Nerup, J., et al., (1974). Proc. R. Soc. Med. 67: 506.*
4. *MacCuish, A.C., et al., (1974). Diabetes 23: 693.*
5. *Irvine, W.J., (1979). In Irvine Medical Immunology, chap. 1. (Teviot Scientific Publications, Edinburgh).*
6. *Irvine, W.J., et al., (1976). Acta Endocr. Copenh. Suppl. 205, 65.*
7. *Bottazzo, G.F., et al., (1974). Lancet ii: 1279.*
8. *MacCuish, A.C., et al., (1974). Lancet ii: 1529.*
9. *Irvine, W.J., (1976). Proc. 9th Congr. Int. Diabetic Federation, Dehli: 260. (Elsevier, Amsterdam 1977).*
10. *Irvine, W.J., et al., (1977). Diabetes 26:138.*
11. *Irvine, W.J., (1979). In Irvine Medical Immunology, chap. 6. (Teviot Scientific Publications, Edinburgh).*

12. Irvine, W.J., et al., (1979). J. Clin. Lab. Immunol. 2:23.
13. Irvine, W.J., et al., (1979). In: The Immunology of Diabetes (Teviot Scientific Publications, Edinburgh).
14. Irvine, W.J., et al., (1979). J. Clin. Lab. Immunol. II (in press)
15. Flier, J.J., (1975). Science 190: 63
16. Irvine, W.J., et al., (1976). Lancet i:638.
17. Rimoin, D.L. and Schmike, R.N. (1971). Genetic disorders of the endocrin glands. (Mosby, St. Louis).
18. Smith, C., et al., (1972). Ann. Hum. Genet. 35:281.
19. Irvine, W.J. (1977). Lancet ii: 325.
20. Morris, P.J. (1979). In: Medical Immunology. Ed. by Irvine, W.J., Chap. 3.
21. Platz, P., et al., (1977). Tissue Antigens 10: 192.
22. Irvine, W.J., et al., (1978). J. Clin. Lab. Immunol. I: 107.
23. Cudworth, A.G., et al., (1977). Lancet i: 385.
24. Irvine, W.J., et al., (1978). J. Clin. Lab. Immunol. I. (in press)
25. Bertrams, J. and Gruneklee, D. (1977). Tissue Antigens, 10: 273.
26. Irvine, W.J., et al., (1978). J. Clin. Lab. Immunol. I: 183.
27. Irvine, W.J., et al., (1977). Clin. Exper. Immunol. 30: 16.
28. Ortved Anderson, O. (1972). Acta Endocr. Copenh. 71: 126.
29. Irvine, W.J., et al., (1978). J. Clin. Lab. Immunol. 1:187.
30. Gamlen, T.R., et al., (1977). Clin. Exp. Immunol. 28:192.
31. Buschard, K., et al., (1978). Lancet i: 908.

DETECTION AND POSSIBLE FUNCTIONAL INFLUENCE OF ANTIBODIES DIRECTED AGAINST THE PANCREATIC ISLET CELL SURFACE

A. Lernmark*, T. Kanatsuna, A.H. Rubenstein
and D. F. Steiner

Insulin-dependent diabetes mellitus seems to be associated with a specific destruction and loss of B-cells. The endocrine pancreas, which represents a complex parenchyma of endocrine cells, remains, however, and islets composed of cells reactive with antibodies against glucagon, somatostatin or pancreatic polypeptide are present (1). The disappearance of B-cells is concomitant with a deterioration in secretory capacity since at the time of diagnosis patients with insulin-dependent diabetes have very low or undetectable levels of serum C-peptide (2). The pathogenesis of the insulin-dependent diabetes is not known. However, recent attention has been paid to immunopathological phenomena. For example, the endocrine pancreas in newly diagnosed patients is frequently infiltrated by mononuclear cells,(1), and leucocyte migration inhibition tests against islet cell antigens suggest the presence of cell-mediated immunity (3). In support of a possible involvement of autoimmune mechanisms humoral organ-specific, non-species-specific antibodies against islet cells are common at the onset of the disease (4,5).

Using suspensions of cells from rat islets we have found that cell surface antibodies are present in serum from many insulin-dependent diabetics (5) or from rabbits immunized with dispersed islet cells (6). It is unclear whether islet cell surface antibodies are of importance in the pathogenesis of insulin-dependent diabetes. The method for detecting these antibodies with functionally intact B-cells makes it possible to test whether antibodies bound to the cell surface affect the function of the cells. In the present study, rabbit and human sera were tested for the presence of islet cell surface antibodies and their effects on the biosynthesis of insulin were investigated.

MATERIAL AND METHODS

Dispersed Islet Cells

Suspensions of cells were prepared from isolated islets of Sprague-Dawley's rats (6). Briefly, pancreatic islets were isolated from 8 rats by collagenase digestion and separation of the islets from the collagenase digest by gradient centrifugation on Ficoll. The islets, individually chosen by the aid of a stereo-microscope, were kept in a modified Swim's S-77 medium (5). The islets were disrupted into single cells by mechanical shaking in Swim's medium supplemented with ethylene-glycol-bis (oxyethylenenitrilo) tetra acetic acid (EGTA) and 10-20 mg/l DNase (5). The cells were washed by centrifugation in Swim's medium without EGTA and DNase. Each preparation usually resulted in approximately $1.5\text{-}2 \times 10^6$ cells. Trypan blue exclusion test indicated that 90-98% of the cells were viable and column perifusion of islet cells showed a biphasic insulin release in response to high concentrations of glucose.

Detection of Cell Surface Antibodies

Antibodies bound to islet cells were detected either by indirect immunofluorescence (5) or by a ^{125}I-Protein A binding assay (6). In the immunofluorescence assay aliquots of cells in 50-100 μl Swim's medium supplemented with 40 g/l BSA were first incubated at room temperature for 60 min in the presence of heat-inactivated (56°C, 30 min) serum. After washing by centrifugation the cell pellet was resuspended in Swim's medium with 40 g/l BSA and fluoresceine isothiocyanate (FITC) conjugated antibodies. After incubation at room temperature for 30 min, the cells were washed by centrifugation, the cell pellet mounted wet and evaluated in the fluorescence microscope equipped with an epifluorescence condenser.

In the protein A-binding assay (6) dispersed rat islet cells were first incubated in serum as above. After washing by centrifugation, the cells were incubated in tracer amounts of ^{125}I-labelled protein A for 30 min. The cells were washed twice by centrifugation and finally counted in a gamma scintillation counter.

Insulin Biosynthesis

The effects of islet cell surface antibodies on insulin biosynthesis was studied in suspensions of rat islet cells. Dispersed rat islet cells prepared as described above, were incubated in an IgG fraction prepared from rabbit sera by DEAE-Sephadex chromatography or from human sera by ammonium sulfate precipitation. After washing by centrifugation the cells were incubated at 37°C for 60 min in Hank's medium supplemented with a mixture of essential amino acids and 100 μCi/ml ^{3}H-leucine at either 3 mmol/l or 30 mmol/l D-glucose. The cells were washed by centrifugation and extracted in acid-ethanol. Acid-ethanol soluble proinsulin and insulin was separated by chromatography on 1x50 cm columns of Biogel P-30 in 3M-acetic acid.

Anti-islet Cell Antiserum

New Zealand rabbits were immunized with 0.5-1x10^6 dispersed rat islet cells in saline. The rabbits were given a primary injection into the popliteal lymph nodes followed by three intravenous booster injections of 1 ml 0.5-1x10^6 cells in saline at weekly intervals. The antiserum used will be referred to as the R2 anti-islet cell antiserum.

RESULTS

Islet Cell Surface Immunofluorescence

Roughly 50-60% of the total number of cells appeared as single cells in freshly prepared islet cell suspensions. The appearance of rat islet cells stained by indirect immunofluorescence after exposure to the R2 anti-islet cell anti-serum is shown in Figure 1. The cell surface immunofluorescence appears as a ring-shaped fluorescent reaction with a dotted appearance after exposure to lower concentrations of the antiserum. High concentrations (5-50%, v/v) induced an intensive fluorescent reaction without any patchy distribution of the fluorescent antibody. There was no fluorescence on living cells exposed to normal rabbit serum or to the FITC-conjugated swine anti-rabbit IgG alone. However, non-viable or damaged cells non-specifically accumulated the fluorescent antibody whether cells were previously exposed to serum or not (Figure 1).

The fluorescent antibody reaction remained unchanged on islet cells exposed to the R2 anti-islet cell serum extensively adsorbed to suspensions of spleen cells and hepatocytes.

Radioassay of cell-bound IgG

Figure 2 shows the binding of ^{125}I-protein A to rat islet cells previously exposed to various concentrations of the R2 anti-islet cell anti-serum or of normal rabbit serum. There seem to be a detectable difference between the two sera even at the lowest concentration tested (0.1%). In separate experiments the

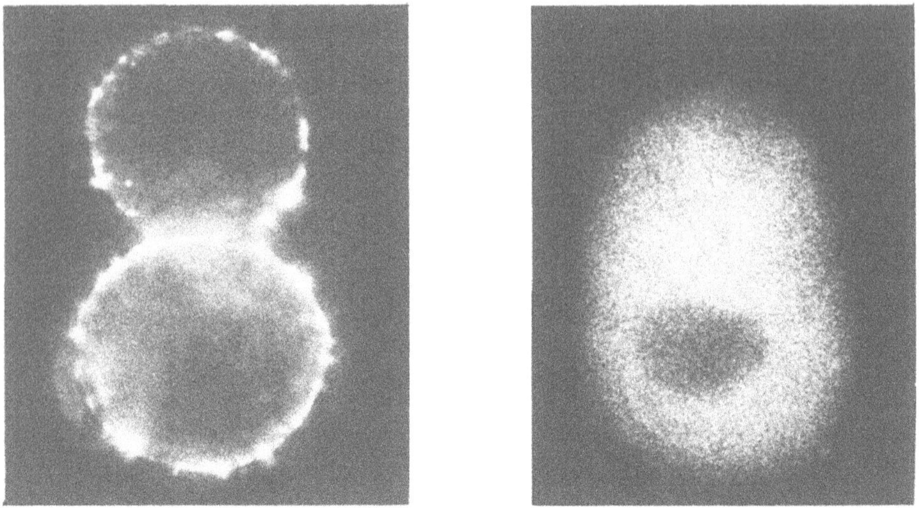

Fig. 1. Cell surface immunofluorescence on rat islet cells exposed to the rabbit anti-rat islet cell antiserum x 3600 (left). Non-specific uptake of fluoresceine-isothiocyanate conjugated swine anti-rabbit IgG in a damaged islet cell (x 4500) (right).

binding of protein A was linear in relation to the number of cells. Moreover, it was found that the Protein A assay could be used in a competition assay (6). The assay is based on incubation of cells with serum followed by washing and an additional incubation at various concentrations of non-radioactive protein A. After washing the cells are finally incubated with the ^{125}I-labelled protein A. It was estimated that after exposing about 10^5 rat islet cells to 5% (v/v) R2 anti-islet cell serum, roughly $3x10^4$ binding sites for protein A were generated.

Effects of Islet-Cell Antibodies On Insulin Biosynthesis

Islet cells in suspension were incubated in the presence of fractionated rabbit or human serum with or without islet cell surface antibodies. By indirect immunofluoresence it was found that the antibodies remained on the cells after washings by centrifugation and a 60 min incubation at 37°C at various glucose concentrations. The ability of islet cells with or without antibodies bound to the cell surface to synthesize proinsulin and insulin is shown in Table 1. When the glucose concentration was increased from 3 to 30 mmol/l there was about a 13-fold increase in the incorporation of ^{3}H-leucine into the combined proinsulin/insulin fractions. In islet cells exposed to anti-islet cell antibodies, the rate of (pro)insulin biosynthesis was decreased.

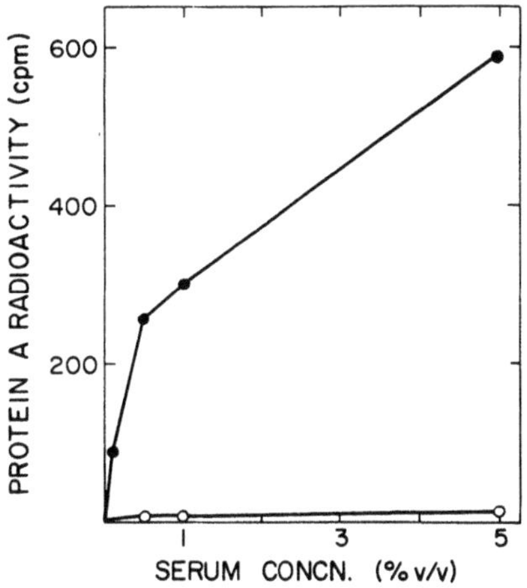

Fig. 2. Protein A radioassay of cell bound IgG. Rat islet cells in suspension were incubated at various concentrations of either normal rabbit serum (O—O) or rabbit anti-rat islet cell antiserum (●—●). The cells were washed by centrifugation before the incubation with ^{125}I-protein A. Radioactive protein A bound to IgG on the cell surface was finally determined after extensive washing of the cells.

There was no difference in the conversion of proinsulin to insulin as analyzed by column-chromatography on Bio-gel P-30.

DISCUSSION

The present study demonstrates that serum from a rabbit immunized with suspensions of rat islet cells, develop a high titer of islet cell surface antibodies. The antibodies are detected by indirect immunofluorescence (5) or in a radioassay using ^{125}I-Protein A (6). It is interesting to note that the antibodies developed after a primary injection of only 0.5-1x10^6 rat islet cells into the popliteal lymphnodes followed by three intravenous booster injections of the same number of cells at weekly intervals. Cell surface antibodies could still be detected after high dilutions of the antiserum indicating that even small numbers of living cells are highly antigenic.

After exposure to the R2 anti-islet cell antiserum all the islet cells developed immunofluorescence, suggesting that the antibodies are not specific for any particular cell type. However, since the rabbits were immunized with rat islet cells, one would expect that antibodies are formed against antigens common to a variety of cell types. Such anti-islet cell antisera in fact contain antibodies reactive with rat spleen cells and hepatocytes (6). However, islet cell reactive antibodies remained after extensive absorption to both spleen cells and hepatocytes (6). Whether the remaining antibody population react exclusively with B-cells or with other endocrine cells as well, cannot be decided until various islet subpopulations have been separated.

The role of islet cell antibodies in the pathogenesis of insulin-dependent diabetes is still unclear. In addition to the high incidence of such antibodies in diabetes of recent onset (4) antibodies are also present in patients treated with sulfonylureas but later requiring insulin for their diabetes (7). Thus, it has been suggested that islet cell antibodies may be regarded as a marker

TABLE 1

EFFECTS OF ISLET CELL ANTIBODIES ON INSULIN BIOSYNTHESIS

Pretreatment of cells	No. of exp.	^{3}H-leucine radioactivity (cpm/10^3 cells) in (Pro)insulin fractions: 3mM D-glucose	30 mM D-glucose	Effect of D-glucose
Control Rabbit serum	5	134± 21	1737± 241	$p < 0.005$
Rabbit anti-rat islet cell anti-serum	5	110± 15	1464± 216	$p < 0.005$
Effect of rat islet cell antiserum		$p > 0.05$	$p < 0.05$	
Healthy controls	8	107± 21	1489± 189	$p < 0.001$
Diabetes islet cell antiserum	9	56± 10	941± 164	$p < 0.001$
Effects of islet cell antiserum		$p < 0.02$	$p < 0.05$	

Mean values ± S.E.

for the development of insulin-dependent diabetes (7). The availability of viable islet cells makes it possible to study directly the effect of cell surface antibodies on the B-cell function. The present studies suggest that anti-islet cell antibodies bound to rat B-cells inhibit the ability of these cells to synthesize proinsulin and insulin.

SUMMARY

Antibodies directed towards determinants on the surface of rat islet cells can be detected qualitatively by the indirect immunofluorescence or quantitatively by a specific radioassay for IgG. Antibodies are found in insulin-dependent diabetics or in rabbits immunized with islet cells. Such antibodies may affect the B-cell function as indicated by the inhibition of incorporation of radioactive leucine into proinsulin/insulin in vitro.

REFERENCES

1. *Gepts, W. and De Mey, J. (1978). Diabetes 27 (suppl. 1), 251*
2. *Rubenstein, A.H., et al·(1977). Rec. Progr. Horm. Res. 33, 435*
3. *Nerup, J., et al.(1971). Diabetes 20, 424*
4. *Irvine, W.J., et al.(1977). Diabetes 26, 138*
5. *Lernmark, A., et al.(1978). New Engl. J. Med. 299, 375*
6. *Lernmark, A., et al.(1979). Irvine, W.J. ed., The Immunology of Diabetes: Proceedings of the Edinburgh International Symposium, Teviot Publications, Edinburg. In press*
7. *Irvine, W.J., et al.(1977) Lancet i, 1025*

Portions of this work were supported by the University of Chicago Diabetes Research and Training Centre (AM-20595), the Swedish Medical Research Council and the Nordic Insulin Foundation.

DISCUSSION

P. RUBINSTEIN: *I have a couple of questions for Dr. Notkins. Was the susceptibility of the different mice strains the same for all the viruses you tested? Secondly, do you have information as to the linkage group of these genetically susceptible mice?*

A. NOTKINS: *We don't have any information on the linkage group. In terms of susceptibility among the various inbred strains of mice, there is really quite a bit of difference. We have some strains that are highly susceptible, others that seem to be completely resistant, and then other strains that seem to be in between with just abnormal glucose tolerance tests and not overt hyperglycemia.*

P. RUBINSTEIN: *But is this the same for all inbred strains?*

A. NOTKINS: *I'm talking now just about EMC virus. We've looked at 24 inbred strains and we find some that are highly susceptible, some that are intermediate, and some that are resistant. In the studies, we selected a highly susceptible and a highly resistant strain.*

P. RUBINSTEIN: *Is the pattern the same for other viruses? Are the same strains susceptible to all the viruses or not?*

A. NOTKINS: *The only other one we looked at is the variant of Coxsackie virus and it appears that many of the strains, which are susceptible to EMC, are also susceptible to Coxsackie. However, there are some exceptions. There are at least a couple of strains now which don't seem to be similar.*

A. S. REDDI: *Dr. Notkins, Dr. Bush from New Orleans has shown that inoculation of mice virus destroys major and minor blood vessels and also produces pericaditis and myocarditis. Did you look into the pathology of blood vessels and other organs besides the endocrine pancreas? In other words, is the destruction of beta cell primarily due to the virus or secondarily to other manifestations?*

A. NOTKINS: *We have looked at some of the other organs, but we've concentrated primarily on the beta cells. There, by the immunofluorescent technique, we can clearly show that the virus in the beta cell is destroying the beta cell.*

M. VRANIC: *Referring to the same question, what about the other islet cell types? Do you have any evidence that the viruses attack only the beta cell? You have shown that, in most of your slides, the virus was on the periphery of the islet where most of the alpha cells are found.*

A. NOTKINS: *I have to take it virus by virus. Let's talk about EMC virus first. In the case of EMC, we've done some collaborative studies with Dr. Orci and, with his morphometric techniques, he observed what's happening to the A and D cells. The alpha cells seem intact. In fact, there seems to be a redistribution of the alpha cells. If you look at the islet a week after infection, you will find that they're filled with alpha cells. Instead of being at the periphery, they've now migrated towards the center of the islet. It's hard to tell whether there is really a reduction in the absolute number of alpha cells, but there is certainly an inversion of the ratio of alpha cells to beta cells, with very little decrease in the glucagon concentration of the pancreas. Now, with reovirus, we haven't looked very carefully. I agree with you that in some of the sections the alpha cells appear attacked. We have not been able to find reovirus type 3, by electronmicroscopy in the alpha cells. However, we can show that reovirus type 1 attacks the alpha cells.*

E. TUTWILER: *Dr. Irvine, in your patients with diabetic retinopathy, have you some thought about the role of immune complexes and platelet aggregation?*

W. J. IRVINE: *No, but I think we can mention we observed increased prevalence of complexes in patients with severe retinopathy.*

R. CAMERINI-DAVALOS: *Dr. Notkins, in humans, can you prevent the action of the virus?*

A. NOTKINS: *Dreaming, but not trying, I think it's a long, long step.*

R. CAMERINI-DAVALOS: *What about infected animals? Can you protect them?*

A. NOTKINS: *I'm sure we can. We could prevent viral-induced diabetes in mice. All you have to do is to take an inactivated virus and immunize the mouse with it; this would prevent the mouse from developing diabetes.*

R. CAMERINI-DAVALOS: *Would any of the three speakers care to comment on the studies in Germany and Denmark about the passive transfer of streptozotocin diabetes and the implication that lymphocytes are involved?*

W. J. IRVINE: *Transferring lymphocytes from type 1 diabetes into mice, who subsequently develop abnormalities of glucose tolerance, is very interesting indeed. There's a great tendency now to think of autoimmunity as caused by humoral antibodies. This could well be antibody-dependent cell-mediated immunity. What has been described in the islet cells is lymphocytic infiltration, not plasma cell infiltration. I believe all of us would think that cell-mediated immunity is likely to be a major factor, if autoimmune mechanisms are important in type 1 diabetes. The leukocyte migration inhibition test is a fairly inaccurate way of determining cell-mediated immunity. The evidence is positive that lymphocytes are sensitized to pancreatic antigen in type 1 diabetics. Therefore, it is possible that lymphocytes, sensitized to islet cells and transferred to a nude mouse who won't reject them, will induce an abnormality of glucose tolerance. Cell-mediated immunity or antibody-dependent cell-mediated immunity is potentially a very exciting experiment.*

M. COHEN: *Dr. Notkins, in stretching the analogy of viral-induced diabetes in mice to the human situation, I think it would be important to know what happens after a longer period of time in some of these infected animals, particularly with respect to the possibility of recovery or regeneration of islet cell function. By the same token, do you have data as to whether this is a cytolytic process and/or a problem in insulin biosynthesis?*

A. NOTKINS: *With regard to the last question, these are highly lytic viruses. Once the virus gets into the cell and starts replicating, it's all over for the cell. The cell doesn't recover. It is destroyed. In fact, if we look very early in the course of the infection, at one to two days, the animals are not hypoinsulinemic. Some of them are hyperinsulinemic due to the fact that the insulin is being released into the circulation. With regard to recovery, the data depends on the particular virus which you're talking about. With EMC virus, we can get 70-80% of the animals to develop hyperglycemia. This number declines over a period of one, two, and three months. Moreover, those animals who return to normal may have abnormal glucose tolerance tests. But the question is why so many recover? I believe at least part of the answer has to do with the initial degree of beta cell damage. If we actually knock out a lot of beta cells, then these animals are more likely to be persistently hyperglycemic.*

J. ANDERSON: *Dr. Irvine, one link of your hypothesis is that diabetes is an autoimmune deficiency or autoimmune disturbance. On the other hand, do you think that the susceptibility to virus infections is also an immune defect of another type?*

W. J. IRVINE: *It could be.*

S. FAJANS: *Dr. Notkins, in your animal model can you detect the virus triggering off any phenomenon that he can interpret as autoimmunity?*

A. NOTKINS: *About two years or more ago, we observed the EMC model after infection and tried to find islet cell auto-antibodies in the circulation of these animals. We weren't able to detect any at that time. Perhaps our techniques were not as good then and this should be done over again. In the patient I discussed, we found some islet antibody in the serum obtained at post. We haven't yet looked at the serum which was obtained on admission.*

A. LERNMARK: *The system we are studying is immensely complex. In autoimmune diseases like myasthenia gravis, everyone thinks an antibody against the acetylcholine receptor causes the disease, and it seems to do so on passive transfer. However, the T lymphocytes are also important. What we are all interested in is the regulation of the cell-mediated system, which is an interaction between macrophages and TMB lymphocytes. Therefore, we would be interested mainly now in the T lymphocytes. The Zink-Analgo-Dort hypothesis says that there is a possible association between the HLA antigens on the cell surface and the recognition of that changed cell surface by T lymphocytes, which would be transferred or differentiated into T killer cells. So, the possibilities are enormous and it will be very important to understand the interaction between beta cells, for example, and lymphocytes of different kinds. I would also like to add that the antibodies we are studying -- for example, cytoplasmic dependent diabetics -- show heterogenity. Consequently, one-third of the patients would have only cytoplasmic antibodies, one-third cell surface antibodies, and one-third both types of anti-bodies. This is from a collaborative study between Dr. Irvine and our laboratory in Chicago.*

P. L. POFFENBARGER: *With respect to the hypothesis that the islet cell surface antibody affects islet cell function, Dr. Lernmark, in your rabbits with the highest islet cell surface antibody, do they indeed have an insulin secretory abnormality?*

A. LERNMARK: *We don't know that. We have not studied the rabbits in detail yet.*

P. L. POFFENBARGER: *Dr. Notkins, with respect to the number of viral receptors on susceptible islet versus non-susceptible islet, you did find EMC or Coxsackie 4B viral receptors on beta cells isolated from non-susceptible mice strains? Is that correct?*

A. NOTKINS: *We did these studies by culturing beta cells from our susceptible SWR strains, both strains that developed diabetes and strains that did not. Then, we measured the binding of infectious virus to these cells and we found two to three times more virus binds to the SWR cell. Those strains are animals who develop diabetes as compared to the C57 Black, which did not.*

P. L. POFFENBARGER: *In that case, would you hypothesize that the infectivity or virulence of the virus is dose-dependent, or would you hypothesize that the fact that the non-susceptible strain has some other additional mechanism involved, such as viral processing or immune response?*

A. NOTKINS: *These experiments are very difficult to do because our beta cell cultures are not pure.*

W. J. IRVINE: *Dr. Lernmark, in relation to your studies on beta cell function and antibody to the cell surface antigen, is the antibody in fact cytotoxic to these cells, or what is the role of complement in that reaction?*

A. LERNMARK: *In those experiments, we were very careful not to have any serum present, because we have found that the serum itself, whether obtained from a healthy or a diabetic individual, will deactivate the process by the alternative complement pathway. Now, with regard to the question whether there is a complement-mediated cytotoxicity of these islet cell antibodies, we have preliminary results, both with the rabbit anti-rat islet cell antiserum and human serum, indicating that cells exposed to the IGG alone, and then to complement source from guinea pigs, will release chromium 51 from these cells. Therefore, you would say these antibodies are cytotoxic in the complement-dependent way.*

HETEROGENEITY OF INSULIN RESPONSES IN MATURITY-ONSET TYPE DIABETES (MOD) AND IN MATURITY-ONSET TYPE DIABETES OF YOUNG PEOPLE (MODY)

S. S. Fajans*

Previously we presented evidence for heterogeneity among maturity-onset diabetes of the young (MODY) pedigrees, particularly in regard to occurence of vascular disease. It is the purpose of this presentation to present evidence for heterogeneity of insulin responses to orally administered glucose in patients with MODY and maturity-onset diabetes (MOD) diabetes. (1,2,3) Our initial studies suggested that MODY or MOD diabetes is characterized by subnormal insulin responses to glucose as compared to healthy control subjects (4) while other investigators have reported increased insulin responses in latent or chemical diabetic patients. (1) When data for 25 MODY patients, age 9 to 17 years at diagnosis, were compared with results of 125 control subjects, mean concentration of plasma glucose for the two groups showed significant differences from fasting through three hours. (3) The diabetics showed a significantly delayed and subnormal insulin response to glucose. A comparison of mean plasma levels of glucose and insulin during glucose tolerance tests of 125 control subjects aged 18 to 25 years and for MODY patients aged 18 to 25 years at diagnosis showed that concentration of plasma glucose were again significantly different from fasting through three hours for the two groups. For all 30 non-obese MODY patients for whom insulin levels are available, the mean level of plasma insulin was significantly lower at 1/2 hour after ingestion of glucose. However, when the sum of all six increments during the glucose tolerance test are considered, six of the 30 patients had responses which were greater than the mean + 1 standard deviation of the sum of increments of the control subjects (3). In the other 24 patients, mean levels of plasma insulin were subnormal and similar to those of the younger patients shown before.

In analyzing insulin responses to an oral glucose load of the 125 control subjects and of a group of 68 nonobese mildly diabetic

MODY and MOD patients, with men ages of 22 and 23 years respectively, it became apparent that both groups displayed a wide spectrum of insulin responses. Twenty-one patients had increments in plasma insulin in response to ingested glucose which were less than 1 SD below the mean of the normal control subjects. (3) They are designated as patients with "low insulin responses". On the other hand, 13 patients had sum of increments in plasma insulin in response to glucose which exceeded those of the control subjects by more than 1 SD and in 12 of the 13, by more than 2 SDs. They were designated as "high insulin responders". The glucose tolerance tests on which the initial insulin determinations were made for the two groups showed significant differences only at 2½ and 3 hours of the test(3). Evidence that we are dealing with heterogeneity of insulin responses and not with the extremes of a spectrum of insulin responses comes first of all from the finding of a familial aggregation of the type of insulin responses. Most diabetic members of typical MODY families have low insulin responses or responses below the mean of the control subjects. In these families, young members with normal or non-diagnostic glucose tolerance tests have had low insulin response to glucose. Two MODY families have members with high insulin responses. Most of the MODY or MOD patients with high insulin responses have had a family history of diabetes, but not a three-generation family history. An example would be a nonobese father and son with glucose intolerance and high insulin responses. In no family did low and high insulin responses appear together.

The strongest evidence of heterogeneity of insulin responses is apparent from an examination of follow-up data of patients in these two groups. Progression to insulin-requiring diabetes, defined as fasting hyperglycemia unresponsive to diet and/or sulfonylurea therapy, after intervals of up to 15 years, occurred only in individuals who had insulin responses which were delayed and low, or lower than the mean response of the control subjects. Greatly decreased insulin responses appear to be the determinant, at least in part, of abnormal carbohydrate tolerance and of progression of carbohydrate intolerance to insulin-requiring diabetes. The MODY patients who have progressed to insulin-requiring diabetes had increments at 30 minutes which were all below the mean −1 SD of the control subjects. The sum of increments were all below the mean of the control subjects.

To date, none of the nonobese patients with MODY or MOD whose insulin responses were supernormal or above the mean of those of the control subjects have progressed to insulin-requiring diabetes, with a follow-up of up to 20 years for glucose and up to 13½ years for insulin levels. On follow-up with therapy, when carbohydrate intolerance improved in these patients, the insulin responses decreased toward or to normal. This suggests that in these latter patients, hyperinsulinemia is secondary or compensatory to factors that cause glucose intolerance. We may be dealing with an insensitivity to endogenous insulin, the hyperinsulinemia being secondary to insulin resistance. One possibility is the release of insulin with impaired biological activity. Another possible mechanism is a decreased number of insulin receptor sites as reported by Olefsky and Reaven in chemical diabetics with high insulin responses (5). Other possible mechanisms, such as defects at post-receptor sites, must be considered as well (3).

The data of other investigators indicate also that among young nonobese diabetic patients, only those patients with low insulin responses progress to insulin-requiring diabetes.(2) None of the nonobese patients with elevated insulin responses have been reported to progress to insulin-requiring diabetes. These findings would support our interpretation, that, in young nonobese subjects, the pattern of insulin responses associated with carbohydrate intolerance has prognostic implications and supports the conclusion that there is a heterogeneity of insulin responses to glucose that may delineate differing syndromes and different mechanisms in the pathogenesis of carbohydrate intolerance in MODY and MOD.

Not all patients with low insulin responses to glucose progress to insulin-requiring diabetes, within a period of 20 years. Two examples will be given. A diagnosis of asymptomatic diabetes was made in an 11-year old boy on the basis of a glucose tolerance test in 1958. He is a member of the large R.W. MODY pedigree, belonging to the third generation of diabetes in which seven of 11 siblings have MODY diabetes (see Chapter on "Familial Patterns of Inheritance of Diabetes Mellitus" and reference 3). He has been treated with diet and sulfonylureas. Since 1965, he has had intermittent fasting hyperglycemia, particularly when chlorpropamide had been discontinued for two weeks,with the highest recorded fasting blood sugar being 264 mg% in 1973. In 1978, he had an elevated fasting blood sugar level while on chlorpropamide but off diet, but normal fasting and postprandial blood sugar levels when on diet as well as chlorpropamide. He has had persistently low insulin responses to glucose. (3) He has had progression of the severity of glucose intolerance which is paralleled by his inability to raise plasma insulin after ingestion of glucose. Nevertheless, the patient can maintain normal fasting and postprandial blood glucose levels on diet and sulfonylurea therapy. It would appear that the very small amounts of insulin which the patient's islets can still release are sufficient for sulfonylureas to produce their extrapancreatic effect. One possibility is that they cause an increase in hepatic insulin receptors, thus causing increased sensitivity to insulin.

On the other hand, obese patients with a delayed but considerable insulin response to glucose may progress to insulin-requiring diabetes with time (3). A.P.S. is a member of the PO. pedigree. She is an example of maturity-onset type diabetes in childhood. When this patient was ten years old, a routine glucose tolerance test was abnormal; it returned to normal with modest weight reduction. Since 1969, from age 15 years on, glucose tolerance has been abnormal. At age 18, she delivered an 11 lb. 8 oz. child, a hallmark of a diabetic mother. The patient has remained obese all of her life. She first developed fasting hyperglycemia at age 28, 18 years after initial diagnosis. In 1976, she was first symptomatic with nocturia and pruritis vulvae. Weight reduction plus chlorpropamide normalized her fasting blood sugar. When she gained weight again, insulin became necessary to correct fasting hyperglycemia 23 years after initial diagnosis.

In 1969 and 1970, she had delayed insulin responses of considerable magnitude during the glucose tolerance test(3). The insulin responses to glucose decreased by 1972, and in particular, by 1977, when insulin became necessary to control fasting hyperglycemia and symptoms. This is an example of the very gradual decrease in insulin reserve in a MODY or MOD diabetic in whom caloric excess and obesity appear to be important aggravating factors in the decreasing insulin reserves after many years of carbohydrate intolerance and the associated onset of progressive fasting hyperglycemia.

Reaven and Olefsky have confirmed the considerable variation of insulin responses to oral glucose among older control subjects and older patients with chemical diabetes, and have supplied further support for the proposal of true heterogeneity of insulin responses in MODY patients(6). These authors found a highly significant inverse correlation between the height of insulin responses and the severity of insulin resistance as determined by their infusion technique. The majority of their patients had supernormal insulin response. The difference in proportion of low and high insulin responders in our series and those reported by Reaven and Olefsky appear to be due more to selection of patients than their age. A large proportion of our patients were members of typical MODY families who are characterized by low insulin responses. The patients studied by Reaven and Olefsky are nonfamilial sporadic clinic patients, some of whom had hypertriglyceridemia,as related by Dr. Reaven by personal communication. Carbohydrate intolerance associated with hypertriglyceridemia is probably a different clinical entity than MODY diabetes. The differences in insulin responses among MODY or MOD patients are probably due to differences in genetic background and differences in superimposed environmental factors.

REFERENCES

1. *Fajans, S.S., et al., (1974). Trans. Assoc. Amer. Phys. 87, 83.*
2. *Fajans, S.S., et al., (1976). Arch. Int. Med. 136, 194.*
3. *Fajans. S.S., et al., (1978). Diabetes 27, 1112.*
4. *Fajans, S.S., et al., (1969). Trans. Assoc. Amer. Phys. 82, 211.*

5. *Olefsky, J.M., and Reaven, G., (1976). J. Clin. Endoc. Metab. 43, 226.*
6. *Reaven, G.M., and Olefsky, J.M., (1977). Diabetologia 13, 201.*

Supported in part by U.S. Public Health Service Grants AM-0888 and AM-02244; NIH-5 M01 RR-42 General Clinical Research Centers; and by Grants from The Upjohn Company, Kalamazoo, Michigan and Pfizer, Inc., New York, New York.

PROGRESSION OF EARLY DIABETES

W. Oppermann, C. A. Velasco, A.S. Reddi,
B. Hanover and R.A. Camerini-Davalos *

The hereditary nature of diabetes has been amply established. Even though the nature of the genetic change is unknown, diabetes is a molecular disease; that is, a disease in which important cellular components are seriously impaired. Eventually, the activities or the products arising from the impairment find expression in various ways, finally culminating in the abnormalities of diabets. Insulin deficiency, one of the landmarks of overt, symptomatic diabetes, was investigated by us in patients at different stages of the disease, in an attempt to elucidate the pathophysiology of the progression of the disease.

MATERIAL AND METHODS

Blood sugar and serum insulin were determined at least twice a year, in a 12 year follow-up of 144 non-treated Caucasian early diabetic patients, 20 to 45 years of age, as part of a long-term ongoing study, and their results compared with 56 age-matched controls.

Blood sugar and serum insulin were determined during the 3 hours oral glucose tolerance test (OGTT). The test was performed in the AM after 3 days on at least a 300 gm carbohydrate diet, by oral administration of 100 gm of glucose in a cold cola-flavored preparation (Koladex) after an overnight 14 hour fast. Three milliliters of blood were drawn for blood glucose determination via an indwelling catheter (Longdwel, N° 18) in the antecubital vein at 0 time, and after glucose load at 30, 60, 120 and 180 minutes. Blood glucose was determined in whole blood in the Autoanalyzer by Hoffman's ferricyanide method (n-2A). Serum immunoreactive insulin levels were determined fasting and following the glucose load, using immunosorbents as solid phase, according to our modifcation of the Axen and Porath method (1). Insulin area (insulin under the curve) was determined according to the formula:

$$\text{Area} = \frac{t_o + 2\ (t_{30} + t_{60} + t_{90} + t_{180}) + 3\ t_{120}}{4}$$

where t_j = insulin in uU/ml at j minutes, and t_o = fasting insulin level.

Early diabetics and control subjects, selected to be included in the analysis were during the entire follow-up period within 15% of the ideal body weight, according to the table of "Average Weights of Adults" from the Society of Actuaries (Build and Blood Pressure Study, Volume 1, Chicago 1959). Sixty-two were prediabetics (normal oral glucose tolerance test) when they entered the study; 82 were chemical diabetics (normal fasting but abnormal tolerance to glucose). Of the 62 prediabetics, 38 were offspring of proven maturity-onset diabetic parents, mother and father (genetic prediabetics); the rest had father or mother (and sometimes other family members) diabetics. Of the 82 chemical diabetics, 49 had both parents diabetics (genetic chemical diabetics); the rest only 1 parent.

RESULTS

Mean blood sugars and serum insulin levels during the OGTT were not significantly different in prediabetics and controls, but higher in chemical diabetics. The significance of the difference was $p < .001$ at each time of the curve for glucose and $p < .02$ and $< .01$ for insulin at 120 and 180 minutes. In chemical diabetics patients with both parents diabetic, a clear relationship was found between fasting blood glucose and 30' increment above fasting. No such relationship was found in the other groups.

Percent increases at 30' over fasting blood glucose levels were analyzed during the first OGTT test in all patients and according to their response, divided into average, low or high glucose responders. A significant difference was found between the means of the 3 groups ($p < .01$ to $< .001$). Mean 30' glucose increase over fasting, over 30' insulin increase ($\Delta BS/\Delta I$) was very similar in pre-and chemical diabetic patients: average (10 and 11), low (31 and 25) or high glucose responders (6 and 7).

During the follow-up period, 30 prediabetics (48%) developed chemical diabetes and 8 (27%) overt diabetes (abnormal fasting). Dividing the prediabetics according to their 30' blood sugar response to glucose (Tab. 1), 60% of those progressing to chemical

TABLE 1 Prediabetics Patients Divided According to Their 30' Blood Sugar Response to Oral Glucose. Average: Average Responders. Low: Low Responders. High: High Responders. A: Genetic Prediabetics (Both parents diabetics). <A: Only 1 parent diabetic. >29 Yr: Patients 29 years of age or older. #: Number of Patients. Prediabetes→Chemical Diabetes→Overt Diabetes: Patients Progressing to the next stage. 10/20: ten chemical diabetics of the Twenty Prediabetics.

RESPONSE TO GLUCOSE	PRE-DIABETES→	CHEMICAL DIABETES→	OVERT DIABETES
AVERAGE	<A 20	10/20	0/10
#26	<A 6	0/6	0
LOW	A 8	5/8	2/5
#11	<A 3	0/3	0
HIGH	A 10	6/10	2/6
#25	<A 15	9/15	4/9
62		30	8
AVERAGE		38%	
LOW		45%	
HIGH	>29 YR.	60% (72%)	40% (83%)

diabetes were high glucose responders. Subdividing the prediabetics according to age, a higher percentage of those progressing were 29 years of age or older. Of the 82 patients who entered the study at the stage of chemical diabetes, 21 (26%) developed overt diabetes, divided almost equally between average and high glucose responders, most of them were 29 years or older (Table 2).

In the follow-up of patients with progression of their disease, it was found that the mean insulin area at the time of last normal OGTT of 20 prediabetics with both parents diabetics (genetic prediabetics) was not significantly different from the one of the 56 controls. The mean insulin area of the same 20 subjects was significantly higher ($p < .001$) during the first abnormal OGTT (genetic

TABLE 2 Chemical Diabetics Who Progressed to Overt Diabetes, Divided According to Their 30' Response to Oral Glucose

RESPONSE TO GLUCOSE	CHEMICAL DIABETES ⟶	OVERT DIABETES
AVERAGE	A 16	4/16
#24	< A 8	2/8
LOW	A 2	-
#2		
HIGH	A 31	6/31
#56	< A 25	9/25

AVERAGE		25%
	> 29 YR.	(83%)
HIGH		27%
	> 29 YR.	(93%)

chemical diabetics). Seven developed abnormal fasting blood glucose (overt diabetes), and the mean insulin area as expected was lower at that time (Figure 1).

Mean insulin area of 20 patients who entered the study with already abnormal OGTT, was higher than the controls ($p < .01$) and higher than the same patients at the time they developed overt diabetes ($p < .001$) (Figure 2). Mean insulin area of the forty chemical diabetics (those who entered the study as prediabetics and those who entered as chemical diabetics) was higher than controls ($p < .001$) and overt diabetics ($p < .001$) (Figure 3).

Immunoreactive insulin increments (from 0 time) at 30' were lower in prediabetics than controls ($p < .02$). Increments of chemical diabetics were higher than prediabetics ($p < .05$) and overt

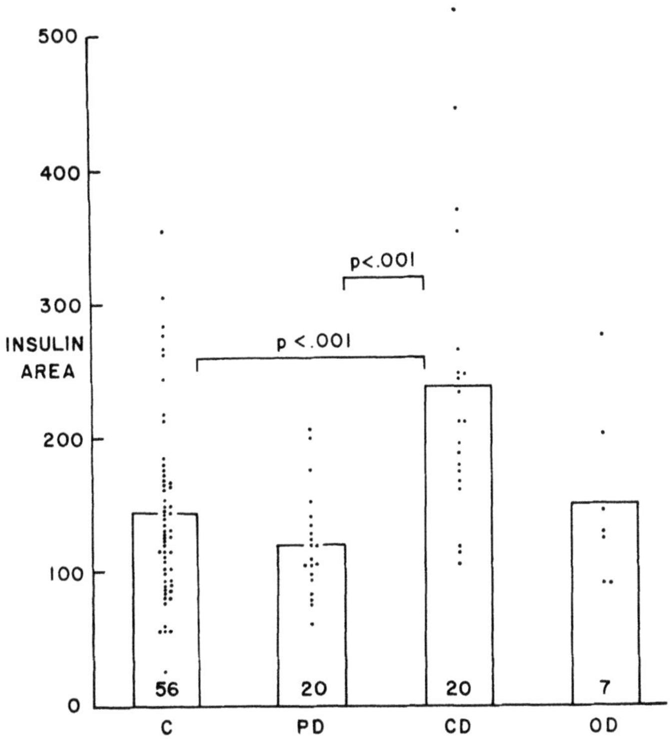

Fig. 1. Insulin area (insulin under the curve during the OGTT). C: controls. PD: genetic prediabetics. CD: chemical diabetics. OD: overt diabetics. 56: number of patients.

diabetics (p <.01) (Figure 4). No difference in the sum of increments was found between controls and prediabetics. Chemical diabetics had sum of increments higher than prediabetics (p <.005) and overt diabetics (p <.001) (Figure 4). As expected, overt diabetics had lower sum of increments.

DISCUSSION

Progression from pre-to chemical diabetes was more frequent in those 29 years or older and with high 30' blood glucose response to oral glucose (60%), probably related to the decrease in the insulin increment at 30' found in prediabetics, even though the sum of increments and the mean insulin levels and area were not different than the controls.

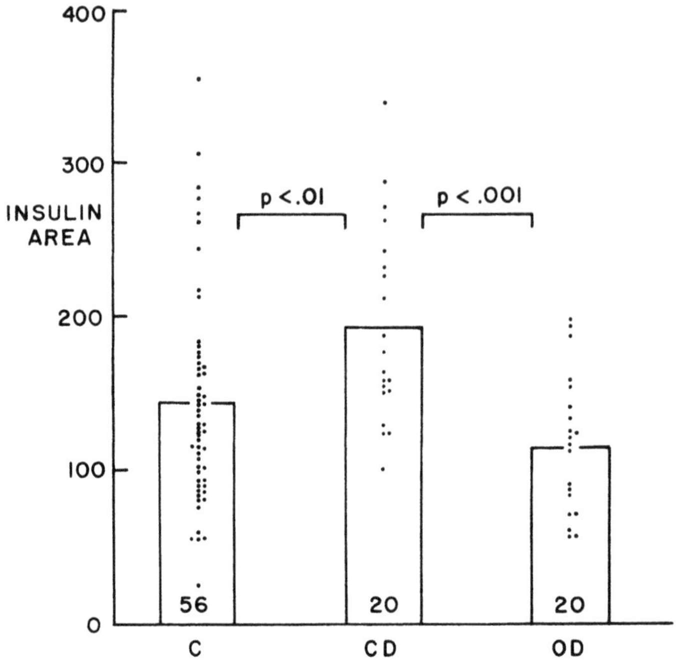

Fig. 2. Insulin area (insulin under the curve during the OGTT). C: controls. CD: chemical diabetics. OD: overt diabetics.

Since we and other investigators demonstrated that, in Caucasian prediabetics, insulin release with almost normal kinetics can be obtained by intravenous administration of tolbutamide (2), glucagon (3), isoproterenol (2), or even by glucose after pretreatment with theophylline (4), the most appealing explanation for this lower insulin increment at 30' would be the one suggested by Luft and Efendic (5) that, in prediabetes, there is a decreased sensitivity of the B cell for the recognition of glucose.

High total insulin area in chemical diabetics, and high increments (at 30' and total sum) suggest a decrease in the efficiency of insulin in the face of hyperglycemia. In fact, looking at the scatogram of Figures 1 and 3, many chemical diabetic patients have insulin area within the range of the controls and prediabetics. We use the term "efficiency" since they seem to have enough circulating insulin (not less than the controls) but still abnormal blood sugars.

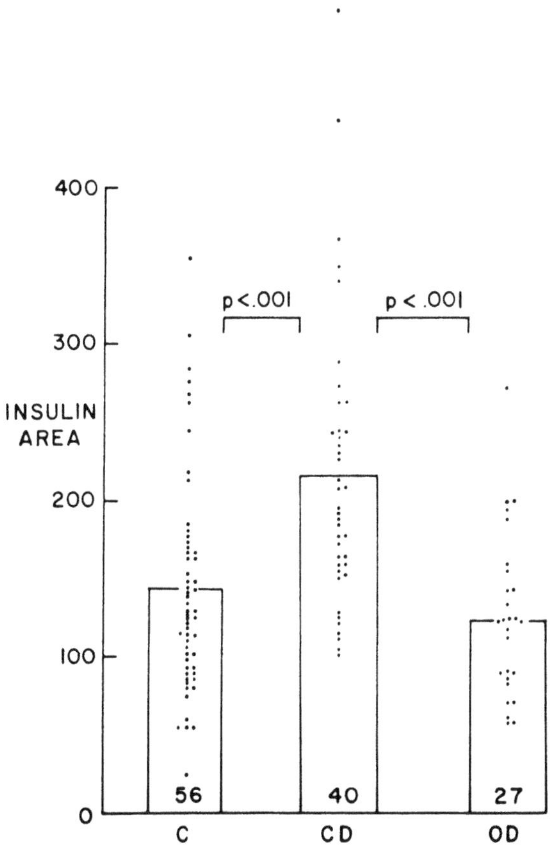

Fig. 3. Insulin area (insulin under the curve during the OGTT). C: controls. CD: chemical diabetics. OD: overt diabetics.

Fajans, et al. (6) had earlier indicated that patients with chemical diabetes could have widely different insulin responses to oral glucose, and emphasized the heterogeneity of this population. But, why do so many have so much insulin? Why, in the progression of diabetes, is decreased availability of insulin at 30' (prediabetes) followed by a period of "overproduction" (chemical diabetes) before the final stage of B cell exhaustion? What pathogenetic mechanism is involved at this stage? If we accept the mechanism suggested by Luft and Efendic (5) for prediabetics, of a decreased sensitivity of the B cell for the recognition of glucose, is that recognition (signal) restored to normal, compensated, or even overcompensated at the stage of chemical diabetes? Why? Our patients were not treated by us, nor did they gain weight.

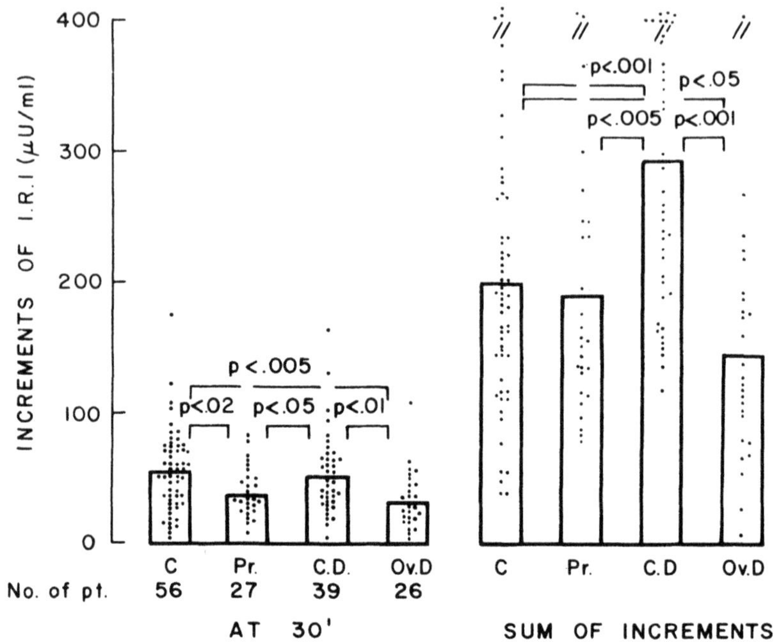

Fig. 4. Immunoreactive insulin in uU/ml increments above fasting. At 30' Sum of increements: increments above fasting during the OGTT. C: controls. PD: prediabetics. CD: chemical diabetics. OD: overt diabetics.

Even though not entirely logical, we can postulate a different mechanism acting at the stage of chemical diabetes. Despite its complexities, we can accept that the biological effect of insulin is a function of the concentration of the hormone-receptor complex. The concentration of this complex depends on several factors, the most important being the concentrations of the hormone and receptor and the affinity of their interrelation. Flier et al. (7) recently listed some factors known at present to affect the concentration and affinity of hormone receptors according to their effect on: a) receptor concentration (genetics, cycle AMP levels, cell differentation, etc.); b) receptor affinity (ionic environment);and c) concentration and affinity (hormone which affects its own receptors, hormone which affects receptor for another hormone, etc.).

Reaven (8) had clearly shown that his chemical diabetic patients had also a decrease in the efficiency of insulin, or, as he prefers to call it, "insulin resistant". Is this less efficient insulin related to changes in the insulin-receptor complex? If this pathogenetic mechanism proves to be correct, which of the factors listed by Flier et al. (7) are responsible? Is this mechanism already acting in Caucasian prediabetics? What interaction do other hormones have on these changes?

REFERENCES

1. *Velasco, C.A. et al. (1973). Clin. Chem. 19, 201.*
2. *Deckert, T., et al. (1972). Dan. Med. Bull, 19, 222.*
3. *Mehtalia, S.D. and Camerini-Davalos, R.A. (1969). Clin. Res. 17, 590.*
4. *Cerasi, E. and Luft, R. (1969). Horm. Met. Res. 1, 162.*
5. *Luft, R. and Efendic, S. (1978). Acta. Diab..Lat. XV, 1.*
6. *Fajans, S.S., et al. (1975). Trans. Assoc. Amer. Phys. 87, 83.*
7. *Flier, J.S., et al. (1979). New England J. Med. 300, 413.*
8. *Reaven, G.M. (1979) in Treatment of Early Diabetes, eds. R. Camerini-Davalos and B. Hanover, Plenum Press, New York, 1979, p. 187.*

INSULIN RESISTANCE AND INSULIN SECRETION IN PATIENTS WITH CHEMICAL DIABETES: IMPLICATIONS CONCERNING THE PATHOGENESIS OF IDIOPATHIC DIABETES MELLITUS

G. M. Reaven*

It has been apparent since the introduction of the radioimmunoassay for insulin that patients with idiopathic diabetes mellitus can be hyperglycemic in the face of normal to elevated levels of plasma insulin (1). On the other hand, there are patients with diabetes mellitus who demonstrate absolute insulin deficiency (1). This issue has been considered in detail (2), and certain generalizations have emerged. Significant numbers of diabetic patients with the mildest form of diabetes (chemical diabetes) are hyperglycemic in spite of circulating insulin levels which are equal to or greater than those seen in normal subjects. As the magnitude of hyperglycemia increases, the insulin response begins to fall off. Lowest plasma insulin concentrations are seen in patients with the most severe degrees of hyperglycemia, and there is agreement that ketosis-prone diabetics are hyperglycemic as the result of absolute insulin deficiency. This relationship between plasma glucose and insulin responses to an oral glucose challenge was explicitly described more than 10 years ago in a Caucasian population (3), and more recently been observed in Pima Indians in the United States (4), and in a Micronesian population in the Central Pacific (5). The apparent universality of this correlation between plasma glucose and insulin responses is noteworthy, and focuses attention on two important issues. In the first place, if patients with minimal glucose intolerance have normal to elevated plasma insulin levels, the possibility arises that hyperglycemia in these subjects is due to loss of normal insulin sensitivity. Secondly, given the described relationship between magnitude of hyperglycemia and insulin response, one unifying view is that the basic defect in diabetes is resistance to the action of insulin, with progression to severe hyperglycemia and insulin deficiency as the pancreas decompensates in an attempt to maintain glucose homeostasis. Evidence from our laboratory which is relevant to both of these issues will be summarized in this presentation.

METHODS

These data have been derived from investigation of 195 non-obese individuals who volunteered to take part in our announced studies of the etiology of diabetes and were admitted to the Stanford Clinical Research Center. None of the subjects were receiving insulin or oral hypoglycemic agents, nor were they taking any medications known to modify carbohydrate metabolism. Relative weights varied between 0.85 and 1.15, and subjects consumed a liquid weight-maintenance formula diet. An oral glucose tolerance test (OGTT) was performed three days after admission using a glucose load of 40 g/m^2 body surface area. Blood samples were drawn before and during the following three hours for measurement of plasma glucose and insulin levels.

Two days later, after a 14 hour overnight fast, all subjects received an intravenous injection of 5 mg of propranolol, followed in five min by a constant intravenous infusion of glucose (6 mg/kg/min), insulin (80 mU/min), epinephrine (6 μg/min) and propranolol (0.08 mg/min). The solution was infused continuously for 150 min into an antecubital vein. Blood samples were drawn from the opposite arm every 5 min from 120 to 150 min. Under these conditions, endogenous insulin secretion is suppressed and steady state plasma glucose (SSPG) and insulin (SSPI) levels are reached by 90 min (6). Since similar SSPI values are achieved in all subjects, this technique allows comparison of the ability of different subjects to dispose of identical glucose loads under the same insulin stimulus. Therefore, the SSPG values are a measure of efficiency of insulin-mediated glucose utilization, i.e., insulin resistance.

Blood for determination of plasma glucose and insulin was drawn into test tubes containing EDTA, the plasma quickly separated, and aliquots stored at -20° C until subsequent analysis for insulin (7) and glucose (8).

Subjects were categorized by their degree of glucose intolerance (Table 1). Individuals were compared on the basis of plasma glucose and insulin levels during the OGTT, total area under the plasma glucose and insulin responses during the OGTT, and SSPG responses during the continuous infusion studies.

RESULTS

I. Evidence that Insulin Resistance Exists in Patients with Chemical Diabetes

Nonobese subjects with fasting euglycemia were classified as being normal or as having chemical diabetes on the basis of results of the OGTT (Table 1a). Twenty-five subjects were recruited to each group, and their mean plasma glucose responses are seen in Figure 1. Mean plasma insulin responses of the two groups are also seen in Figure 1, and indicate that patients with chemical diabetes had insulin levels which were as high, or higher, than those of normal subjects. Similar results have been described by several research groups (2).

Table 1. DIAGNOSTIC CRITERIA

Study	Group	Plasma glucose concentration (mg/100 ml)		
		Fasting	1 hour	2 hour
a	Normal	<110	<165	<135
	Chemical diabetes	<110	>185	>145
b	Normal	<110	<185	<145
	Chemical diabetes	<110	>185	>145
	Fasting hyper-glycemia	>110	-	-

Individual insulin responses for each subject were obtained by calculating the area under the plasma insulin response curve during the OGTT, and these results are seen in Figure 2. These data indicate that the mean insulin response of patients with chemical diabetes is greater than that of normal subjects. However, it is clear that a good deal of heterogeneity exists, and this has also been noted by Fajans et al (9). Qualitatively similar data were obtained when other methods of estimating insulin response were used, i.e., different time-points, incremental increases, etc.

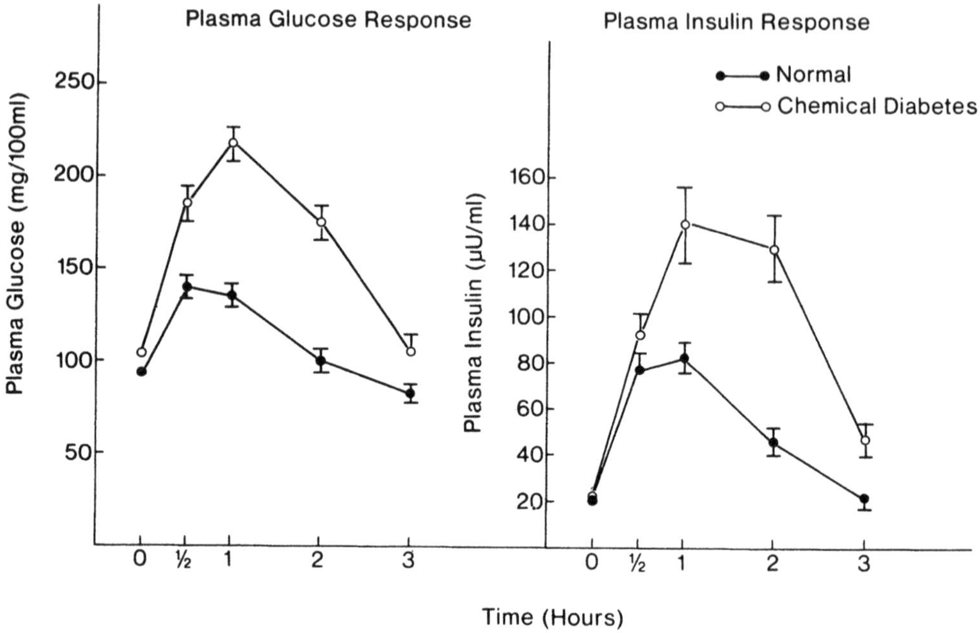

Fig. 1. Mean ± SEM plasma glucose and insulin responses during the OGTT in two groups of subjects. (25 in each group).

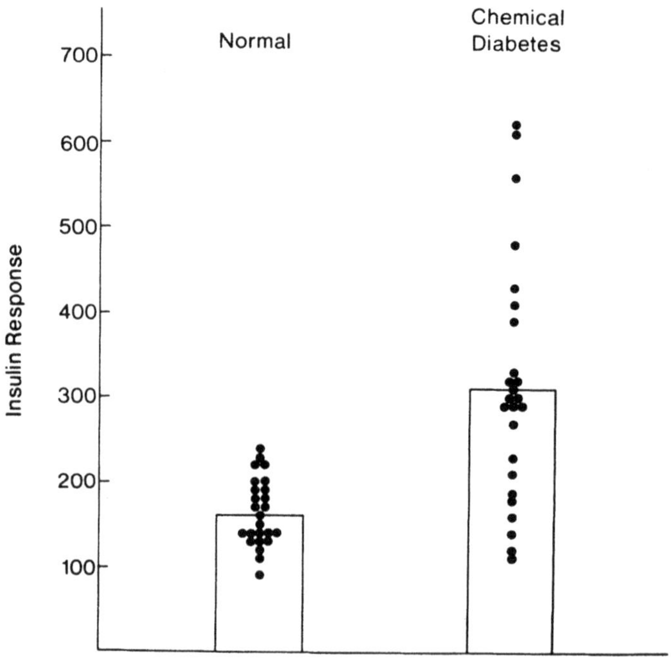

Fig. 2. Individual area under the plasma insulin curve during the OGTT. The mean response is given by the height of the bar.

The combination of hyperglycemia and hyperinsulinemia suggests that some degree of insulin resistance is present in subjects with chemical diabetes. We have attempted to provide direct evidence for this hypothesis by determining the SSPG response during a continuous infusion of glucose, insulin, epinephrine, and propranolol as described in the Methods. The results of these measurements are seen in Figure 3, and indicate that patients with chemical diabetes, as a group, are more insulin resistant than subjects with normal glucose tolerance. However, it is obvious that some patients with chemical diabetes are not particularly insulin resistant. Thus, heterogeneity also exists in terms of insulin sensitivity.

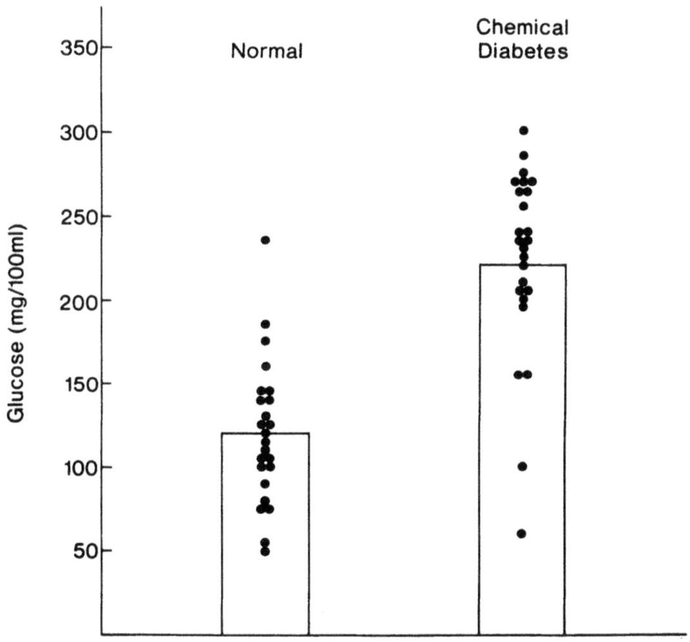

Fig. 3. Individual steady state plasma glucose (SSPG) responses during the infusion of epinephrine, propranolol, glucose and exogenous insulin. The mean response is given by the height of the bar.

In order to define the relationship between insulin response and insulin resistance within a given individual, the correlation between these two variables was examined. These data appear in Figure 4, and indicate that the majority of patients with chemical diabetes were both hyperinsulinemic and insulin resistant as compared to the majority of normal subjects. However, a few patients with chemical diabetes were neither hyperinsulinemic nor insulin resistant. These data suggest that there may be two kinds of patients with chemical diabetes, in which different metabolic defects lead to abnormal glucose tolerance.

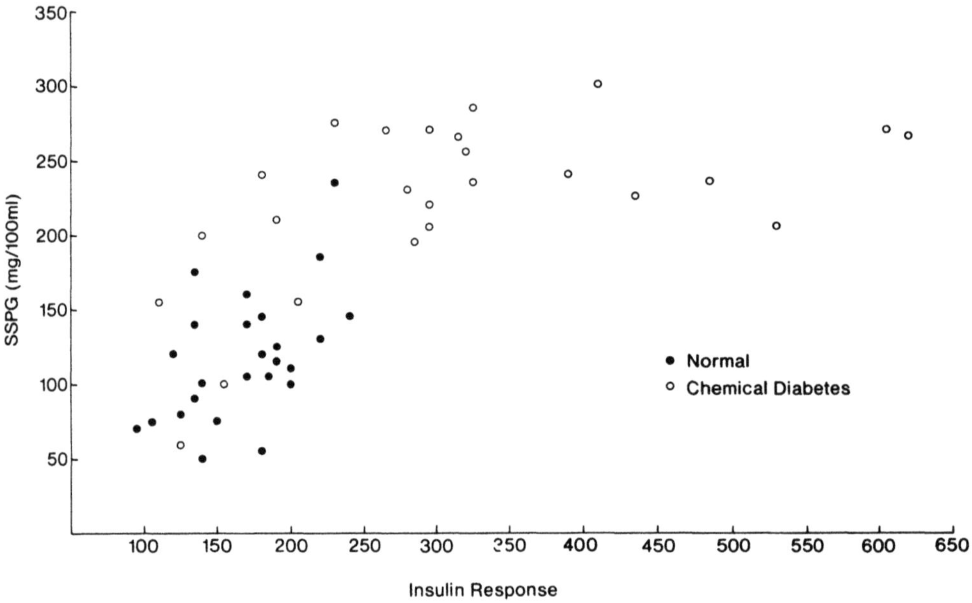

Fig. 4. The relationship between insulin response (area under the plasma insulin curve during the OGTT) and insulin resistance (SSPG) in all subjects studied.

II. Role of Patients with Chemical Diabetes in the Syndrome of Diabetes Mellitus

The insulin response during the OGTT of 145 subjects with widely varying degrees of glucose tolerance is seen in Figure 5. These data, obtained on a different patient population, again indicate that the mean plasma insulin response of subjects with chemical diabetes is not lower than that of normal subjects at any time interval. On the other hand, the plasma insulin response to a glucose challenge of patients with fasting hyperglycemia is less than that of normal subjects, and the more severe the fasting hyperglycemia, the more reduced the insulin response.

A two-dimensional scattergram of the relationship between the total plasma glucose and total plasma insulin responses to oral glucose is seen in Figure 6. For comparison, Figure 7 is a scattergram made of data from 125 patients studied by Reaven and Miller approximately ten years ago (3). Even though the 125

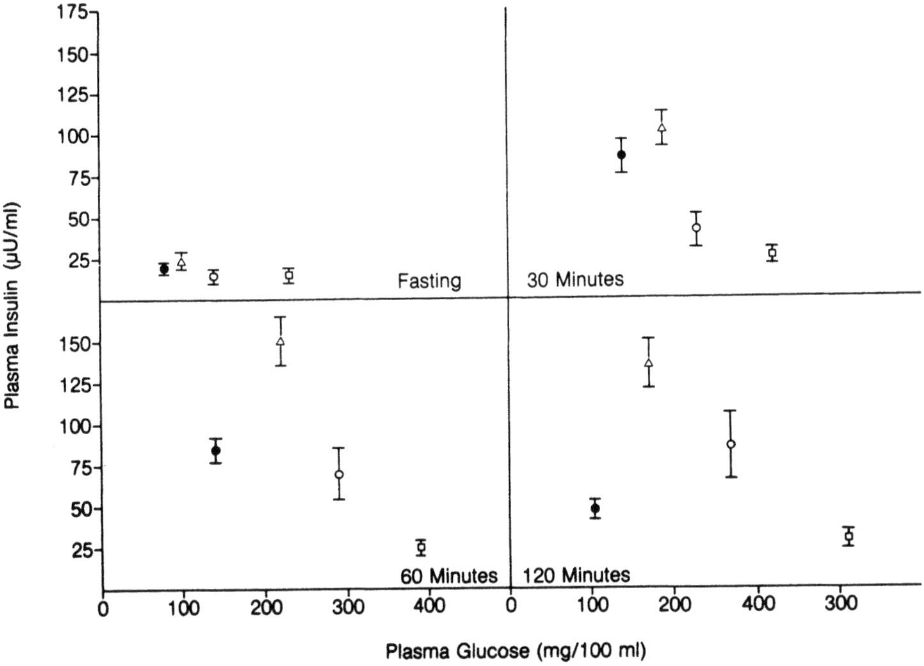

Fig. 5. The relationship between mean (± SEM) plasma glucose and insulin concentrations at various time intervals during the OGTT in the following four groups of subjects: normal (●), chemical diabetes (Δ), fasting plasma glucose concentration 110-150 mg/100 ml (O), and fasting plasma glucose concentration >150 mg/100 ml (□).

subjects in the previous study were completely different from the 145 subjects in the current study, and were investigated more than ten years ago, the scattergram patterns are practically identical - both have central cores with one wing extended upwards and another wing down and to the right.

Although there is ample evidence in support of this relationship (3-5), its significance remains unclear. In an attempt to pursue the issue further, the 145 patients were divided into three groups (normal, chemical diabetes, fasting hyperglycemia) on the basis of the criteria in Table 1-b. They were then compared on the basis of three metabolic variables: total glycemic response to a glucose challenge, total insulin response to a glucose challenge, and insulin sensitivity.

The data in Figure 8 depict the relationship between glucose and insulin responses in the three groups of patients. By and large patients with chemical diabetes seem to be going off in a

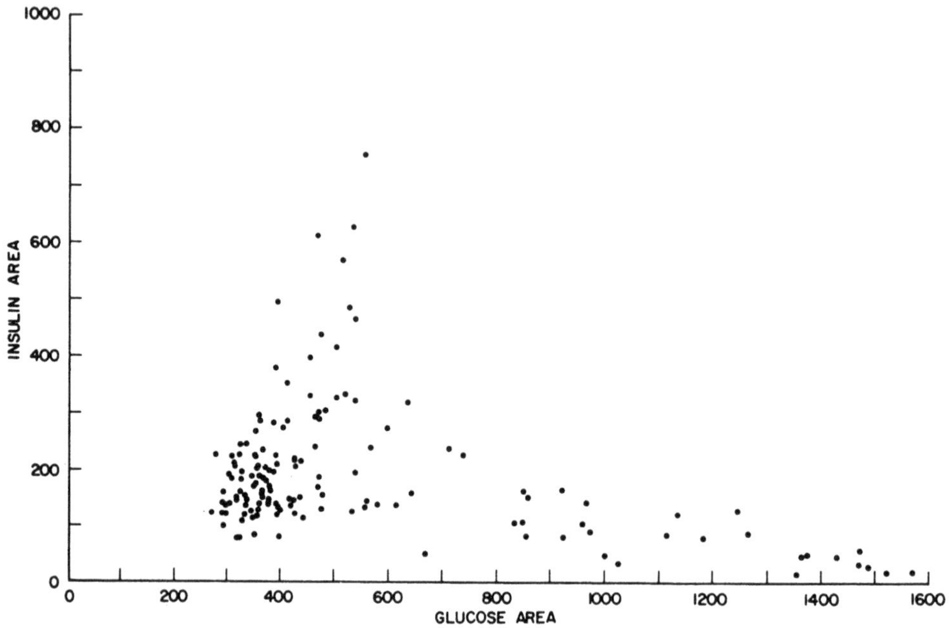

Fig. 6. Relationship between the plasma glucose (mg/100 ml. hr) and insulin (μU/ml. hr) responses during the OGTT for all 145 subjects.

different direction (up) as compared to subjects with fasting hyperglycemia (down and to the right). On the other hand, inspection of the data indicates that there are exceptions to this generalization.

Figure 9 displays the relationship between insulin response and insulin resistance (SSPG) in the three groups. As in Figure 8, patients with chemical diabetes and fasting hyperglycemia seem to be going off in different directions, i.e., upwards and to the right, and upwards and to the left, respectively. Again, there are individual exceptions.

Figure 10 depicts the relationship between glucose response and SSPG in the three groups and this relationship has a different appearance than that seen in Figures 8 and 9. In this instance, there is no evidence of a clustering of the experimental groups

DISCUSSION

For over 50 years diabetes has been viewed as a homogenous disorder, due to a primary failure of insulin secretion, in which

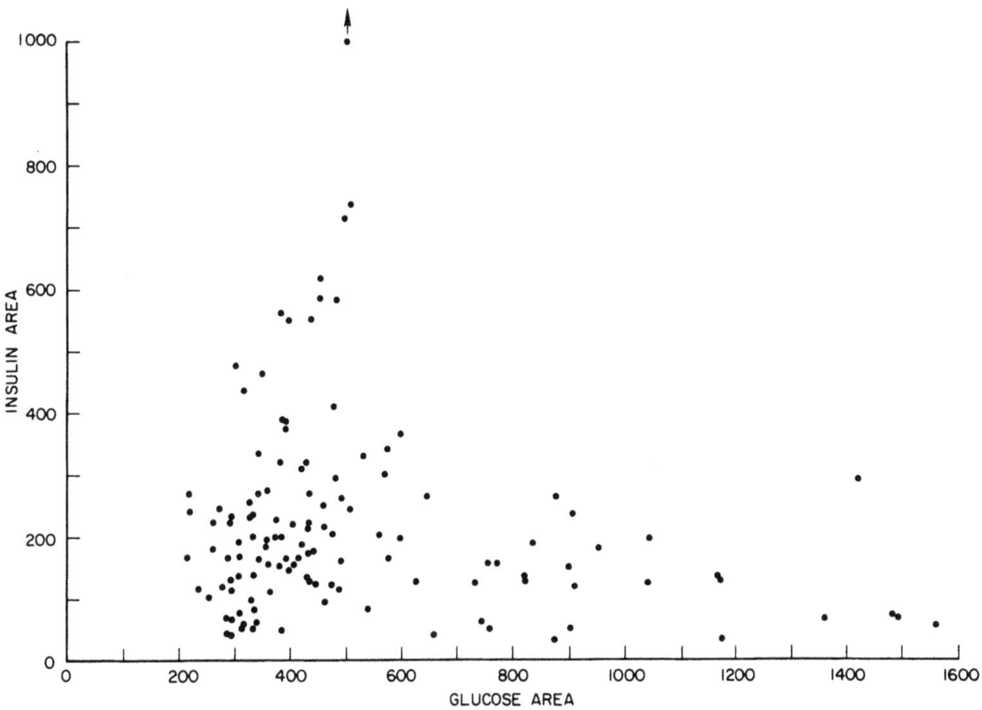

Fig. 7. Relationship between the plasma glucose (mg/100 ml. hr) and insulin (μU/ml. hr) responses during an OGTT for 125 subjects studied by Reaven and Miller in 1968.

the severity of the carbohydrate intolerance is directly related to the degree of insulin deficiency. In this formulation there is a continuum of patients with diabetes, ranging from individuals with the mildest discernable degree of glucose intolerance to subjects who are dependent upon exogenous insulin to prevent death from ketoacidosis. Within this context, patients with the smallest detectable abnormality of glucose intolerance (chemical diabetes) play a pivotal role. Can these patients be viewed as representing the beginning of a disease, characterized by progressive degrees of insulin deficiency, which at the other end of the spectrum consists of patients with insulin-dependent diabetes? The results that have been presented strongly suggest that this formation is an unlikely one.

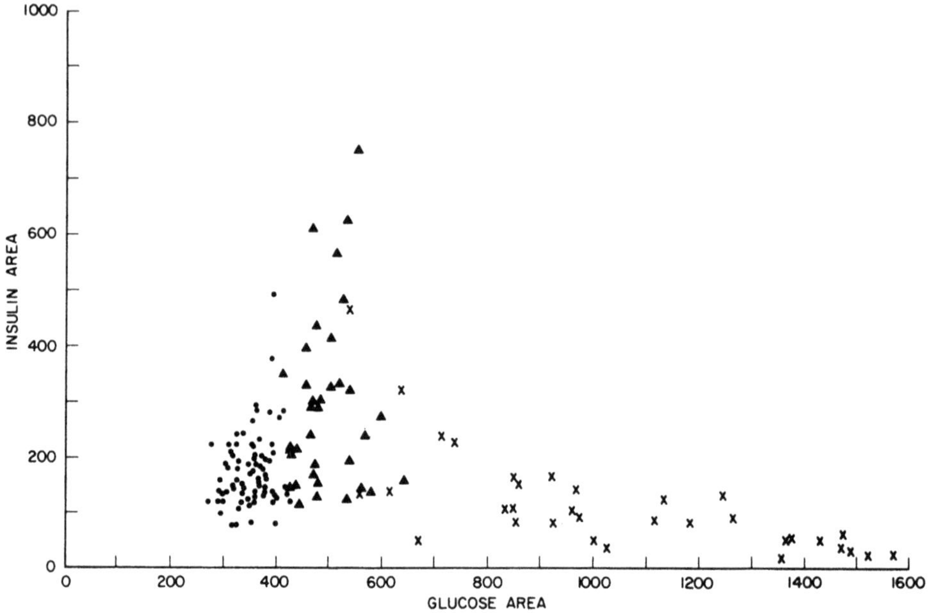

Fig. 8. *Relationship between the plasma glucose (mg/100 ml. hr) and insulin (μU/ml. hr) responses during the OGTT for all 145 subjects. Subjects have been defined as being normal (●), or as having either chemical (Δ) or overt (X) diabetes on the basis of the criteria given in Table 1.*

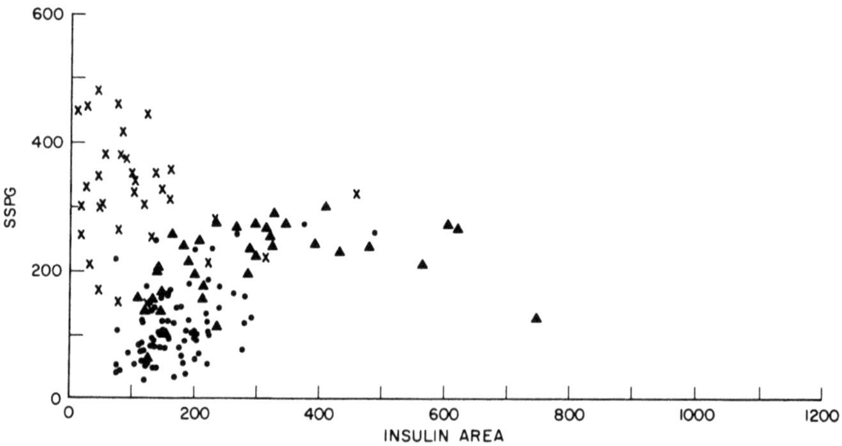

Fig. 9. *Relationship between the plasma insulin response (μU/ml.hr) during the OGTT and SSPG (mg/100 ml) for all 145 subjects Subjects have been defined as being normal (●),or as having either chemical (Δ) or overt (X) diabetes on the basis of the criteria given in Table 1.*

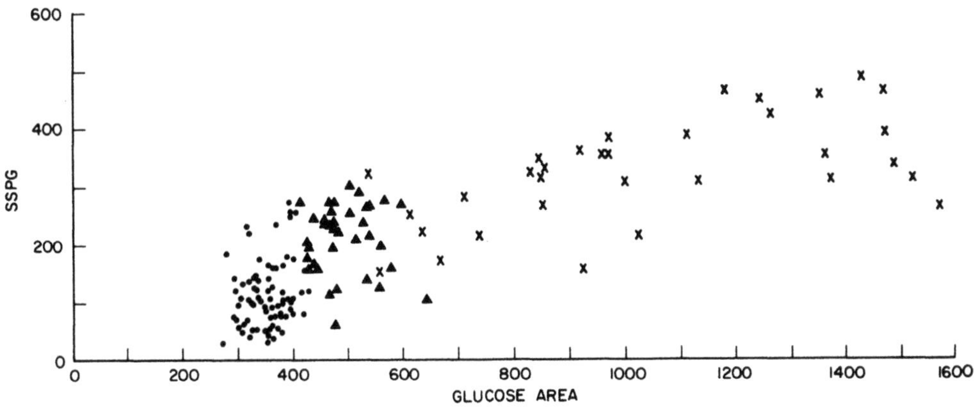

Fig. 10. Relationship between the plasma glucose response (mg/100 ml.hr) during the OGTT and SSPG (mg/100 ml) for all 145 subjects. Subjects have been defined as being normal (●), or as having either chemical (Δ) or overt (X) diabetes on the basis of the results of criteria given in Table 1.

The simplest issue in this regard relates to the mechanism of glucose intolerance in patients with chemical diabetes. The results presented indicated that most patients with chemical diabetes were more insulin resistant, and had, in general, greater total insulin responses to oral glucose than did normal subjects. As such, these data are consistent with previous observations (2). On the other hand, not all patients with chemical diabetes were insulin resistant, nor did they all demonstrate an increased insulin response. Furthermore, it appears that the patients who were the least insulin resistant, were also the individuals with the least insulin response. Thus, it appears possible to subdivide patients with chemical diabetes into at least two subgroups on the basis of divergent metabolic characteristics. In one group of patients who comprised the majority in this study, it would appear that glucose intolerance is due to loss of normal insulin sensitivity, and develops in the face of circulating insulin levels which are at least equal to those of normal subjects. There is no evidence of increased insulin resistance in the other group of patients with chemical diabetes, and their insulin response is at the lower end of the normal range. In these patients, the glucose intolerance may be secondary to deficient insulin secretion. Fajans et al (9) had earlier indicated that patients with chemical diabetes could have widely different insulin responses to oral glucose, and emphasized the heterogeneity of this population. Indeed, the only differences in our conclusions lies in the relative proportion of the two forms of chemical diabetes. In contrast to the current results, Fajans and associates found that the majority of their patients with chemical diabetes had a somewhat lower insulin response than did normal subjects. The explanation for this difference is not clear, but most likely represents differences in patient selection.

The significance of the relationship between the metabolic defects in patients with chemical diabetes and those with severe hyperglycemia presents a more difficult problem. For the reasons discussed earlier, it seems necessary to reject the notion that diabetes is one disease, characterized by increasing degrees of insulin deficiency, in which the severity of the hyperglycemia is directly related to the insulin deficiency. Having done this, we are left with at least two viable hypotheses. Diabetes could still be considered to be one disease, in which the basic defect is loss of normal insulin sensitivity. The homeostatic response to the loss of insulin sensitivity would be to increase insulin secretion, but only up to a certain point. Beta cell exhaustion would eventually supervene, resulting in a progressive decrease of insulin secretion and increasing severity of hyperglycemia. Thus, one could view the natural history of diabetes as representing a "Starling Curve". Alternatively, one could consider patients with chemical diabetes and those with more severe hyperglycemia as having basically different and unrelated causes for their glucose intolerance. Thus, some patients may be primarily insulin resistant, while others are primarily insulin deficient. Under these conditions the "Starling Curve" may be more apparent than real, and the relationship between the plasma glucose and insulin responses to an oral glucose load is a function of the metabolic heterogeneity of the diabetic population.

The data presented in Figures 5-7 take into account two metabolic variables - degree of glucose intolerance and insulin response to an oral glucose challenge - and inspection of these results suggests that they are compatible with either hypothesis. However, when a third metabolic variable is also taken into consideration, specifically the efficiency with which insulin disposes of a glucose load (insulin sensitivity), the situation seems quite different. Thus, inspection of the combined data in Figures 8 and 9 suggests that patients with chemical diabetes form a population whose metabolic characteristics are quite disparate from those patients with fasting hyperglycemia. Given the fact that the two groups cluster so independently, it becomes difficult to imagine that all patients with overt diabetes have evolved from patients with chemical diabetes.

It is obvious that the above conclusions are based upon the view that glucose intolerance in patients with chemical diabetes is associated with a loss of insulin sensitivity, without a primary defect in the insulin secretory response to oral glucose. It is apparent from the current results that not all patients with chemical diabetes share these metabolic characteristics, and it has previously been pointed out that the glucose intolerance in some patients with chemical diabetes is associated with a defect in the plasma insulin response to glucose (2). As such, these patients may well represent the small proportion of patients with chemical diabetes who progress to more severe hyperglycemia (10). On the other hand, most patients with chemical diabetes do not develop overt diabetes (10), and this is not surprising when the metabolic characteristics of these patients are taken into consideration.

Finally, these differences between the metabolic characteristics of patients currently classified as having diabetes may well represent the metabolic corollary of the differences in inheritance and immune response that are now known to exist in diabetic patients. Thus, it has recently been suggested that idiopathic diabetes mellitus can be divided into at least two general disease processes on the basis of differences in autoimmunity (11). Using this classification patients with chemical diabetes who are insulin resistant (and not hypoinsulinemic) would be classified as having Type II diabetes. On the other hand, patients with chemical diabetes who are not insulin resistant (but hypoinsulinemic) would have Type I diabetes. This formulation is consistent with the recent observation (12) that 13 of 20 (65%) newly diagnosed patients with relatively mild diabetes at the onset, and positive pancreatic islet cell antibodies, progressed to insulin requiring diabetes. In contrast, only 14 of 1959 (9%) of similar patients, without islet cell antibodies, progressed in a similar fashion during the period of observation. If the existence of islet cell antibodies can be considered to be indicative of insulin deficiency (either present or future), these data would explain both the metabolic heterogeneity of patients with chemical diabetes, as well as their eventual clinical course.

REFERENCES

1. *Yalow, R.S. and Berson, S.A. (1960). J. Clin. Invest. 39, 1157.*
2. *Reaven, G.M. and Olefsky, J.M. (1978). Adv. in Metab. Disorders 9, 313.*
3. *Reaven, G.M. and Miller, R. (1968). Diabetes 17, 560.*
4. *Savage, P.J., et al. (1975). Diabetes 24, 362.*
5. *Zimmet, P., et al. (1978). Diabetologia 15, 23.*
6. *Shen, S.W., et al. (1970). J. Clin. Invest. 49, 2151.*
7. *Desbuqois, B. and Aurbach, G.D. (1971). J. Clin. Endo. Metab. 33, 732.*
8. *Kadish, A.H., et al. (1968). Clin. Chem. 14, 116*
9. *Fajans, S.S., et al. (1975). Trans. Assoc. Amer. Phys. 87, 83.*
10. *O'Sullivan, J.B. and Mahan, C.M. (1968). New Engl. J. Med. 278, 1038.*
11. *Irvine, W.J. (1977). Lancet 1, 638.*
12. *Irvine, W.J., et al. (1977). Lancet 1, 1025.*

This work was supported in part by grants from the National Institutes of Health, #HL 08506, and #RR-70 from the Clinical Research Centres Branch, and from the Research Services of the Veterans Administration.

INQUIRIES INTO THE PATHOGENESIS OF GESTATIONAL DIABETES

Boyd E. Metzger* and Norbert Freinkel

Except for insulin-dependent diabetes of acute onset, it is usually difficult to time the duration of glucose intolerance with any degree of accuracy. Gestational diabetes may be one of the few exceptions. Herein glucose homeostasis is challenged by increased requirements for insulin and contrainsulin hormones which exert their maximal impact by the end of the second trimester and persist unabated throughout the third. Consequently, glucose intolerance is first recognized between 24 and 32 weeks of gestation. Thus, pregnancy may be the ideal time in which to evaluate the determinants of early diabetogenesis in the "maturity onset" or "not insulin-dependent" type of diabetes.

This review summarizes some of the inquiries that we and our colleagues have been conducting in this regard for several years. Our interests in gestational diabetes have also been stimulated by certain additional considerations. First, despite some controversy, even mild abnormalities of glucose homeostasis seem to convey an increased risk for perinatal complications including macrosomia, neonatal hypoglycemia and even perinatal deaths. Secondly, since glucose intolerance during pregnancy is frequently reversed in the immediate postpartum period but subsequently progresses to permanent chemical or overt diabetes, it is one of the few situations in which identifiable potential diabetics can be followed prospectively. Although we are attempting to identify the factor(s) responsible for the perinatal complications of gestational diabetes and are securing prospective follow-up of women with glucose intolerance of pregnancy, this report is directed specifically toward those factors which might be related to the diabetogenic process.

We define gestational diabetes as asymptomatic glucose intolerance with onset during pregnancy. The diagnosis is made by oral tolerance test with 100g of glucose using the criteria of O'Sullivan and Mahan (1) to define abnormalities. For the purposes of the studies reported here, and to minimize contributions from secondary metabolic alterations, we have specifically focused on those gestational diabetics with the mildest impairment of glucose tolerance, i.e. subjects whose fasting plasma glucose was within the normal range for pregnancy but oral glucose tolerance was abnormal.

PLACENTAL EFFECTS ON HORMONES

The metabolic alterations of pregnancy are not manifest with equal intensity throughout gestation. Rather, there is a characteristic temporal progression in which the increasing demands for insulin (and resistance to insulin action) parallel the growth of the conceptus. Indeed, in the immediate postpartum period, the exuberant insulinogenic response to secretory stimulation in normal subjects disappears, normoglycemia may supervene in gestational diabetics, and the therapeutic insulin requirements may precipitously decline in patients with established diabetes mellitus. Several properties of placental function have been implicated in the gestational alterations of insulin economy. Can any be specifically implicated in gestational diabetes?

Nearly two decades ago, Freinkel and Goodner demonstrated that throughout gestation the placenta of rats and humans contains systems for degrading insulin into cleavage products devoid of hypoglycemic properties and that the added potential for insulinolysis parallels total placental mass (2). It was shown with labeled insulin that fractional rates of insulin removed from the circulation in the rat near term were increased approximately 30% and reverted to non-gravid levels following expulsion of the conceptus. Although the magnitude of impact of insulin degradation in the placenta upon overall insulin kinetics in humans remains uncertain, Freinkel and Goodner were unable to demonstrate any greater breakdown of insulin by placenta from diabetics than with placenta from women with normal carbohydrate metabolism.

Is placental biosynthesis and release of hormones with contrainsulin properties implicated in gestational diabetes? We have used human placental lactogen (HPL) as an index of such placental hormonogenesis (3). Table 1 shows the values for plasma, HPL, a known insulin antagonist, and human chorionic gonadotropin (HCG) secured after 14 hour overnight fast during weeks 30-40 of pregnancy in 33 women with normal carbohydrate metabolism and 13 gestational diabetics. Although "steady state" glucose was significantly higher in the gestational diabetics, neither HPL nor HCG differed in the two groups.

Metabolic hormones of nonplacental origin are regulated by nutrient feedback signals. Early reports stressed the constancy of HPL concentrations and the lack of metabolic feedback regulation of this peptide. However, several later reports have provided evidence for some reciprocal relationships between excursions in plasma HPL and glucose. Thus increases in plasma HPL have occurred in association with hypoglycemia induced by fasting or administration of insulin. We have observed significant decrements in plasma HPL and HCG following 100g oral glucose loads (3) (Table 1). However, the decrements in HPL are the same in gestational diabetics and gravida with normal carbohydrate metabolism. When the data for the two groups are pooled, the integrated 180 min glucose areas correlate significantly with the HPL decrements at 60 min (r=0.346; p .05).

TABLE 1

PLASMA HPL AND HCG+

	Basal	Changes from basal +30	Changes from basal +60
	HPL(μg/ml)		
Normal Pregnancy (33)	8.4±0.4	-0.35±0.11**	-0.24±0.11*
Gestational Diabetes (13)	8.8±0.6	-0.38±0.12**	-0.58±0.18**
p	ns	ns	ns
	HCG (IU/ml)		
Normal Pregnancy (33)	12.9±1.6	-0.20±0.15	-0.63±0.25*
Gestational Diabetes(13)	12.3±3.3	-0.08±0.23	-0.25±0.34
p	ns	ns	ns

+ Concentrations of HPL and HCG were measured during weeks 30-40 of pregnancy in plasma obtained under basal conditions after 14 hour overnight fast. "Changes from basal" denotes the absolute deviations from basal plasma values 30 and 60 min following oral glucose. "p" denotes significance of differences between normal pregnant and gestational diabetic subjects. Significant changes from basal for each group on basis of paired "t" test are indicated by asterisks: * <.05; ** <.01; ns denotes p>.05.

Changes in HPL of comparable magnitude have been observed after intravenous glucose loads but others have been unable to demonstrate changes in HPL after the ingestion of meals of mixed composition. Thus, although the physiological importance of these small changes in HPL and HCG are uncertain, it is clear that generalized abnormalities in basal secretion or in the feedback regulation of these placental hormones cannot be invoked in the pathogenesis of gestational diabetes. These observations do not exclude the possibility that augmented secretion of HPL or other placental hormones might be implicated in individual cases of gestational diabetes.

PANCREATIC ALPHA CELL FUNCTION

Primary or secondary abnormalities in the feedback between alpha and β-cell have been invoked as contributory to the pathogenesis of diabetes mellitus (4). To test this possibility we have compared insulin/glucagon relationships in non-gravid women, normal pregnant subjects and gestational diabetics (5). Our studies, and subsequent confirmatory reports by others (6,7) indicated that basal insulin/glucagon rations, suppression of circulating glucagon following oral glucose administration and stimulation of glucagon secretion by proteins or amino acids are preserved in normal third trimester pregnancy. Thus, alterations of alpha cell response do not appear to contribute to the insulin resistance which prevails in the last half of gestation. Table 2 shows the relationships among basal plasma glucose, immunoreactive insulin (IRI) and glucagon under "steady state" conditions in 25 normal subjects and 13 gestational diabetics. Plasma glucose, IRI and glucagon are all significantly higher in the gestational diabetics. However, the IRI/glucose and IRI/glucagon ratios are the same or higher than in the women with normal carbohydrate metabolism.

The dynamic changes in plasma glucagon following 100g oral glucose during late pregnancy are summarized in Table 3: Absolute decrements in plasma glucagon are of similar magnitude in normals and gestational diabetics; relationships are also similar when the changes in glucagon are expressed as % decline from basal. Taken together, these results, as well as the confirmatory findings of Kuhl and Holst (7), indicate that abnormalities of alpha cell-β-cell feedback cannot be implicated in gestational diabetogenesis.

PANCREATIC BETA CELL FUNCTION

Early reports of immunoreactive insulin (IRI) secretion during oral glucose tolerance test established that gestational diabetics, like most maturity-onset diabetics, are not severely insulin deficient. Indeed, it was reported that integrated IRI release in gestational diabetics may equal or exceed that in non-diabetic subjects during the course of a three hour glucose tolerance test. Contributions of obesity to the increased elaboration of insulin may not have been appreciated in some of these early reports and may have accounted, in part, for the seemingly "normal" secretion of insulin.

TABLE 2

RELATIONSHIPS AMONG BASAL PLASMA GLUCOSE, IMMUNOREACTIVE INSULIN (IRI) AND GLUCAGON+

	Normal Pregnancy (n = 25)	Gestational Diabetes (n = 13)	p
Glucose (mg/dl)	80.2±1.5	95.7±4.5	.001
IRI (μU/ml)	13.0±1.0	21.1±2.5	.001
Glucagon (pg/ml)	59.6±3.0	97.5±17.1	.01
IRI/Glucose (μU /mg)	16.3±1.2	22.2±2.5	.05
IRI/Glucagon (molar ratio)	5.6±0.5	7.4±1.7	ns

+ Plasma glucose, IRI and glucagon were measured under basal conditions after 14 hours overnight fast during weeks 30-4o of gestation in 25 subjects with normal carbohydrate metabolism and 13 gestational diabetics. "p" denotes significance of the differences between the groups.

Until recently, the nature of the circulating immunoreactive insulin products had not been examined. Since proinsulin and proinsulin-like intermediates react with insulin antibodies but are biologically much less potent than insulin, an increased proportion of such precursor molecules would overestimate the biological effectiveness of the circulating IRI. Thus, we utilized gel filtration to characterize circulating insulin immunoreactivity in pregnancy (8). We found that insulin immunoreactivity in our mild gestational diabetics exhibited insulin/proinsulin relationships which did not differ from pregnant subjects with normal carbohydrate metabolism. These results indicate that it is unlikely that circulating immunoreactive insulin in gestational diabetes consists of an increased proportion of products with diminished biological activity. Others have also failed to find disturbed IRI/proinsulin relationships in pregnancy(9).

The acute release of insulin following nutrient secretagogue stimulation is a more sensitive parameter of β-cell sensitivity than integrated secretion measured over several hours. However, there are

TABLE 3

CHANGES IN PLASMA GLUCAGON AFTER ORAL GLUCOSE+

	Δ Glucagon (pg/ml)+		
	60 min	120 min	180 min
Normal Pregnancy (25)	-7.4±2.8*	-12.3±2.5**	-14.7±2.6***
Gestational Diabetes (13)	-11.5±4.7*	-16.2±4.7**	-16.5±6.5*
p	ns	ns	ns

+"ΔGlucagon" denotes the net deviations from basal plasma glucagon concentration (shown in Table 2) which were seen at 60 and 120 min following 100g oral glucose loads. "p" denotes comparisons between normals vs. gestational diabetics. Significant changes from basal within each group (on the basis of paired "t" test) are indicated by asteriaks: * < .05; ** < .01; *** < .001.

few studies of "early" insulin release during glucose tolerance testing in gestational diabetes. In a recent study (7), Kühl and Holst reported no absolute diminution of plasma insulin values during a 50 g OGTT performed in late pregnancy in a group of 14 normal weight pregnant women designated "gestational diabetic" on the basis of criteria established in their laboratory from nonpregnant healthy women. However, ΔInsulin/ΔGlucose ratios were significantly reduced during the first 60 minutes of the OGTT.

For our assessments of the kinetics of acute IRI release we have been focusing specifically on those gestational diabetics with the mildest impairment of glucose tolerance; all have fasting plasma glucose within the normal range, i.e. < 105mg/dl. To secure an index of acute β-cell response, the first sample is secured 15 min after 100g oral glucose administration. As a group, the gestational diabetics manifest a "sluggish" pattern of response with a delayed peak (10). The dyskinesis of early insulin secretion is even more apparent when the changes in insulin and glucose at 15 min are examined in more detail. The mean ratio of insulin/glucose increments in gestational diabetics is only 60% of that found in pregnant subjects with normal carbohydrate metabolism.

Is the sluggish insulin release a true feature of gestational diabetes or are other characteristics of the population implicated?

Many groups have reported that gestational diabetics are more obese and older than the overall population of pregnant women and both age and weight are variables known to influence insulin/glucose relationships. However, when our gestational diabetics are compared to non-diabetics of comparable age and weight, they still exhibit a diminution of acute insulin response to oral glucose challenge. Although the majority of gestational diabetics manifest this defect, this does not imply the same mediation in all cases. In fact, nearly 20% show acute responses that are above the mean $\Delta I/\Delta G$ response of the non-diabetics. It is tempting to speculate that heightened resistance to insulin as a result of gestational factors may be especially important in these subjects.

CONCLUSIONS

The gestational diabetic does not appear to be "blackmailed" by disproportionately high levels of gestational contrainsulin factors. She also does not respond to secretory stimulation by releasing inappropriately partitioned secretory products. Rather, when challenged by increased demands for insulin, her β-cells display their limited reserve by a sluggish rate of insulin release. The lesion is not present uniformly and can only be demonstrated in about 80% of cases. From what we know about the mechanisms involved in insulin secretion even the 80% are probably heterogeneous and the sluggish insulin release may only represent the final expression of a variety of disturbances in earlier steps of islet stimulus-secretion coupling. Other aspects of heterogeneity of the population will undoubtedly be demonstrated as family pedigrees, genetic studies and long-range follow-up are secured. For example, further evidence for heterogeneity has already become apparent in that glucose tolerance returns fully to normal postpartum in only 60% of our cases and the normalization does not appear to be related to antepartum patterns of insulin secretion.

REFERENCES

1. *O'Sullivan, J.B. and Mahan, C.M. (1964). Diabetes, 13, 278*
2. *Freinkel, N. and Goodner, C.J. (1962). Arch. Intern. Med., 109, 235*
3. *Surmaczynska, B.Z., et al.(1974). Isr. J. Med. Sci., 10, 1481*
4. *Unger, R.H. (1976). Diabetes, 25, 136*
5. *Daniel, R.R., et al.(1974). Diabetes, 23, 771*
6. *Luyckx, A.S., et al. (1975). Diabetologia, 11, 549*
7. *Kühl, C. and Holst, J.J. (1976). Diabetes, 25, 16*
8. *Phelps, R.L., et al.(1975). J. Clin. Endocrinol. Metab., 41,1085*
9. *Kühl, C. (1976). Diabetologia, 12, 295*
10. *Metzger, B.E., et al.(1975). Clin. Res., 23, 445A*

Supported in part by Research Grants AM-10699 and HD-11021 and Training Grants AM-05071 and AM-07169 from the NIH, Bethesda, Md., a Research Grant from The Kroc Foundation, and Research Grant 6-136 from The National Foundation March of Dimes.

EFFECT OF INTRAVENOUS GLUCOSE, LEUCINE AND ARGININE ON CONCENTRATION OF INSULIN IN MATERNAL AND UMBILICAL CORD SERUM

S. Grasso*, G. Palumbo, S. Rugolo, R. Vigo
and G. Tumino

Glucose rapidly crosses the placenta in the presence of a concentration gradient between mother and fetus and the fetal plasma glucose may be controlled indirectly via the maternal endocrine system. Although insulin is present in the fetal pancreas as early as the 12th gestational week, little information is available about the secretion of insulin by the fetal pancreas or its physiological effect (1). However, it is widely accepted that glucose is an important stimulus of B-cells growth and function. In fact the hyperplasia and hypertrophy of the endocrine pancreas and the high levels of insulin in the cord blood of a fetus born to a diabetic mother are attributed to maternal and consequent fetal hyperglycemia (2).

In normal pregnant women plasma glucose remains remarkably constant over the 24 hour period (3). It was reported that the mean concentration of hourly samples taken over 24 hours is 81 ± SD 5 mg per 100 ml in early pregnancy and 85 ± SD 5 mg per 100 ml in late pregnancy. The concentration of fetal blood glucose mirrors that of the mother and is slightly lower (1). Early in gestation the human fetal pancreas is relatively insensitive to glucose infused to the mother, but the fetus at term is capable of responding to maternal hyperglycemia with an elevation of serum insulin. It is also known that neither maternal nor fetal insulin cross the placenta (4). We reported (5) that after infusing 50 gm of glucose or saline for 60' to healthy mothers at term, undergoing caesarean section, the serum insulin level after glucose rose from 17 ± 3 to 82 ± 12 μU/ml while the blood glucose increased from 77 ± 3 to 237 ± mg/100 ml. At delivery, maternal serum insulin was 55 ± 11 μU per ml and blood glucose was 207 ± 11 mg per 100 ml. In the umbilical blood, serum was 46 ± 8 μU per ml while the blood glucose was 187 ± 13 mg per 100 ml. The maternal infusion of saline did not cause any significant change in either mother or fetus. Similar data have been reported by several authors (4) and prove the theory postulated by Pedersen (2) that the hyperinsulinism of the infant of diabetic mother is due to maternal hyperglycemia. However the facts that control insulin secretion in the fetuses of healthy mothers still remain obscure.

The study presented here suggests that some amino acids, such as l-leucine or l-arginine with glucose may contribute to the normal regulation of fetal insulin secretion. Due to the functioning of the placenta, it is well established, that amino acid concentrations in the fetal blood are higher than in maternal blood. In fact the placenta can selectively transfer the natural L-isomer more rapidly than its D-isomer and also establishes a gradient where fetal concentration is higher than the maternal one (6). It has also been demonstrated that in the adult (8) and preterm infant (7) glucose and amino acids are synergistic in their insulin stimulatory action.

Fetal insulin and glucose response in utero were evaluated by infusing saline, glucose (25 g), L-leucine (15 g), or L-arginine monochloride (15 g) with or without glucose (25 g) to normal pregnant women at term undergoing cesarean section. The infusion lasted 60 minutes and was synchronized so that birth occurred 10 minutes after it ended. Venous blood samples were taken from the mother throughout the infusion and simultaneously at delivery from both maternal and umbilical vein.

The pregnant women were neither obese nor with history or evidence of diabetes mellitus and underwent cesarean section for pelvic disproportion. They were chosen because the fetus didn't undergo the stress of labor. Glucose was estimated by glucose oxidase reagent. Insulin was measured by standard immunoassay technique (5). The results of our study are shown in Table 1.

The simultaneous administration of glucose with leucine or glucose with arginine monochloride is followed by a marked increase of cord blood serum insulin and a slight one of glucose. The fetal insulin levels produced by these combinations are similar to those seen after the maternal infusion of 50 g of glucose, while the cord blood glucose levels are higher and statistically different ($p < o.01$) from those seen in mothers who received saline. In the mothers the infusion of these mixtures causes an increase in serum insulin greater than does the separate infusion of these substances. Furthermore, as in normal subjects (8), the synergistic effect is greater for arginine-glucose than for leucine-glucose. However, this difference is not evident in the fetuses and is probably due to the different placental transfer

TABLE 1. Comparison of maternal and fetal blood glucose and serum insulin (Mean ± SEM) in pregnant women at term infused for 60 min. with saline, glucose (25 g), leucine (15 g), arginine monochloride (15 g), glucose (25 g) with leucine (15 g), or glucose (25 g) with arginine monochloride (15 g).

	0'	30'	60'	70'	Cord Blood
MATERNAL INFUSION OF SALINE (n=10) b.w.[1] Kg 3.285±98					
Blood Glucose[2]	70±3	73±2	75±2	78±4	60±5
Serum Insulin[3]	17±2	17±3	18±2	15±2	14±2
MATERNAL INFUSION OF GLUCOSE (n=10) b.w. Kg 3.400±121					
Blood Glucose	61±2	106±4	132±13	103±8	84±7
Serum Insulin	7±2	49±9	48±7	24±6	17±4
MATERNAL INFUSION OF LEUCINE (n=8) b.w. Kg 3.350±127					
Blood Glucose	68±3	76±4	77±9	79±4	70±5
Serum Insulin	13±2	34±5	29±3	19±5	16±1
MATERNAL INFUSION OF ARGININE (n=4) b.w. Kg 3.225±166					
Blood Glucose	73±3	73±1	87±5	88±3	73±2
Serum Insulin	17±2	24±3	33±3	22±1	12±3
MATERNAL INFUSION OF GLUCOSE WITH LEUCINE (n=7) b.w. Kg 3.628±149					
Blood Glucose	75±4	102±6	117±6	117±7	84±4
Serum Insulin	15±2	54±10	85±13	68±14	58±9
MATERNAL INFUSION OF GLUCOSE WITH ARGININE (n=6) b.w. Kg 3.523±95					
Blood Glucose	74±4	99±4	120±5	122±6	88±6
Serum Insulin	21±1	86±20	139±14	100±28	47±6

1 - Body weight of the infants
2 - Mg/100 ml
3 - uU/ml

rate for the individual amino acids. One study of placental transport of free amino acids in animals (9) has demonstrated that the branched-chain amino acids, such as leucine, belonging to the "L-preferring" group of Christensen, are the most readily transported across the placental membrane.

The data concerning the role of amino acids on insulin secretion in the fetus are conflicting. It has been reported that isolated human fetal pancreatic tissue from 14 to 20 weeks gestation releases insulin when incubated with leucine or arginine but not with glucose (10). Furthermore amino acids but not glucose enrichment of the culture medium favors the growth of fetal rat pancreatic rudiments (11). Contrastingly the infusion of arginine (0.75 g per minute from 27 to 60 minutes) to pregnant women at term during active labor causes no signifcant serum insulin rise in their fetuses (12). In the present study the maternal infusion of leucine or arginine alone causes a slight increase only of maternal insulin.

The reasons for the lack of response of fetal B-cells to leucine and arginine alone remain unknown. In the case of arginine the low blood glucose concentration of the normal fetus may be a factor that determines the absence of insulin response. In vitro studies have shown that arginine initiated insulin release is dependent upon the presence of adequate glucose concentration in the medium (13). In the adult it has been shown that hypoglycemia inhibits,whereas hyperglycemia stimulates, arginine induced insulin release (14).

In conclusion our study shows that fetal hyperinsulinemia could result from augmented fetal plasma amino acid levels in absence of fetal hyperglycemia. However, we suspect that rising levels of certain amino acids and glucose, after a mixed protein carbohydrate meal, in both mother and fetus regulate the insulin secretion in the fetus. In normal non-pregnant adult (15) protein feeding induces an increase in plasma insulin.

REFERENCES

1. *Cornblath, M. and Schwartz, R. (1976). Vol. III, Philadelphia, W. B. Saunders.*
2. *Pedersen, J. (1954). Acta Endocr. 16, 330.*
3. *Gilmer, M.D.G., et al. (1975). Br. Med. J. 3, 399.*
4. *Obenshain, S.S., et al. (1970). New Engl. J. Med. 283, 566.*
5. *Grasso, S., et al. (1976). Diabetes, 25, 545.*
6. *Prenton, L. and Young, M. (1969). J. Obstet. Gynaec. Brit. Cwlth. 76, 404.*
7. *Grasso, S., et al. (1973). Diabetes, 22, 349.*
8. *Floyd, J.C., Jr., et al. (1970). Diabetes, 19, 109.*
9. *Hopkins, L., et al. (1971). J. Physiol. 215, 11.*
10. *Milner, R.D.G., et al. (1972). J. Endocr. 52, 497.*
11. *De Gasparo, M., et al. (1978). J. Endocr. 77, 241.*
12. *King, K.C., et al. (1971). New Engl. J. Med. 285, 607.*
13. *Edgar, P., et al. (1969). Endocrinology 84, 835.*
14. *Effendic, S., et al. (1971). Metabolism 20, 568.*
15. *Floyd, J.C., Jr., et al. (1966). J. Clin. Invest. 45, 1479.*

DISCUSSION

R. CAMERINI-DAVALOS: *Dr. Reaven, I wonder if you would consider the possibility that some of your chemical diabetics, those you find in the normal range, are those who regress their abnormalities? I think that we, Steve (Fajans) and probably you as well as many others, found that the stages of diabetes are not necessarily progressive and some patients do come back to normal blood sugars. In fact, many of our chemical diabetics, at one time or other during a 16 year follow-up, were found to have normal blood sugars, and in some cases, the insulin levels were not what we expected at that time.*

G. M. REAVEN: *We don't have much information, in terms of following patients over time. What we're trying to do is to relate the existing glucose intolerance to the problem of insulin secretion versus insulin action.*

R. CAMERINI-DAVALOS: *Yes, but do we really have two groups of chemical diabetics, one with non-resistance, and the other with resistance? Or, is it that we have different stages of chemical diabetes?*

G. M. REAVEN: *When I show you two patients, whose glucose tolerances are essentially the same, and insulin response and insulin resistance in one is up there and in the other down there; all I can say is, at that particular moment in time, those patients' glucose tolerances, or intolerances, had different mechanisms.*

S. FAJANS: *I can answer that question more definitively, because we've been following the same patients for 17 years. Those with lower insulin responses stay high, so we're very definitely dealing with two different groups of patients with carbohydrate intolerance. I'd like to ask Dr. Camerini again how many of his "genetic prediabetics" developed chemical diabetes? About four years ago, Tattersall reported on 199 offspring, each from two diabetic parents, whom we followed, tested and extrapolated up to the age of 60. Sixty-one percent developed chemical diabetes or overt diabetes. In other words, 40% did not. The next question, Dr. Camerini, did I hear correctly that 93% of your chemical diabetics went on to fasting hyperglycemia? Dr. Reaven, I think we all agree that carbohydrate intolerance is non-specific and not necessarily diabetes. How many of your patients have a family history of diabetes and how many of your patients have hypertriglyceridemia? The last point, Dr. Metzger, I was very interested in the delay of insulin release in gestational diabetes. Dr. Rull, who is in the audience, with us some years ago reported exactly the same phenomenon in patients with negative glucose tolerance-*

just a family history of diabetes, but positive cortisone glucose tolerance.

R. CAMERINI-DAVALOS: *The 93% relates to prediabetics, 29 years or older, and high glucose responders, who developed abnormal glucose tolerance. If we take the total group of prediabetics now and determine how many went into chemical diabetes, whether high, low or average responders, our percentage is 52%. This is close to the number reported by Soldner in Boston at the ADA meeting, where he found 43%. We had 33% chemical diabetics who went to overt diabetes (fasting hyperglycemia). Soldner reports only 2% in adult onset diabetics, but in families with juvenile diabetes, 18%.*

E. PFEIFFER: *None of you reported on normal control subjects, subdivided into low and high responders.*

R. CAMERINI-DAVALOS: *Yes, in 1974, (Acta Diabet. Lat. XI, 4), we published high, low and average glucose responses in 134 controls. We had insulin levels on 56, 14 of whom were low insulin responders. Of the 14, we were able lately to retest 7, all of whom remained normal.*

E. PFEIFFER: *Eight days ago in Ulm, Dr. Luft reported that 3 low insulin responders became chemical diabetics and one became an overt diabetic.*

R. CAMERINI-DAVALOS: *In subjects with no family history for diabetes.*

E. PFEIFFER: *Normal population. He is convinced this is a kind of marker.*

G. M. REAVEN: *Our entire purpose was to look at the world in general, not unique subgroups. I would agree with the notion that there is a specific syndrome of hyperinsulinemia and hypertriglyceridemia. I think that a situation which is characterized by a loss of insulin sensitivity, hyperinsulinemia, and then hypertriglyceridemia, is an almost inevitable event. This is true of all kinds of rodent species, both genetic and acquired.*

B. METZGER: *I'll just respond to Steve (Fajans) earlier comment. I agree that cortisone glucose tolerance testing produces a similar deterioration as gestational diabetes. When administered to women with previous gestational diabetes, either cortisone or HPL, or the sex steroids, at least the synthetic ones, all produce decompensation similar to that seen in gestational diabetes. Usually, not quite as high a percentage. In pregnancy, a large percent of the population performs a stress event on themselves and, if identified and followed prospectively, we have the opportunity to identify the potential diabetics in a large percentage of the female population.*

N. FREINKEL: *Dr. Grasso, I think it's extremely intriguing that minor limitations in insulin availability should be translatable into oscillations of fuels other than glucose. We have been testing that for a number of years by taking some of the gestational diabetics, described by Dr. Metzger, and doing around-the-clock, 24 hour sampling. These are patients who then have, at most, minimal disturbances in insulin and no discernible disturbances in the fasting state. With these patients, we've been able to delineate not only abnormalities in glucose, but also abnormalities in amino acids, free fatty acids and triglycerides around the clock. It's the basis of this heightened oscillation of all the nutrients that made us propose that the determinant of insulin secretory maturation of the fetus must be the oscillation of all fuels, and that the oscillation of all of these fuels, exaggerated in the gestational diabetic, should eventuate in the hypersecretion of insulin in the neonate. Neonates of mild gestational diabetics do have a heightened insulin secretory mechanism. At the CIBA symposium, on the basis of this, we suggested that perhaps the Pedersen hypothesis requires expansion and can no longer be phrased in terms of just hyperglycemia, hyperinsulinism, but hyperfuel presentation, with hyperinsulinism as the determinant of neonatal hypersecretion.*

J. HOET: *Dr. Metzger, have you an idea about the weight gain during pregnancy and do you assess the dietary intake of your patients? Secondly, have you checked the recovery of that sluggishness after pregnancy in your gestational diabetics?*

B. METZGER: *The weight gain of our pregnant subjects, as well as our gestational diabetic subjects, is ascertained by history and by documentation of prepregnancy weight. The gain is no greater than that of the normal pregnant subjects. We have no precise quantitative breakdown of their dietary intake. That's a very difficult area to get reproduceable, reliable information. Regarding recovery of sluggishness, we now prospectively try to check all of them. We have limited numbers of patients tested post partum for their insulin secretion. Whether or not their sluggishness was present, antepartum study does not seem to identify those who will return to normal in postpartum. However, if they are normal postpartum, their peak insulin response appears to be early rather than late in the postpartum tests.*

E. TUTWILER: *Dr. Fajans, is there heterogeneity in terms of the response of insulin in either the high or low insulin responders, or in chemical versus overt diabets if you use secretogogues other than glucose? Do you see a change in the order of secretogogue potential between arginine, leucine, tolbutamide and glucose and the relationship of those three or four to each other when you go from one form of diabetes to another, or between what we're defining as high or low insulin responders?*

S. FAJANS: *Our data is very scanty along those lines. My impression would be that a high glucose responder is also a high arginine responder and a low glucose responder is a low arginine responder.*

R. CAMERINI-DAVALOS: *Dr. Reaven, would you like to comment on your studies on the insulin receptors in patients with early diabetes?*

G. M. REAVEN: *As a group, patients with chemical diabetes have decreased binding at every insulin concentration, along with insulin resistance, and the decrease in binding is due to a decrease in number of receptors with change in affinity. In general, the chemical diabetics have higher fasting insulin levels and less binding to the monocytes, but there are chemical diabetics with normal binding and low fasting insulin. We see people who have glucose intolerance with normal fasting insulin levels, normal number of insulin receptors, and respond to glucose with a low insulin response, and we have the opposite. Therefore, I think it's consistent with what we see.*

E. PFEIFFER: *I missed, in all of the reports, the percentage of regression from overt to chemical diabetes and from chemical diabetes to the normal situation.*

R. CAMERINI-DAVALOS: *A very good question. I do not have the figures with me, but I can give you my impression. I have the feeling that 50% of our chemical diabetics, including all, obese and nonobese, revert to at least one normal glucose tolerance test.*

S. FAJANS: *I think many of us, Dr. Camerini, Dr. Soeldner, and our own group have pointed out for many years that part of the natural history of early diabetes is fluctuation, even at the same weight, from normal to abnormal glucose tolerance, and there is no question that minor changes in body weight can be followed by definite changes in one direction or another. I'd like to make one comment that compounds the heterogeneity. I believe Dr. Reaven's data are fascinating, about the decreased number of insulin receptors in chemical diabetes. In his talk, he referred to the Pima Indians and these results were similar on hyperinsulinemia. However, Dr. Savage showed us some data yesterday where, in the Pima Indians there was no change in insulin receptors with the same hyperinsulinemia. So again, we are dealing with different groups of carbohydrate intolerance, and I think the picture isn't going to get any easier. It's only going to become more complicated, as we're going to get into different groups of carbohydrate intolerance.*

J. HOET: *I would like to come back to the presentation of Dr. Grasso and really also to stress the fact of what Dr. Freinkel said, to implement the Pedersen hypothesis, one has to take into account also the maturation of the gastrointestinal tract during fetal life. Over the last two years, we have been able to demonstrate that the fetal gastrointestinal tract matures, especially in the rat, during the last two days. This means that glucose, which appears into the gastrointestinal tract in the fetus, is available to the fetus at 21 days, for instance, but not at 19 days. As soon as the blood sugar of the fetus increases just 10 or 20 mg, the fetus immediately has a major glycosuria and that brings about an increase in the glucose of the amniotic fluid. In about one hour, the fetus swallows this and increases the amount of glucose in his stomach and in his gastrointestinal tract. That glucose can then be mobilized when you fast the mother, increase her intake of glucose, withdraw the amniotic fluid of the fetus -- all these changes are able to modify the blood glucose of the fetus predominantly at 21½ days or 21 days and not at 19, showing that really the Pedersen hypothesis has to be implemented for the maturation of the gastrointestinal tract.*

BETA CELL DYSFUNCTION IN MATURITY-ONSET DIABETES: REVERSIBLE LOSS OF GLUCOSE-INDUCED INSULIN SECRETION WITH RETENTION OF RESPONSE TO ARGININE

P.J. Savage*, L.J. Bennion, E.V. Flock
and P.H. Bennett

While spontaneous recovery from severe diabetes is an unusual event, weight reduction and restriction of carbohydrate intake in maturity-onset diabetes often leads to satisfactory control and improvement in endogenous insulin secretion in response to a glucose load (1-3). Furthermore, infusions of insulin sufficient to induce normoglycemia in mild maturity-onset diabetics for 40-60 hours result in enhanced endogenous insulin responses to intravenous glucose (4). Since the beta cell recovers its ability to secrete insulin when hyperglycemia is relieved by such interventions, it has been suggested that hyperglycemia itself might contribute to the decreased insulin secretion which characterizes overt maturity-onset diabetes (3). In an attempt to elucidate the mechanism of insulin secretory failure in maturity-onset diabetes we have investigated glucose and arginine-induced insulin secretion before and after weight loss. The findings indicate that recent-onset fasting hyperglycemia is characterized by a failure of the beta cell to secrete insulin in response to glucose, while the response to arginine stimulation is retained. This failure of beta cell function can be substantially improved by periods of a low carbohydrate hypocaloric diet.

PATIENTS AND METHODS

Six obese Pima Indian subjects, 2 men and 4 women, with symptomatic diabetes of 1-24 months duration were studied. They ranged in age from 20-56 years (Mean $\pm$ SEM 33 ± 5.5 yr) and their percent desirable weight (5) was initially 135-247% (194 ± 16.3%). They had initial fasting plasma glucose levels of 243-409 mg/dl

(281±26). None were taking medications.

All were admitted to a clinical research unit for the duration of the study (Range 35-138 days; Mean±SEM 73±15 days). Initially each was placed on a weight maintaining 300 gm carbohydrate diet and after 3 days received a 100 gm oral glucose tolerance test. On subsequent days, five received an intravenous (IV) glucose tolerance test (25 gm glucose infused over 3 minutes), and an intravenous arginine infusion (5 mg/Kg/min L-arginine monohydrochloride for 40 minutes). Each subject then started a 500 calorie 50 gm carbohydrate diet with daily iron and vitamin supplements. Potassium chloride was given as needed to prevent hypokalemia. Fasting glucose levels were determined weekly and the study continued until fasting glucose levels were stable for one month. Each was then given a 1500 calorie, 300 gm carbohydrate diet for four days which was sufficient to maintain weight in all subjects. The initial sequence of studies was then repeated. Results of the initial and final series of tests are reported.

Plasma glucose concentrations were measured on the AutoAnalyzer using the ferricyanide method (6). Immunoreactive serum insulin concentrations were measured by a double antibody immunoprecipitation technique (7).

Changes in glucose and insulin levels before and after diet intervention were evaluated by paired t-tests.

RESULTS

The fasting glucose levels fell from an initial mean (±SEM) of 281±26 mg/dl to a final level of 102±6 mg/dl ($p < 0.01$) and percent desirable weight fell by an average of 22% to 172±14.8% (11.8±1.54 Kg) ($p<0.01$). Fasting insulin levels decreased but did not change significantly. Insulin response following oral glucose, which was initially absent, increased to reach a three-hour post-load level of 126±31 μU/ml ($p<0.05$) (Figure 1). Glucose tolerance and insulin secretion were restored to the pattern seen in mild carbohydrate intolerance without fasting hyperglycemia.

In response to IV glucose infusion there was initially no demonstrable acute phase insulin response. After weight loss and restoration of fasting normoglycemia, a significant acute phase insulin response was found 4 to 6 minutes after the challenge (Table 1). Although the rate of glucose disappearance improved significantly ($p<0.05$), it remained abnormal.

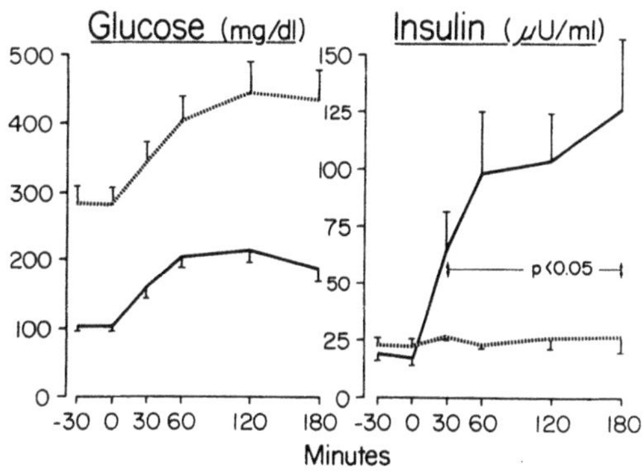

Fig. 1. Mean (±SEM) plasma glucose and serum insulin levels fasting and following a 100 gm oral glucose load before (interrupted line) and during (continuous line) diet-induced remission in six adults with recent-onset diabetes. The paired differences in glucose levels before and during remission were statistically significant at all time points ($p<0.01$). Fasting insulin levels were similar, but post-load insulin levels were statistically significantly different, ($p<0.05$) at all times.

Table 1

MEAN (±SEM) INSULIN LEVELS (μU/ml) AND GLUCOSE CLEARANCE (Kg) IN DIABETICS (N=5) DURING IV GLUCOSE TOLERANCE TESTS BEFORE AND AFTER WEIGHT LOSS

	Time (mins)								Clearance (Kg)
	0	3	4	5	6	10	30	60	
Before	25±9	24±7	23±9	21±6	17±5	14±3	28±8	26±7	0.39±0.02
After	17±2	42±53	42±20	43±18	38±13	32±11	36±6	46±6	0.61±0.06
P	NS	NS	<0.05	<0.05	<0.05	NS	NS	NS	<0.05

In contrast to the glucose response, insulin secretion in response to an IV arginine infusion, shown in Figure 2, was initially brisk, increasing from 22±5 to 69±21 μU/ml within 5 minutes ($p<0.05$). The response did not change significantly after weight reduction and restoration of fasting normoglycemia.

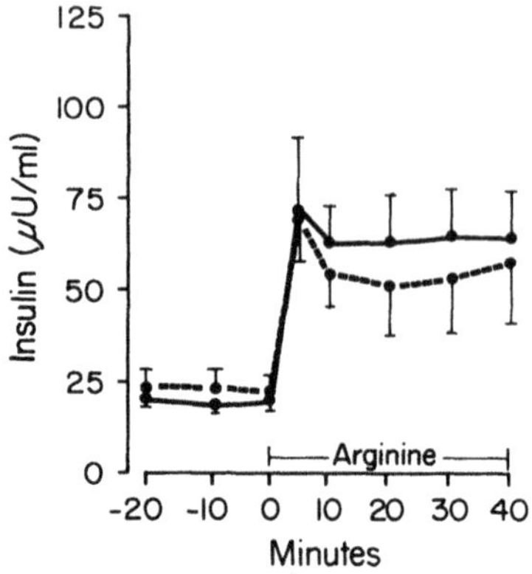

Fig. 2. Mean (±SEM) serum insulin levels before and during a 40-minute L-arginine infusion in five diabetic subjects before (interrupted line) and during (continuous line) diet-induced remission were not statistically different at any time point.

Sequential studies in three of these subjects have shown that the fall in fasting glucose levels occurred promptly with caloric and carbohydrate restriction. In contrast, glucose-induced insulin secretion returned more gradually over several weeks after restoration and maintenance of fasting normoglycemia. Fasting glucose levels have remained stable on followup six to ten months after discharge in those subjects who did not regain weight.

DISCUSSION

The present study confirms that caloric and carbohydrate restriction in recent onset, symptomatic, ketosis-resistant diabetes results in normalization of fasting glucose levels and a marked increase in insulin secretion in response to oral glucose administration. Prior to dietary intervention, all subjects had unequivocal fasting hyperglycemia and failed to increase insulin above fasting levels in response to either oral or intravenous glucose. At this time when the pancreas was completely refractory to glucose, a brisk insulin response occurred following arginine infusion confirming that the pancreatic beta cells retained the ability to manufacture and secrete insulin even during the period of fasting hyperglycemia.

The preservation of beta cell responsiveness to a non-glucose stimulus at a time when glucose induced insulin secretion is blunted has been demonstrated previously with isoproterenol (8) tolbutamide (9), glucagon (10) and arginine (11) in maturity-onset diabetics of other races and suggests that a specific loss of glucose-induced insulin secretion is a characteristic of ketosis resistant diabetes.

Despite the restoration of fasting normoglycemia and beta cell responsiveness to glucose following dietary intervention, glucose clearance remained abnormally slow and late hyperinsulinemia occurred. This observation is consistent with some component of extra pancreatic resistance to the action of insulin. Previous studies in both "genetic", i.e., non-diabetic offspring of two diabetic parents and "true", i.e., non-diabetics who have subsequently developed unequivocal diabetes, prediabetic Pima Indians have failed to demonstrate any impairment of insulin release in response to either intravenous or oral glucose prior to the onset of diabetes (12,13). Furthermore, in the Pimas, mild glucose intolerance with normal fasting glucose levels is accompanied by hyperinsulinemia following oral glucose, while more severe glucose intolerance with fasting hyperglycemia is characterized by hypoinsulinemic responses to glucose (14).

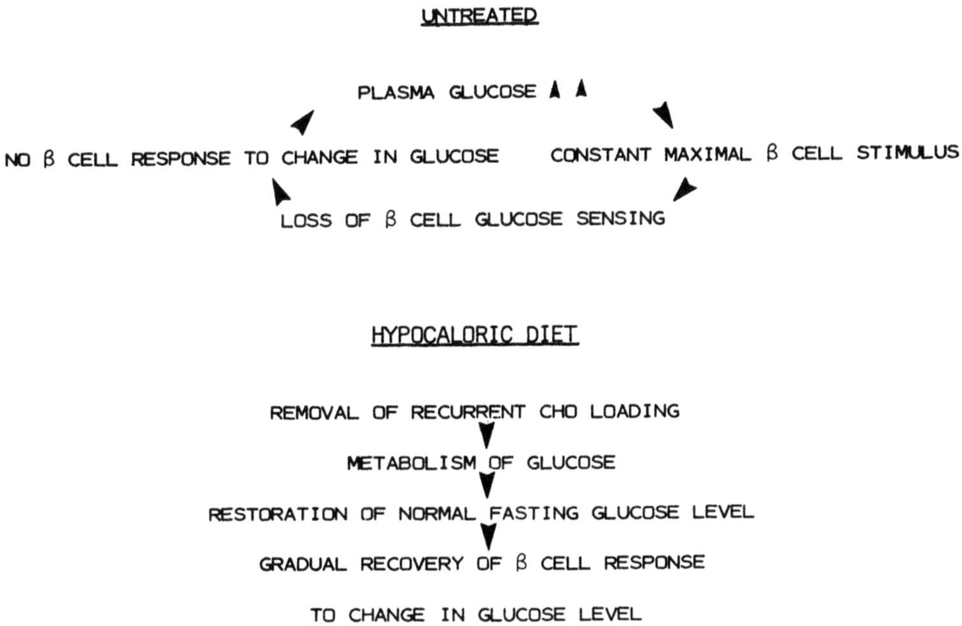

Fig. 3. Proposed mechanisms of beta cell decompensation and restoration of beta cell function by diet. See text for explanation.

Figure 3 shows a proposed scheme of how hyperglycemia develops. Much remains unknown about the cause of the initial increase in glucose levels. This may occur secondary to either a subtle pancreatic secretory defect or an increase in extra pancreatic insulin resistance. The increased insulin resistance described in borderline diabetics is consistent with the second mechanism (15). Once glucose levels have become elevated, there is progressive loss of beta cell sensitivity to changes in glucose concentration and secondary beta cell insulin secretory failure which leads to a major increase in hyperglycemia and symptomatic diabetes. There is some experimental evidence for this in man. Seltzer has reported that a continuous intravenous glucose infusion in six non-insulin requiring diabetics with fasting hyperglycemia resulted in increasing hyperglycemia with falling plasma insulin levels over a five day period (16).

It is also possible that sustained hyperglycemia may lead to more permanent damage. Experimental data in animals are consistent with this hypothesis. Dohan and Lukens (17) demonstrated that intraperitoneal glucose administration in cats can lead to permanent hyperglycemia with changes in the pancreatic islets.

Figure 3 also shows our formulation of how a hypocaloric diet works. In subjects with some residual insulin secretion much of their hyperglycemia is secondary to exogenous food intake. When this is curtailed, fasting glucose levels gradually fall into the normoglycemic range. With several weeks of normal fasting glucose levels a substantial amount of the secondary beta cell failure is reversed, at least in recent onset diabetics, and recovery of insulin secretion in response to a carbohydrate challenge produces improved glucose tolerance.

The therapeutic value of restoring beta cell responsiveness to glucose in the management of uncontrolled hyperglycemia is emphasized by the results of six to ten months' followup of patients in the present study. All have remained asymptomatic. In three, fasting plasma glucose levels have remained about 100 mg/dl, and in two, who have regained much of their weight, fasting plasma glucose levels have increased slightly but remain more than 125 mg/dl below their initial fasting levels. Until safe and more effective methods to induce and maintain fasting normoglycemia are found, intensive dietary management remains the treatment of choice for obese, ketosis resistant, recent onset diabetics.

REFERENCES

1. Rudnick, P.A. and Taylor, K.W. (1965). Brit. Med. J., 1,1225
2. Hadden, D.R., et al.(1975). Brit. Med. J., 3,276
3. Doar, J.W.H., et al.(1975). Lancet, 1,1263
4. Turner, R.C., et al.(1976). Brit. Med. J., 1,1252

5. *Recommended Dietary Allowances (1964). Publication 1146. Report of Food and Nutrition Board. Washington, D.C., National Research Council, National Academy of Sciences*
6. *Technicon Methodology File N-2b (1965). Technicon Instrument Corporation, Tarrytown, New York*
7. *Hales, C.N. and Randle, P.J. (1963). Biochem. J. 88,137*
8. *Robertson, R.P. and Porte, Jr. D. (1973) J. Clin. Invest. 52,870*
9. *Varsano-Aharon, N.E., et al (1970). Metab. Clin. Exp. 19,409*
10. *Kosaka, K., et al.(1974) Diabetologia, 10,775*
11. *Palmer, J.P., et al.(1976) J. Clin. Invest. 58,565*
12. *Aronoff, S.L., et al.(1977) Diabetes 26,827*
13. *Savage, P.J., et al.(1975) Lancet, 1,300*
14. *Savage, P.J., et al.(1975). Diabetes 24,362*
15. *Reaven, G.M., et al.(1976) Am. J. Med. 60,80*
16. *Seltzer, H.S. and Harris, V.L. (1964) Diabetes 13,6*
17. *Dohan, F.C. and Lukens, F.D.W. (1948) Endocrinology 42,244*

We wish to thank the Pima Indian patients who volunteered for this investigation, together with Ms. Judy Brown, Linda Phillips, and Mary Barham for technical assistance, and Ms. Jean Koopman and the nursing staff of the Phoenix Clinical Research Section, and Ms. Janet Clark for secretarial assistance.

Supported in part by National Institutes of Health Contract N01-A-06-2219.

IMPROVEMENT OF INSULIN SECRETION IN DIABETICS BY A PROSTAGLANDIN SYNTHESIS INHIBITOR

R. P. Robertson*, M. Chen, J. R. McRae and
S. A. Metz

Loss of first phase insulin secretion (the acute insulin response) which normally occurs 3-5 minutes after an intravenous glucose pulse is characteristic of patients with fasting hyperglycemia (1). This observation is of interest for several reasons. The acute insulin response (AIR) is probably lost relatively early in the pathogenesis of diabetes since it is absent when circulating glucose levels are only slightly elevated and at a time when basal insulin and second phase insulin secretion are probably normal. A second reason is that the loss of the AIR in hyperglycemic, non-insulin-dependent diabetics is only to glucose stimulation. Acute responses to intravenous isoproterenol and arginine, for instance, remain intact (2,3) despite absent responses to glucose. This suggests a defect related to an abnormality in glucose recognition by the beta cell rather than inadequacy of insulin synthesis or stores in the islet, i.e., the postulated "glucoreceptor" defect. A third reason this defect is of interest lies in the fact that absent first phase insulin secretion is restorable by alpha adrenergic blockade with phentolamine (4). These studies with phentolamine evolved from the observations that alpha adrenergic agonists inhibit the AIR (5) and that circulating catecholamines are elevated in some diabetics (4). They led to the hypothesis that diabetes might be characterized as a state of increased endogenous alpha adrenergic activity.

A similar line of reasoning involving prostaglandins led to the studies described in this manuscript. We had previously demonstrated that prostaglandins (PG) E_1 and E_2 inhibited insulin secretion in vivo in dogs (6). This inhibition was independent of alpha adrenergic activity since phentolamine failed to reverse the inhibitory properties of PGE_1. These findings have subsequently been confirmed by several investigators (7,8). Based upon our results in dogs, we have pursued similar studies in human volunteers and in patients with hyperglycemic, non-insulin-dependent diabetes.

THE EFFECTS OF PGE_2 AND INHIBITION OF PGE_2 SYNTHESIS IN HUMAN VOLUNTEERS

Prostaglandin E_2 was infused intravenously at a rate (10mcg/min) previously shown to increase circulating PGE_2 levels three-fold (9). During the infusion, a small but statistically significant increase in circulating glucose was observed (Table 1). The acute insulin response measured 3-5 minutes after an intravenous glucose pulse was decreased by nearly 50%. This inhibition was accompanied by a significant decrease in glucose disappearance rates following the glucose challenge. During control infusions with saline, rather than PGE_2, none of these changes were observed. In contrast to this inhibitory effect of PGE_2 upon glucose-induced AIR, PGE_2 has no effect upon AIR's to intravenous arginine or isoproterenol (Table 2).

Sodium salicylate was infused to inhibit endogenous PGE_2 synthesis. This infusion rate (40mg/min) increased the serum salicylate levels to approximately 25mg/dl. Sodium salicylate caused a two-fold increase in circulating insulin levels and augmented glucose-induced AIR's (Table 1).

Table 1. The effect of infusions in normal humans of PGE_2 (10mcg/min), saline and sodium salicylate (40mg/min) on circulating glucose (GLU), insulin (INS), acute insulin response (AIR) and glucose disappearance rate (K_G). Pulse 1 (glucose, 5g IV) was given before and pulse 2 was given during the infusion. "p" values refer to comparisons between data before and during infusions. Data = $\bar{x}$ ± SE.

Pulse 1	PGE_2 (n=10)	Saline (n=10)	Sodium Salicylate (n=6)
GLU, mg/dl	96 ± 2	100 ± 2	92 ± 3
INS, μU/ml	12 ± 3	12 ± 2	8 ± 2
AIR, % basal	593 ± 104	518 ± 115	313 ± 62
K_G, %/min	0.73 ± 0.07	0.79 ± 0.10	0.78 ± 0.11
Pulse 2			
GLU, mg/dl	102 ± 1**	99 ± 2	90 ± 3
INS, μU/ml	11 ± 2	11 ± 5	15 ± 3
AIR, % basal	312 ± 55***	464 ± 102	660 ± 86****
K_G, %/min	0.49 ± 0.06*	0.80 ± 0.06	0.89 ± 0.06

*p<.025
**p<.01
***p<.005
****p<.001

Table 2. The effect of PGE_2 infusion on responses to arginine and isoproterenol. Data = $\bar{x} \pm$ SE.

Control	Arginine 2g IV (n=5)	Isoproterenol 2mcg IV (n=6)
GLU mg/dl	102 ± 3	103 ± 3
INS, μU/ml	17 ± 5	13 ± 2
AIR, % basal	592 ± 164	243 ± 48
PGE_2		
GLU, mg/dl	105 ± 3	106 ± 3
INS, μU/ml	19 ± 5	16 ± 3
AIR, % basal	590 ± 118	168 ± 33

THE EFFECT OF SODIUM SALICYLATE UPON INSULIN SECRETION IN DIABETICS

Diabetics were infused with sodium salicylate using the same protocol as that used with normal volunteers. The mean fasting plasma glucose level was 196 ± 19mg/dl and the mean glucose disappearance rate was 0.56 ± 0.05%/min (Table 3). There was no AIR to a control glucose injection. Sodium salicylate infusion increased the circulating insulin level and, in marked contrast to the control injection, the second glucose pulse given during the sodium salicylate infusion stimulated an acute insulin response. This response was accompanied by an almost two-fold improvement in glucose disposal. There were no increases in circulating insulin levels or glucose disappearance rates, nor was there a restoration of the acute insulin response during control studies in which saline rather than sodium salicylate were infused.

Table 3. The effect of sodium salicylate and saline infusion on responses in diabetics.

Pulse 1	Sodium Salicylate (n=12)	Saline (n=6)
GLU, mg/dl	196 ± 19	231 ± 29
INS, μU/ml	18 ± 4	15 ± 3
AIR, % basal	5 ± 6	-13 ± 7
K_G, %/min	0.56 ± 0.05	0.65 ± 0.08
Pulse 2		
GLU, mg/dl	174 ± 21	208 ± 32
INS, μU/ml	38 ± 7****	14 ± 4
AIR, % basal	97 ± 24***	11 ± 10
K_G, %/min	1.02 ± 0.17****	0.72 ± 0.09

***p<.005
****p<.001

POSSIBLE INTERRELATIONSHIPS BETWEEN THE EFFECT OF PHENTOLAMINE AND SODIUM SALICYLATE

Since we had previously reported that phentolamine partially restored the AIR (although to a lesser extent than sodium salicylate), we speculated that there may be a relationship in the pancreatic islet between the effects of alpha-adrenergic antagonism and inhibition of PGE_2 synthesis. To test the hypothesis that endogenous PGE_2 synthesis. To test the hypothesis that endogenous PGE_2 synthesis might be required for the full expression of alpha-adrenergic effects on the beta cell, we investigated whether sodium salicylate would block the ability of epinephrine to inhibit the acute insulin response. Epinephrine was infused intravenously (3mg/min) in normal volunteers. Compared to the control, epinephrine caused a significant inhibition of the AIR to glucose (Table 4). When sodium salicylate and epinephrine were infused simultaneously, however, the AIR to glucose was two-thirds recovered. This finding was consistent with the hypothesis that endogenous PGE synthesis contributes to alpha-adrenergic events in the islet.

Table 4. Partial reversal by sodium salicylate of alpha-adrenergic inhibition of glucose-induced AIR.

	Control	Epinephrine (3mcg/min IV) n=6	Epinephrine and Sodium Salicylate (40mg/min IV) n=6
GLU, mg/dl	93 ± 3	129 ± 6	122 ± 6
	└── $p<.02$ ──┘		
INS, μU/ml	11 ± 3	14 ± 2	19 ± 4
AIR, % basal	463 ± 149	97 ± 38	339 ± 137
	└── $p<.02$ ──┘	└── $p<.02$ ──┘	
K_G, %/min	1.87 ± 0.41	0.60 ± 0.12	0.72 ± 0.13
	└── $p<.02$ ──┘		

SUMMARY AND CONCLUSIONS

These studies with PGE_2 and an inhibitor of PGE_2 synthesis (sodium salicylate) suggest that PGE_2 in humans caused inhibition of glucose-induced acute insulin responses. This inhibition appears to be specific for glucose stimulation because the responses to the non-glucose insulin secretogogues, arginine and isoproterenol, were not affected by PGE_2. Restoration by sodium salicylate of absent AIR to glucose in the diabetic subjects was accompanied by substantial improvement in glucose disposal. The only other pharmacologic agent that has been shown to do this is phentolamine, an alpha-adrenergic antagonist. The magnitude of restoration with sodium salicylate is substantially greater than that reported with phentolamine (4). Furthermore, there is no improvement in glucose disposal or second phase insulin secretion with phentolamine whereas there is a four-fold improvement in this phase during sodium salicylate treatment (9-11). The study in which sodium salicylate and epinephrine infusions were given simultaneously has raised the interesting possibility that endogenous PGE_2 synthesis at the pancreatic level may contribute to the alpha-adrenergic activity of epinephrine.

In conclusion, we wish to emphasize that investigation of abnormal first phase insulin secretion in diabetics is a valuable metabolic approach with which to clarify the incompletely understood pathogenesis of defective insulin secretion. Moreover, the demonstration that absent acute insulin responses to glucose can be at least partially restored by pharmacologic agents such as phentolamine and sodium salicylate raises the possibility of a new approach to the therapy of diabetes, namely, improvement of defective glucose recognition by the beta cell.

REFERENCES

1. *Brunzell, J.D. et al. (1976). J. Clin. Endocrinol. Metab. 42, 222.*
2. *Robertson, R.P. et al. (1973). J. Clin. Invest. 52, 870.*
3. *Lerner, R.L. and Prte, D., Jr. (1971). Clin. Res. 19, 478.*
4. *Robertson, R.P. et al. (1976). J. Clin. Invest. 57, 791.*
5. *Porte, D., Jr. and Robertson, R.P. (1973). Fed. Proc. 32, 1792.*
6. *Robertson, R.P. et al. (1974). J. Clin. Invest. 54, 310.*
7. *Sacca, L. et al. (1975). Acta Endocrinol. 79, 266.*
8. *Dodi, G. et al. (1978). Surgery 83, 206.*
9. *Robertson, R.P. and Chen, M. (1977). Trans. Assoc. Am. Phys.90, 353.*
10. *Robertson, R.P. and Chen, M. (1977). J. Clin. Invest. 60, 747.*
11. *Chen, M. and Robertson, R.P. (1978). Diabetes 27, 750.*

DISCUSSION

P. SAVAGE: *One thing that appears quite clear from the results of our studies is that there is some form of secondary beta cell deterioration and we seem to be able to reverse it. However, in the shortest restoration there was approximately a month of normal fasting glucose levels, and despite this, the two hour glucose did not become completely normal. Therefore, we think we're reversing some sort of a secondary failure, but what the underlying event is, and whether or not severe diabetics can be brought back to the normal state, is a question that we have not been able to prove yet.*

G. M. REAVEN: *We had the same kind of patients in the hospital: fasting glucoses very comparable to what Dr. Savage described, and obesity. We took away their food for approximately two weeks and we quickly normalized their fasting glucose concentration. At the end of two weeks, we put them back on food. At that time, they still maintained some advantage in terms of glucose concentration, but their insulin secretion, which was at the beginning, poor, remained poor. So, in a two-week normalization of plasma glucose concentration, we were incapable of restoring insulin response to normal. Two questions: what are the differences between Pimas and Caucasians, and between 2 weeks and several months of dieting?*

P. SAVAGE: *We also tried a period of 7-10 days of fasting and refeeding in a couple of subjects, but they did not respond as well as the people who were on the diet for a month. Another factor, which I think might be quite important, is the duration of the diabetes. The preliminary data indicates that there's no difference whatsoever between the Caucasians and the Pima Indians, provided they're selected in the same way. They both seemed to respond quite well to several months of dieting, but I think the question of duration of diabetes might be a key one, and one of the other important points is the length of time to restore fasting glucose levels to normal. There may be some minimal time required before insulin secretion starts to recover. We arbitrarily picked the time of our studies. We may have been fortunate in picking a long enough time to show the difference.*

R. CAMERINI-DAVALOS: *Dr. Savage, in 1977, at the American Diabetes Association meeting, your group showed that one of the first changes in prediabetics subjects was increased appetite.*

P. SAVAGE: *The data I showed yesterday, that the children of two diabetic parents were heavier, would be consistent with either an increase in appetite or an increased efficiency of utilizing food and storing it. Obesity is clearly one of the potentially modifiable risk factors we've identified in the Pimas. Obesity clearly stands out with any type of study, with just a simple correlation analysis or with all sorts of complicated multivariant computer modeling. What obesity does is to increase resistance to whatever insulin is available. In that sense, it clearly fits into this scheme, and increasing obesity would precipitate secondary beta cell decompensation.*

B. METZGER: *Others have reported hyperinsulinemic responses to arginine in maturity onset diabetes, and Dr. Grasso pointed out this morning that arginine and glucose are synergistic when one is studying insulin response. Have you made any correction for the difference in glucose levels during the two tests in evaluating the arginine?*

P. SAVAGE: *As far as I know, we have not. Also, if you notice, on that slide of response to arginine, although the levels are very similar, the level of insulin reached at the end of the period of dietary restriction is slightly higher, and that is reached at a glucose level several hundred milligrams lower. So, there could be some increase in response to arginine which is not detectable.*

B. METZGER: *I wonder, if one were testing at the same glucose levels, one wouldn't also see impairment of insulin secretion response to amino acids. In other words, when we compare maturity onset diabetics, or you take the after-weight-loss group and elevated their glucose to 300, adding arginine to that, wouldn't we demonstrate a reduction of responsiveness to amino acids during the hyperglycemic phase?*

P. SAVAGE: *One of the intriguing questions is whether the response to different secretogogues can be used to assess residual beta cell potential and beta cell response. We're in the process of expanding these studies to see if we can get more information as to whether diabetics have normal or diminished insulin response to arginine, even though it's clearly different than the insulin response to glucose in the severely diabetic state. Whether you can use it to measure residual beta cell capacity and even use it to indicate the worth of caloric restriction, is something we'd like further information on.*

M. VRANIC: *Don't you think it's unlikely that the glycemic change is responsible for unresponsiveness of the beta cells? Because, if you take animal studies subjecting the beta cells to similar glycemic levels, you really don't see much degranulation. In order to see degranulation of beta cell, I think you have to have much more pronounced hyperglycemia. In addition, if you subject rats to periods of hyperglycemia infusing glucose, you actually make the beta cell more responsive. Therefore, why postulate glucose? Why not postulate an unknown factor?*

P. SAVAGE: *That's a possibility, but I think there's a difference between most of the animal studies that have been conducted and the situation that we're looking at here. These individuals have been hyperglycemic for periods of up to two years. Most studies conducted in animals are relatively short periods of hyperglycemia. There's a paper which I think does indicate that glucose can cause decompensation in humans, and that's a paper written in 1965 by Dr. Seltzer, in which he took a group of normals, a group with impaired carbohydrate tolerance, and a group with overt carbohydrate intolerance and infused glucose into them for periods of up to seven days. At the end of seven days, the normals were still hyperinsulinemic, putting out large amounts of insulin; the overt diabetics had little insulin response at any time during the glucose infusion; and the borderline initially responded with increased insulin secretion, which fell at the end of that period. So, the issue of whether you could take a normal person with a perfectly normal pancreas, raise their glucose level for a period of time, and cause them to decompensate, remains unknown. However, I think, in people with impaired glucose tolerance, there is evidence you can have this desensitization of the beta cell, or whatever you'd like to call it.*

J. HOET: *There is the work of Ogilvie in Edinburgh, 10 or 15 years ago, which showed that, in the obese with normal glucose tolerance curve, there was a hyperplasia of the islets of Langerhans. But, as soon as there was an impaired glucose tolerance curve, there was a reduction of islet cell mass.*

K.G.M.M. ALBERTI: *The question is what effect does the treatment have on that impaired or reduced islet cell mass?*

S. FAJANS: *In relation to Dr. Metzger's comment, I think we need to distinguish between the arginine response in diabetic patients before and after caloric restriction and the comparison between diabetic and normal in response to arginine. We've shown that diabetic patients have a decreased insulin response to arginine, as compared to normal control subjects, but that the phase one response is decreased much less than the second phase insulin response.*

EFFECT OF DIET LIMITATION ON DEVELOPMENT OF DIABETES IN NON-HYPERPHAGIC PREDIABETIC CHINESE HAMSTERS

C. Gerritsen* and M. C. Blanks

There is little doubt that the interrelation between food intake, obesity, abnormal carbohydrate metabolism, and abnormal pancreatic hormonal secretion is complex. The subject has been reviewed many times, recently by Woods and Porte (1). It is clear that obesity contributes to abnormal carbohydrate metabolism and abnormal insulin secretion in animals (2) and man (3) and conversely, weight reduction tends to correct these abnormalities (4).

It is not known if correction or prevention of obesity by limiting caloric intake will retard or prevent onset of diabetes in prediabetic humans. However, it was shown that limiting food intake to 2.5 grams per day will prevent onset of diabetes in hyperphagic, prediabetic Chinese hamsters born to ketonuric dams and sires (5). Subsequently, it was possible to inbreed sublines of hamsters to the point where all animals develop diabetes. Prediabetics from these highly inbred sublines have diabetic but not ketonuric parents and do not eat significantly more food than their nonprediabetic controls. It was of interest to determine if limiting of food to 2.5 grams per day would alter the development of diabetes in the nonhyperphagic prediabetic Chinese hamsters.

METHODS

Weanling Chinese hamsters, approximately 3 weeks of age, were used. Prediabetics were selected from lines in which all animals became glycosuric by 8 weeks of age. These prediabetics had diabetic but not ketonuric parents and were not significantly hyperphagic. Nonprediabetic hamsters matched for age and sex were used as controls.

All animals were fed Purina Mouse Chow containing 11% fat, 17% protein and 51% carbohydrate. Half of each litter were restricted to 2.5 grams of food per day while their siblings were allowed food ad lib. Animals were tested daily for glycosuria by TesTape[R]. Food consumption of ad lib fed animals was measured by weighing food in and out at 7 day intervals and the average daily food consumption calculated. Two and one half grams of diet were given to diet limited animals each morning. Nonfasting blood glucose and plasma insulin levels were measured at intervals shown in Tables 1 and 2.

All animals were killed by exsanguination in the nonfasted state at nine weeks of age. The tail of the pancreas was removed immediately, fixed in Bouin's, prepared for paraffin embedding and sections stained with aldehyde fuchsin. The remainder of the pancreas was assayed for insulin and glucagon. Blood glucose, plasma insulin and glucagon were determined.

RESULTS

Data from the first eight weeks of diet restriction to 2.5 grams per day for prediabetic Chinese hamsters are presented in Table 1. During the first week post-weaning, food consumption of ad lib

Table 1

EFFECT OF DIET LIMITATION ON DEVELOPMENT OF DIABETES IN PREDIABETIC CHINESE HAMSTERS[a]

Measurement	Diet (g/d)	Age - weeks 3	4	5	6	7	8
Food consumption (g/d)	2.5	-	2.5	2.5	2.5	2.5	2.5
	Ad Lib	-	4.8	3.5	3.1	3.2	3.2
Body weight (g)	2.5	16	13	15	17	17	19
	Ad Lib	17	19	21	21	22	22
% Glycosuric	2.5	0	0	33	33	33	33
	Ad Lib	0	0	50	66	100	100
Blood Glucose (mg/dl)[b]	2.5	115	-	146	-	169	-
	Ad Lib	122	-	209[c]	-	227[c]	-
Plasma Insulin μU/ml)[b]	2.5	-	-	24	-	-	-
	Ad Lib	-	-	106[c]	-	-	-

[a]Means of six prediabetics per group; [b]Nonfasting values; [c]2.5 g/d vs. ad lib; $p<0.01$

prediabetics was high (4.8 g/d) but tapered off to a mean daily consumption of 3.5 to 3.2 g/d. This was slightly higher than consumption of the diet limited prediabetics but similar to food consumption of ad lib fed nonprediabetic controls who ate from 3.0 to 3.7 g/d.

Although body weight of prediabetics was similar at weaning, diet limited prediabetics were significantly lighter after one week. This significant difference in weight persisted for the duration of the experiment. Although not shown in Table 1, there was no difference in body weight of ad lib fed prediabetics compared with ad lib fed nonprediabetics. Weight of ad lib fed nonprediabetics ranged from 19.6-21.0 g.

During the second week, 3/6 ad lib fed prediabetics spontaneously developed glycosuria (4+ TesTape) while 2/6 prediabetics never showed glycosuria. By contrast all of the ad lib fed prediabetics showed glycosuria (4+ TesTape) by the fourth week.

At the beginning of the experiment, there was no difference in nonfasting blood glucose of either prediabetics or nonprediabetics. However, nonfasting blood glucose of ad lib fed predia-was significantly elevated at 5 and 7 weeks compared with the diet limited prediabetics. Nonfasting blood glucose levels of nonprediabetic diet limited (105 ± 10) and ad lib fed (115 ± 3) hamsters was significantly lower than limited prediabetics.

Ad lib prediabetic hamsters had significantly higher plasma insulin levels than their diet-limited prediabetic siblings or nonprediabetic ad lib fed (56 ± 17) or limited (66 ± 5) controls.

The animals were killed after 6 weeks of diet restriction or ad lib feeding. The data are presented in Table 2. Body weight of ad lib fed prediabetics was significantly greater than their prediabetic siblings fed 2.5 g/d. Their body weight was not different than nonprediabetics fed ad lib. Blood glucose of diet limited prediabetics was normal but ad lib fed prediabetics had significantly higher blood glucose levels. The ad lib fed prediabetics were still markedly hyperinsulinemic compared with either their diet limited siblings or nonprediabetic controls. It should be emphasized that diet limited prediabetics had normal plasma insulin levels. No differences in glucagon levels were observed in either plasma or pancreas. The level of insulin in the pancreas of diet limited prediabetics appeared to be higher than their ad lib fed siblings but the difference was not significant due to small numbers and large variation. Histology of these pancreata was consistent with the biochemical data (Figure 1). The islet on the left is representative of the nonfasted nondiabetic islet and had normal granulation. The center islet represents the food limited prediabetic with moderate granulation, and the right islet is representative of the ad lib fed prediabetic group, which shows marked degranulation.

Table 2

EFFECT OF NINE WEEKS OF DIET LIMITATION ON CHINESE HAMSTERS[a]

Measurement	Diet (g/d)	Animal Type[b] Prediabetic	Nonprediabetic
Body weight (g)	2.5	20 ± 0.7	19 ± 1.3
	Ad Lib	24 ± 0.9[c]	21 ± 2.0
Blood Glucose (mg/dl)	2.5	105 ± 1.7	119 ± 4.5
	Ad Lib	177 ± 7.2[c]	125 ± 15
Plasma Insulin μU/ml	2.5	17 ± 6.2	13 ± 4.1
	Ad Lib	125 ± 23	20 ± 7.8
Plasma Glucagon pg/ml	2.5	74 ± 30	121 ± 3.4
	Ad Lib	104 ± 22	153 ±13.5
Pancreatic Insulin μU/g	2.5	0.69 ± 0.21	0.83 ±0.16
	Ad Lib	0.45 ± 0.03	0.87 ±0.36
Pancreatic Glucagon μU/g	2.5	5.6 ± 1.3	4.6 ±0.5
	Ad Lib	4.2 ± 0.6	4.6 ±0.4

[a]Terminal values obtained in the nonfasted state.
[b]Prediab. on 2.5 g/d, $\bar{X}$=4; Prediab. fed ad lib $\bar{X}$=6; Nonpred. on 2.5 g/d, $\bar{X}$=3; Nonprediab. fed ad lib, $\bar{X}$=2.
[c]2.5 g/d vs. ad lib control, $p<0.01$

DISCUSSION

Unfortunately, there are no conclusive data in man which demonstrate that regulation of food intake or maintenance of ideal body weight will prevent or retard the onset of diabetes, but it has been observed that the incidence of diabetes decreased during periods of caloric restriction such as wars. It has been suggested that excessive caloric intake of infants might contribute to obesity and ultimate development of diabetes (6,7).

Our data suggest that dietary limitation of prediabetic Chinese hamsters did prevent onset of glycosuria. It is important to note that these animals were not hyperphagic compared with non-prediabetic controls, but it is conceivable that they contained more body fat than their prediabetic siblings limited to 2.5 g/d. The data also suggest that these prediabetic Chinese hamsters were hyperinsulinemic at the time they were beginning to show glycosuria. Is it possible that these animals, like man and other animals, may go through a hyperinsulinemic phase prior to beta cell exhaustion and death?

Due to small size of the weanling Chinese hamster, plasma insulin could not be measured at weaning when blood glucose was normal. Therefore, it is not known if hyperinsulinism was present prior to hyperglycemia in these animals. Unfortunately, there is no a priori method to establish the cause and effect relationship between obesity, abnormal insulin levels and abnormal carbohydrate metabolism in man. Very carefully planned experiments on the prediabetic hyperinsulinemic Chinese hamster may help provide insight into the complex interrelationships between obesity, hyperinsulinism and hyperglycemia.

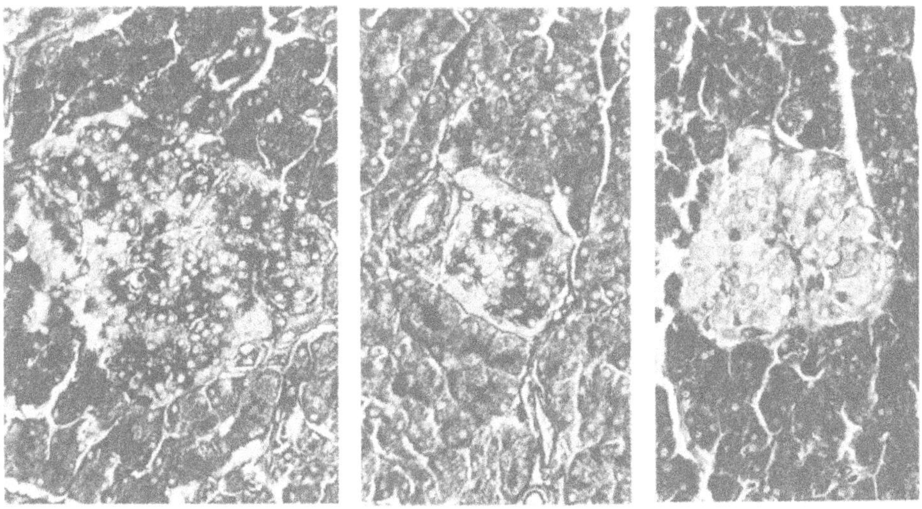

Fig. 1. Islets representative from normal, restricted prediabetic and ad lib fed prediabetic Chinese hamsters.

REFERENCES

1. Woods, S.C. and Porte, D., Jr. (1978 in Advances in Metabolic Disorders, Volume 9, Levine, R. and Luft, R. eds., Academic Press, New York, p. 283
2. Herberg, L.J. and Coleman, D.L. (1977). Metabolism 26, 59
3. Woods, S.C. et al. (1975). Psychol. Rev. 82, 1965

4. *Grodsky, G.M. and Benoit, F.L. (1969). Proceedings, VI Congress of the International Diabetes Federation, Ostmann, J. ed., Excerpta Medica, Amsterdam, p. 540*
5. *Gerritsen, G.C. et al. (1974). Diabetologia 10, 559*
6. *Porter, A.M.W. (1972). Lancet 2, 1250*
7. *Yudkin, J. (1972). Lancet 2, 1424*

The authors gratefully acknowledge the invaluable assistance of M.G. Soret and E.M. Block on the histology and its interpretation.

THE ROLE OF RIBOFLAVIN IN CARBOHYDRATE METABOLISM

A. S. Reddi*, P.K. Ho and
R. A. Camerini-Davalos

Riboflavin, in its coenzyme forms, flavin adenine dinucleotide (FAD) and flavin mononucleotide (FMN), plays an important role in intermediary metabolism (1,2). Its deficiency causes both structural and functional abnormalities (1-3).

A relationship between riboflavin deficiency and carbohydrate metabolism was suggested by earlier investigators in dogs (4,5) and rats (6). In riboflavin-deficient dogs, both lower (4) and higher (5) fasting blood sugar levels were reported. In those with higher fasting blood sugars, the response to oral glucose was impaired as in diabetic animals (5). In riboflavin-deficient rats, both normal and lower fasting blood sugar levels were reported (6). In these rats, the tolerance to oral glucose was normal (6). However, no study has yet been reported on circulating insulin levels in riboflavin-deficient animals.

The purposes of the present investigation were to study: 1) glucose tolerance, 2) circulating insulin levels, 3) insulin response to oral glucose load and 4) insulin sensitivity in Swiss albino mice fed either a normal diet ad libitum or a riboflavin-deficient diet or a normal diet restricted in quantity to the amount ingested by the deficient animals.

MATERIAL AND METHODS

Experimental Material

Male Swiss albino mice (40-day-old) were used in the study. They were divided into three groups. One group was fed the Old Guilford mouse chow (The Emory Morse Co., Guilford, Conn.). The second group was placed on a riboflavin-deficient diet (ICN Life Sciences Group, Cleveland, OH). The third group was fed the old Guilford mouse chow, but pair-fed to riboflavin-deficient mice. All groups of mice were fed the respective diets for 45-55 days. The mice were maintained in plastic cages with sanichips as bedding.

The mice on riboflavin-deficient diets were divided into three groups based on their signs of deficiency and weight. Those that lost weight and had severe signs of deficiency and ocular manifestations were classified as severely-deficient mice. Those that did not lose weight, but showed moderate signs of deficiency and no ocular manifestations were called moderately-deficient mice. Those mice that neither lost weight nor showed signs of deficiency were classified as non-deficient.

Both moderate and severely-deficient mice were supplemented with riboflavin in food (4 mg/lb) and by intraperitoneal injections, after 55 days of feeding the deficient diet. Each mouse received 150 ug of riboflavin in 0.9% saline per day for 21 days.

Oral Glucose Tolerance Tests

These tests were done between 10 A.M. and 1 P.M. The mice were fasted for 18 hours with free access to water. After collecting blood from the eye at 0 min., the mice were given 3 g/kg (0.1 ml/10g) of glucose by mouth using a gastric catheter. Subsequent samples were collected at 30, 60, 120 and 180 min.

Insulin Response to Oral Glucose Load

After an 18 hour fast, blood was collected from the orbital plexus into capillary tubes. The mice were then given 3 g/kg of glucose and subsequent samples were collected at 60 and 180 min. Serum was separated and kept frozen at -25°C until immunoreactive insulin levels (IRI) were determined.

Insulin Sensitivity Tests

The mice were fasted for 6 hours with free access to water from 7 A.M. to 1 P.M. After collecting blood at 0 min., they were injected intraperitoneally with 1U/kg of bovine crystalline insulin and subsequent blood samples were collected at 15, 30, 60, 120 and 240 min. as described before for the determination of blood sugar levels.

Analytical procedures

Blood sugars were determined by potassium ferricyanide method of Hoffman on the Technicon Autoanalyzer (7). Serum insulin levels were determined by a radioimmunoassay, using an immunosorbent as described by Velasco et al. (8).

Statistical Analysis

Student's t test for unpaired and paired samples was applied to calculate the significance of the difference between means of observations. The probability levels above 0.05 were considered non-significant.

RESULTS

Body Weights

The mice fed a regular chow diet ad libitum gained weight P<0.01) whereas the paired-fed controls neither gained nor lost weight. The severely-deficient mice did not show any change in their body weight. The non-deficient mice continuously gained weight as those of control mice (P<0.05). On supplementation with riboflavin, both severely and moderately-deficient mice gained weight as those of control mice.

Oral Glucose Tolerance

The blood sugar response to an oral glucose load in various groups of mice is shown in Fig. 1. The blood sugar levels following glucose load were significantly lower in severely-deficient mice, when compared to either group of controls, non-deficient or moderately-deficient mice. On the other hand, the blood sugars were significantly higher at 60, 120 and 180 min. after glucose load in moderately-deficient than in control (ad libitum) mice. Between the control mice, significantly higher blood sugar levels were found at 30, 60 and 120 min. following oral glucose in pair-fed animals. In non-deficient mice, the blood sugars were significantly lower only at 120 and 180 min. than in control (ad libitum) mice.

When both severely and moderately-deficient mice were supplemented with riboflavin, their tolerance to glucose returned to normal.

Serum IRI Response to Glucose

The serum IRI levels were significantly lower (P<0.005) in pair-fed controls than in mice fed ad libitum only at 180 min. following glucose load (Fig. 2). A significant increase (P<0.001) in IRI levels was found in severely-deficient mice at 60 min. after glucose, when compared to both groups of control mice. By contrast, a significant decrease was observed in moderately-deficient mice. Although the IRI levels at 180 min. were not significantly different between control (ad libitum) and moderately-

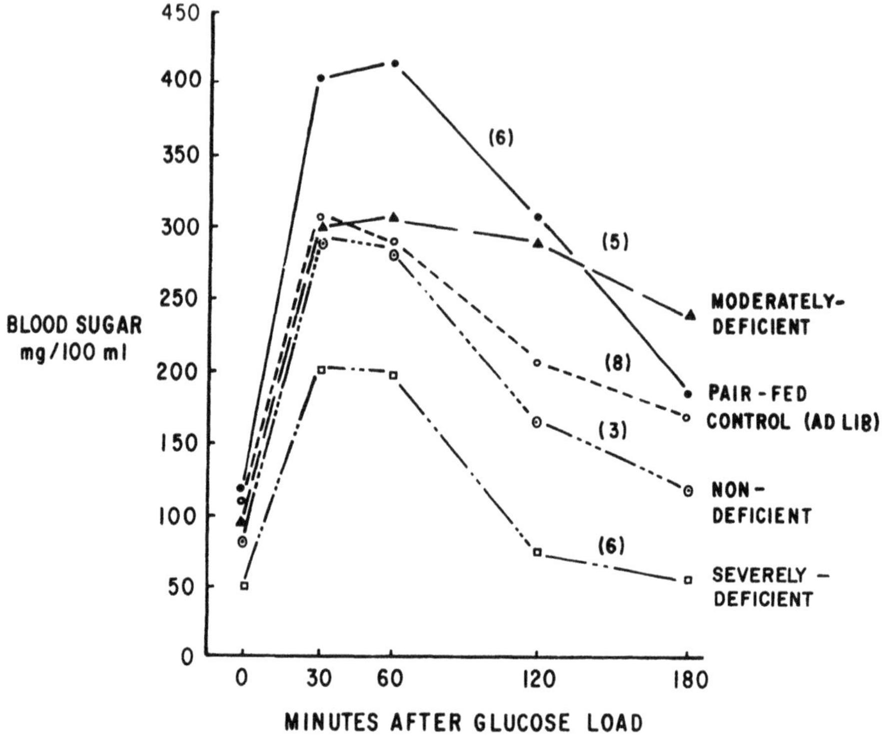

Fig. 1. Oral glucose tolerance tests in various groups of mice after an 18 hour fast. Figures in parentheses indicate number of mice in each group.

deficient mice, a significant decrease ($P<0.02$) was found in pair-fed controls when compared to moderately-deficient mice. The IRI response to glucose was similar in both control(ad libitum) and riboflavin repleted mice. On the other hand, the IRI levels were significantly lower ($P<0.005$) at 180 min. in pair-fed controls than in riboflavin repleted mice. There were no differences in IRI levels between pair-fed controls and non-deficient mice. However, in the latter group, significantly decreased IRI levels were found when compared to control mice fed ad libitum.

Insulin Sensitivity

Fig. 3 shows the percentage decrease of blood sugar levels after insulin administration in various groups of mice. The percentage decreases in blood sugar levels were significantly higher at 15, 30, 60 and 120 min. in severely-deficient mice than in control mice fed ad libitum or non-deficient mice.

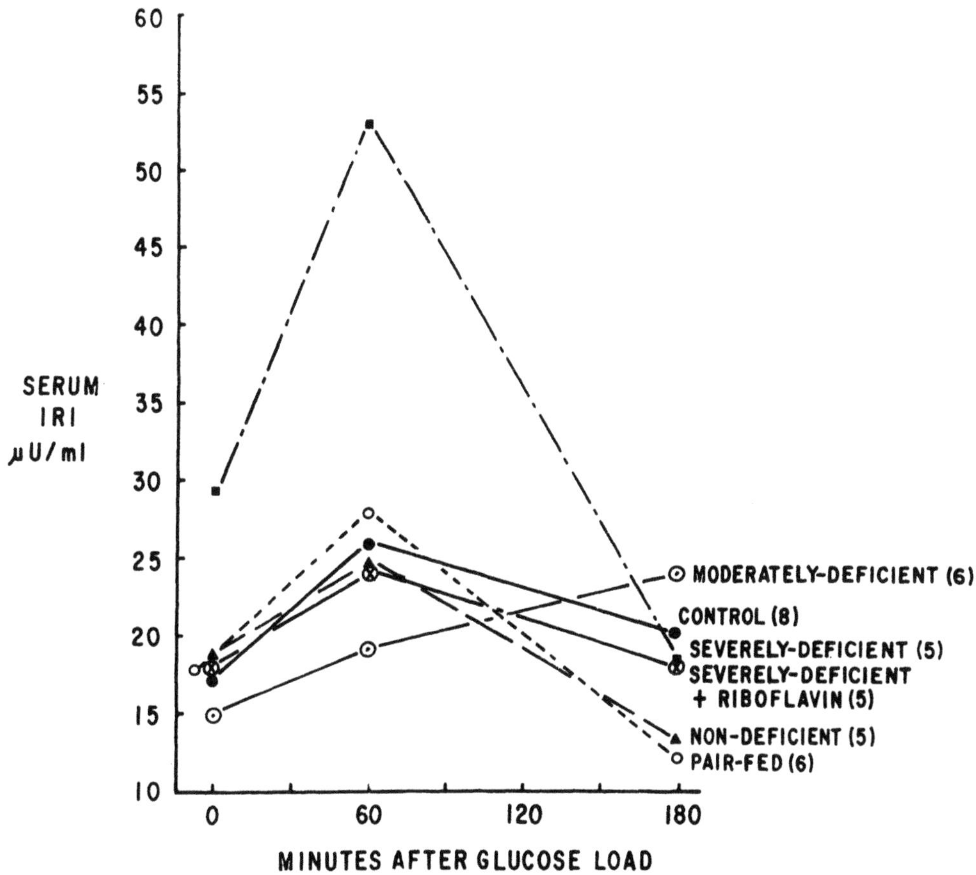

Fig. 2. Insulin response to an oral glucose load in various groups of mice after an 18 hour fast. Numbers in parentheses represent number of animals.

However, this difference was not found between severely-deficient and pair-fed control mice. Also, no difference between control (ad libitum) and non-deficient mice was observed. Supplementation of riboflavin to severely deficient mice restored the blood sugar response to insulin to normal. A comparison of blood sugar response to insulin between the two groups of control mice showed a significant increase in pair-fed mice.

DISCUSSION

The present study demonstrates that riboflavin deficiency in mice causes disturbances in circulating glucose and insulin

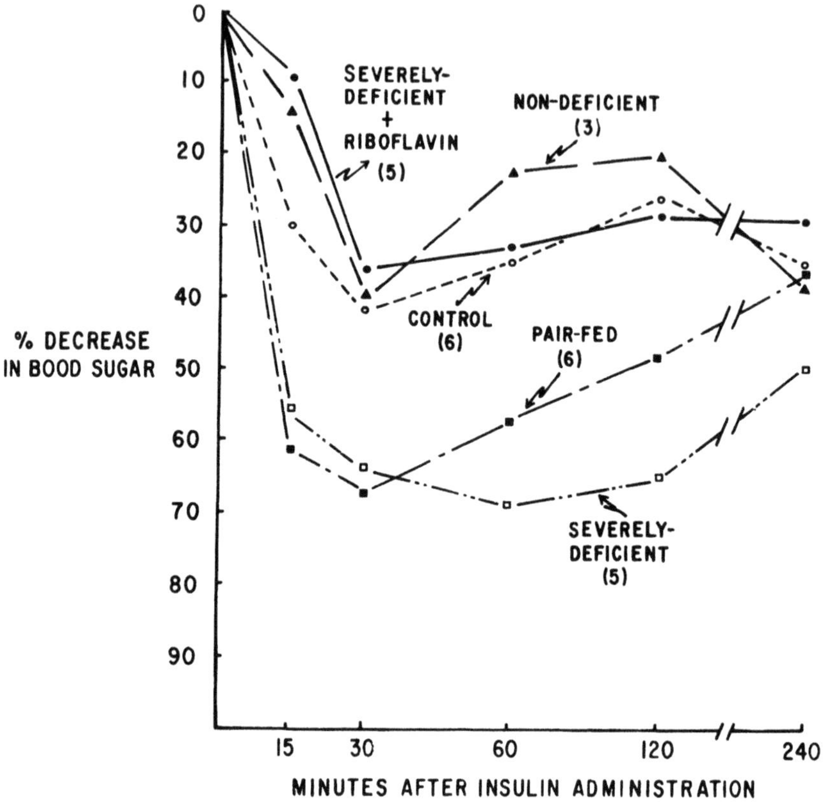

Fig. 3. Blood sugar response (% decrease) to an intraperitoneal injection of bovine crystalline insulin (1U/kg) in various groups of mice after a 6 hour fast. Number of animals in each group is shown in parentheses.

levels. These changes are related to the degree of the severity and not to the duration of the feeding of a deficient diet. The blood sugar response to an oral glucose load was different in three groups of mice fed a riboflavin-deficient diet. In severely-deficient mice, the blood sugars were significantly lower at all periods of the study. In moderately-deficient mice, elevation in blood sugars was observed. These data suggest that riboflavin deficiency causes hypo-and hyperglycemia in mice. The blood sugar response to glucose in non-deficient mice was similar to that of control mice fed ad libitum. The differences observed in blood sugars in all three groups of mice may be due to the severity of the deficiency state, and this may account for the discrepancy of data reported by the earlier investigators.

When both moderately and severely-deficient mice were repleted with riboflavin, their disturbances in tolerance to glucose returned to normal. This suggests the potential importance of riboflavin in the regulation of glucose metabolism.

The low response of blood sugars in severely-deficient mice does not appear to be due to chronic starvation, since the pair-fed controls showed elevated rather than low blood sugar levels. The diabetic response in pair-fed controls may be attributed to malnourishment, and this finding is consistent with the observations of Weinkove et al (9), who reported glucose intolerance in malnourished rats.

The insulin response to oral glucose in moderately-deficient mice was different from that of severely-deficient or non-deficient mice. The insulin levels 60 min. after glucose load were significantly decreased. This finding together with elevated blood sugar levels following glucose load suggests that mild riboflavin deficiency causes impairment in insulin release. In general, the blood sugar and serum insulin response to glucose appear to be undisturbed in non-deficient mice.

Insulin sensitivity, as judged by decrease in blood sugars, was increased in severely-deficient mice. These observations support the findings of Ershoff (6) in rats. A similar increase in insulin sensitivity was also observed in pair-fed controls. This may be due to under-nutrition, since increased insulin sensitivity was reported in malnourished rats (9).

Riboflavin repleted mice showed normal response to insulin administration. This finding, together with normalization of blood sugars and insulin levels, provides an evidence that riboflavin is involved in the regulation of glucose homeostasis. The observation that non-deficient mice had normal carbohydrate metabolism further supports this suggestion.

This study raises several possibilities as to the mechanism of glucose regulation in riboflavin deficiency. Although pertinent data are not available, a possible explanation for low blood sugar levels in severely-deficient mice may be due to low levels of glucagon in the presence of high circulating insulin concentrations. Conversely, the elevated blood sugars and the associated low insulin response to glucose in moderately-deficient mice may be due to elevated glucagon levels. The possible involvement of growth hormone, catecholamines and glucocorticoids should also be considered. Measurements of these hormone levels in riboflavin deficient mice are underway.

Since glucose tolerance has been reported to be impaired in vitamin A-deficient rats (10) and administration of vitamin B_6 to gestational diabetic women improves their tolerance to glucose (11), it would be of interest to study the role of vitamins and their deficiencies in the regulation of glucose homeostasis.

REFERENCES

1. *Rivlin, R. S.: (1970). N. Engl. J. Med. 283: 463*
2. *Goldsmith, G.A.: (1975). Riboflavin, p. 221. Plenum Press.*
3. *Reddi, A.S. (1978). Metabolism 27: 531*
4. *Axelrod, A.E., et al.(1941). Am. J. Physiol, 133: 555*
5. *Axelrod, H. E., et al.(1951). Am. J. Physiol, 165: 604*
6. *Ershoff, B.H. (1954). Metabolism 3: 357*
7. *Hoffman, W.S. (1937). J. Biol. Chem., 120:51*
8. *Velasco, C. A., et al.(1973). Clin. Chem. 19: 201*
9. *Weinkove, C. , et al. (1976). Clin. Sci. & Mol. Med. 50: 153*
10. *Blaizot, S.J. Bonmort (1976). Exerp. Med. 34(Abstract)*
11. *Bennink, H.J.T.C., W.H.P. Schreurs (1975). Br. Med. J. 3:13*

This study was supported in part by the General Research Support Grant RR-05398 from the General Research Support Branch, Division of Research Resources, National Institutes of Health, Hope for Diabetics Foundation, New York, and the Diabetes Research Fund, New York.

DISCUSSION

W. MALAISSE: *Dr. Gerritsen, I'd like to underline data which can be derived from your measurements. Based on both the level of circulating insulin and the insulin content you found in the pancreas at the end of the experiments, in fasting animals the turnover of pancreatic insulin is more than 10 times higher than in animals who had a restricted access to food. I think this is very important to take into consideration, because it is a measurement which is usually not available in human patients.*

E. TUTWILER: *Dr. Gerritsen, there was an increase in blood glucose in those restricted in diet through the seven weeks' period. While it might not have been significant, what happened after months on the restricted diet; do they still develop overt diabetes? Secondly, while there is no body weight difference between the prediabetic and non-prediabetic, is there a difference in terms of content of body fat?*

G. GERRITSEN: *In this particular group of animals we have not yet measured body fat. I suspect that there probably is a difference. In some of our earlier studies we studied the animals who were obviously hyperphagic. We showed, on carcass analysis, an increase in the body fat. But, when we returned them to an ad lib feeding regime, whatever we did by limiting the diet seemed to program their appetite control mechanism so they no longer displayed hyperphagia. As long as they ate a normal amount of food, they remained clinically asymptomatic. Whether that would occur in this study, I really don't know. I rather doubt it, because they do not appear to have the hyperphagia that the animal born from the ketonemic uterus has.*

D. E. SCHTEINGART: *Did you observe your Chinese hamsters' islets to see if there were any changes in D cells or deficiencies of somatostatin-producing cells? Dr. Unger's group suggested that, in the obese hyperglycemic mice, a deficiency of somatostatin-production might explain the hyperinsulinemia and, that changes in nutrient absorption explains the hyperphagia. I wonder if, with your Chinese hamsters, there was a reduction in somatostatin, and if changes in food intake might have caused an increase in somatostatin, and therefore changes in food intake, as well as in insulin occurred?*

G. GERRITSEN: *That's a very good point. We have blocks fixed for EM, so that we'll be able to look at the D cells.*

J. BARBOSA: *Dr. Reddi, in the carbohydrate intolerance of women taking birth control pills, it has been postulated it might be related to vitamin deficiencies, and I think riboflavin has also been implicated. Any comments on that?*

A. S. REDDI: *No.*

K.G.M.M. ALBERTI: *Would you like to speculate at all, Dr. Reddi, on what is going on in the liver of these deficient mice? Have you looked in any detail to see what is going on with respect to, say, glucose production?*

A. S. REDDI: *No, we didn't look into that.*

EFFECT OF VARIATIONS IN CARBOHYDRATE INTAKE ON PLASMA GLUCOSE, INSULIN, AND TRIGLYCERIDE RESPONSES IN NORMAL SUBJECTS AND PATIENTS WITH CHEMICAL DIABETES

G. M. Reaven*

Previous reports from our laboratory have indicated that plasma glucose, insulin and triglyceride responses vary as a function of amount and kind of ingested carbohydrate (1-4). Given the many observations that elevations of plasma glucose, insulin and triglyceride (TG) concentrations may predispose individuals to develop atherosclerotic heart disease, the importance of dietary control of hyperglycemia, hyperinsulinemia, and hypertriglyceridemia is self-evident. This approach is of particular relevance in the treatment of patients with chemical diabetes, a syndrome characterized by all three metabolic abnormalities. Our laboratory has been particularly interested in studying the effect of variations in carbohydrate intake on plasma glucose, insulin and TG responses in normal subjects and patients with chemical diabetes, and this presentation will summarize some of our recent efforts.

METHODS

The data to be presented have been derived from investigation of 137 individuals. None of the subjects had ever received insulin, nor were they taking medications known to modify carbohydrate metabolism. There was no clinical or laboratory evidence of hepatic or cardiovascular disease, and no patients were obese (relative weight $<$ 115%). Inpatients were fed a liquid, weight-maintenance (35 cal/kg) formula diet for at least three days following admission. In some instances this diet was consumed throughout the study, in other instances it was modified. Outpatients consumed a weight-maintenance solid food diet that included at least 200 g of carbohydrate each day of the study.

After at least three days on these basic diets, subjects were given an oral glucose load of 40 gm per sq. meter body surface area, and blood samples were drawn for measurement of plasma glucose (5) and insulin levels (6). The fasting sample was also used for measurement of TG concentration (7). Patients were classified as normal or having chemical diabetes according to the criteria of Fajans and Conn (8), adjusted for measurement of plasma glucose. Patients with fasting plasma glucose levels $>$ 110 mg/100 ml were excluded. Following this, patients were studied according to one of several protocols.

RESULTS

I. Plasma Glucose, Insulin and TG Responses in Control Subjects and Patients with Chemical Diabetes

Mean ($\pm$ SEM) plasma glucose and insulin responses of 15 normal subjects were compared with those of 15 patients with chemical diabetes. These results appear in Figure 1, and indicate that the subjects with chemical diabetes were both hyperglycemic and hyperinsulinemic. Fasting plasma TG was also measured, and these comparisons are seen in Figure 1. It is apparent that patients with chemical diabetes also had a significant ($p < 0.01$) elevation in their mean fasting plasma TG level. There were no differences in either the mean age or relative weight of the two experimental groups.

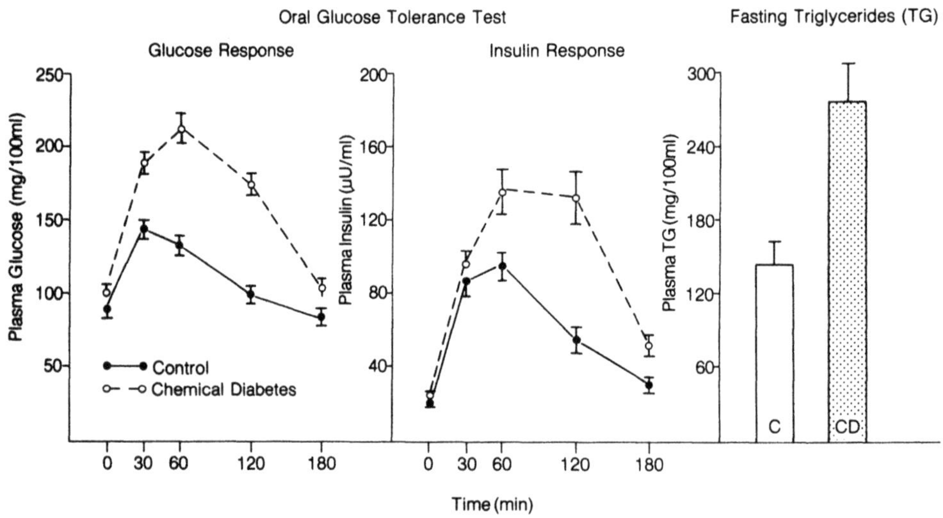

Fig. 1. Mean ($\pm$SEM) plasma glucose and insulin concentrations during an oral glucose tolerance test in 15 control subjects (C), and 15 patients with chemical diabetes (CD). Mean ($\pm$SEM) fasting triglyceride concentrations of the two groups are also illustrated in this figure.

II. Effect of Differences in the Manner of Carbohydrate Ingestion on Plasma Glucose and Insulin Responses

These studies were carried out in 35 inpatients - 14 classified as having chemical diabetes and 21 as having normal glucose tolerance. Patients were maintained on the basic formula diet, and received their daily caloric intake in four equal formula feedings: 8 AM, 11 AM, 2 PM and 5 PM. Each formula was consumed over 30 minutes in order to simulate normal eating conditions. Blood was drawn at 11 AM (just before starting their formula), and then at noon, 1 PM and 2 PM. This procedure was performed on two separate occasions. Plasma glucose and insulin responses to these formula feedings were then compared to those observed during the oral glucose tolerance test. The amount of carbohydrate given in the two circumstances was essentially identical, e.g., a patient 70 inches tall, weighing 70 kg would receive 66 g of carbohydrate in the formula and 68 g during the tolerance test.

Plasma glucose responses to the two oral carbohydrate challenges are seen in Figure 2. Plasma glucose levels of patients with chemical diabetes were significantly elevated ($p < 0.01$) as compared to normal subjects at every time interval during the glucose tolerance test. In marked contrast, plasma glucose levels of the two groups were not significantly different after receiving a comparable amount of carbohydrate during the formula feeding.

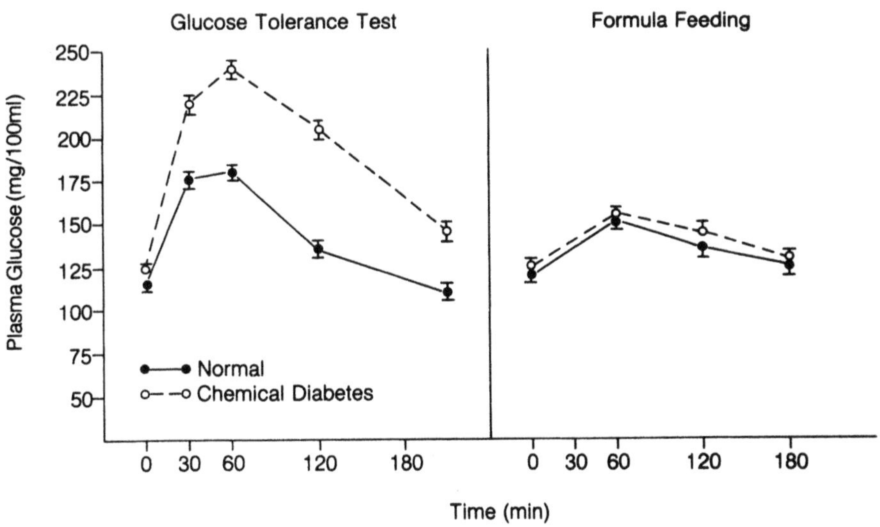

Fig. 2. Mean (±SEM) plasma glucose responses to equivalent amounts of carbohydrate given as an oral glucose tolerance test or as part of a mixed-formula feeding to 21 normal subjects and 14 patients with chemical diabetes.

The plasma insulin responses to the two different forms of carbohydrate ingestion are seen in Figure 3. During the glucose tolerance test the plasma insulin response of the patients with chemical diabetes was significantly greater ($p < 0.01$) than that of the normal subjects at the 60, 120 and 180 min time interval. A similar difference in insulin response was also observed during the formula feeding, and patients with chemical diabetes had significantly elevated ($p < 0.05$ - $p < 0.01$) plasma insulin levels at every time point following the meal feeding.

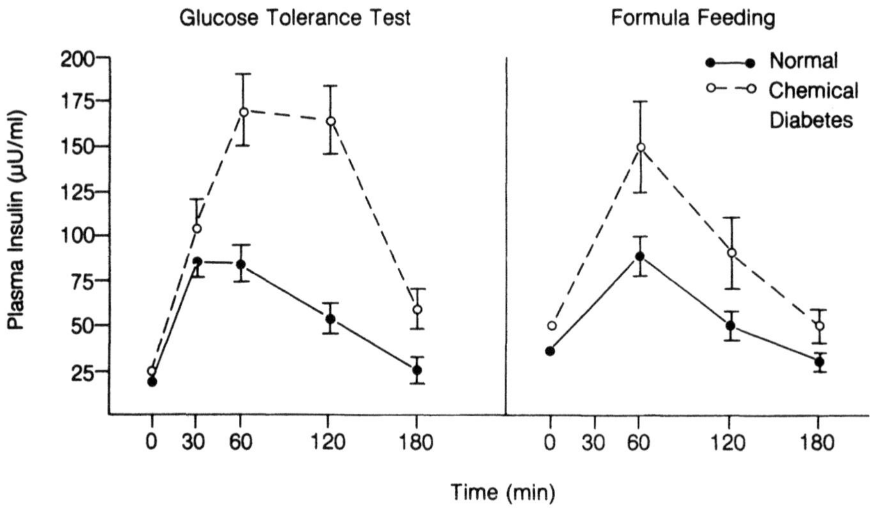

Fig. 3. Mean (±SEM) plasma insulin responses to equivalent amounts of carbohydrate given as an oral glucose tolerance test or as part of a mixed-formula feeding to 21 normal subjects and 14 patients with chemical diabetes.

III. Effect of Differences in the Amount of Ingested Carbohydrate on Plasma Glucose, Insulin and Triglyceride Responses

These studies were carried out in 27 inpatients. Following the three day period on the basic diet, patients were studied on two different isocaloric formula diets - one containing 40% carbohydrate, the other 55% carbohydrate. The sequence in which the test diets were given was randomly determined, and each diet was consumed for one week. The 40% carbohydrate diet contained (as percent of total calories) 40% carbohydrate, 45% fat, and 15% protein. The 55% carbohydrate diet contained 55% carbohydrate, 40% fat and 15% protein. The dietary carbohydrate intake was comprised of dextrins, maltose, lactose and sucrose. The same absolute amounts of sucrose were present in both diets, consisting of 25% of the carbohydrate calories of the control diet. Both diets had a polyunsaturated: saturated fat ration of 1:1. The subjects consumed 35 Kcal/kg body weight/day in portions of 1/5, 2/5 and 2/5 calories served at 8 AM, 12 noon and 6 PM.

On the morning of the seventh day of each diet, fasting blood was obtained for measurement of plasma TG concentrations. Blood samples were also obtained on this day just prior to the 12 noon formula feeding and at 1 PM, 2 PM and 3 PM for determination of the plasma glucose and insulin responses to noon formula. Fasting blood samples were again obtained the following morning for measurement of plasma TG levels. The mean of the two measurements of fasting TG concentration at the end of each diet period were used as the value for that period. Daily weights were obtained in all subjects and were stable throughout the two-week study period.

The results of these studies are illustrated in Figure 4. Mean plasma glucose levels were slightly higher in response to the meal containing 55% of total calories as carbohydrate, but the differences were only significant at 2 PM and 3 PM ($p<0.01$, paired t-test). The difference between the insulin responses to the two diets was more dramatic, and significantly ($p<0.01$) higher plasma insulin levels were seen at each time interval following consumption of the 55% carbohydrate diet. Figure 4 also demonstrated that significant hypertriglyceridemia results from eating a diet containing 55% carbohydrate for one week. The mean plasma TG level of the group increased 41% on the 55% carbohydrate diet ($p<0.001$) and 26 of the 27 subjects had elevations in their fasting plasma TG levels after eating the 55% carbohydrate diet. When the group was divided into thirds on the basis of the height of their plasma triglyceride levels on the 40% carbohydrate diet, the percent increment in all three groups was comparable. However, the greater the basal TG level, the greater the absolute increment. On the other hand, the absolute effect of the 55% carbohydrate diet was great enough in 9 of the 18 subjects with normal values on the 40% carbohydrate diet to result in the induction of hypertriglyceridemia (TG levels > 150 mg%).

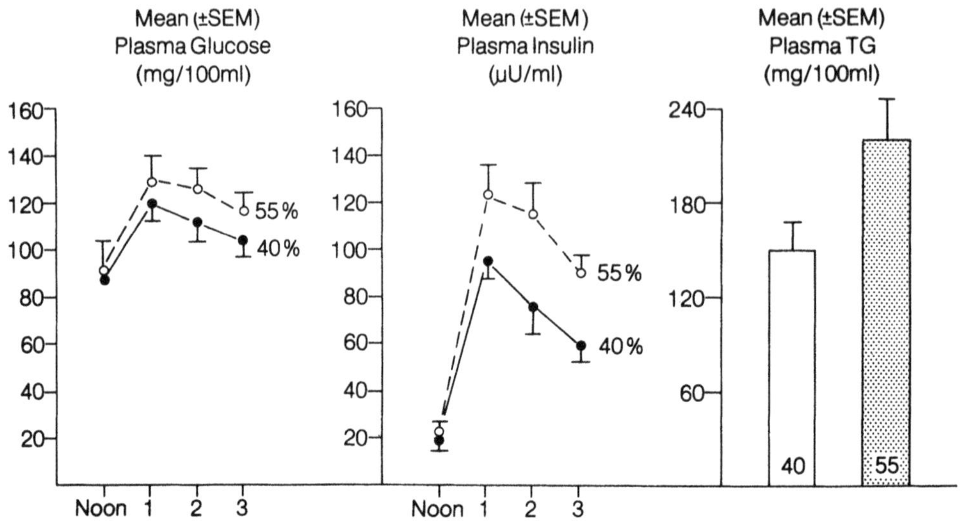

Fig. 4. Mean (±SEM) plasma glucose and insulin responses in 27 subjects to isocaloric diets containing (as percent of total calories) 55% carbohydrate (30% fat and 14% protein) and 40% carbohydrate (45% fat and 15% protein). Mean (±SEM) fasting plasma triglyceride concentrations to the two diets are also seen in this figure.

IV. Effect of Variations in the Type of Dietary Carbohydrate on Plasma Glucose and Insulin Responses

a) In these experiments, the effect of three different sources of carbohydrate (glucose, sucrose and starch) on plasma glucose and insulin responses was studied in 19 outpatients with normal glucose tolerance. The test loads were calculated so that the amount of administered glucose was equal, i.e., 50 gm of glucose, starch (amylopectin) and 100 g of sucrose. In addition to the carbohydrate, the test load consisted of 20 g of corn oil and 20 g of powdered egg albumin. The total volume of the test meals was adjusted to 500 ml, given at 8 AM, and consumed over a 15 min period. Blood was drawn before the meal was given, and for the next three hours.

The results of these studies, which are seen in Figure 5, indicate that there is no difference in the plasma glucose response to a glucose or sucrose meal. The plasma glucose response to a starch meal is flattened in the first hour compared with glucose and sucrose meals, but is somewhat higher at 60, 120, and 180 minutes. The insulin responses, following both the glucose and sucrose meals, were significantly elevated at 30 minutes as compared to starch, but fell rapidly thereafter.

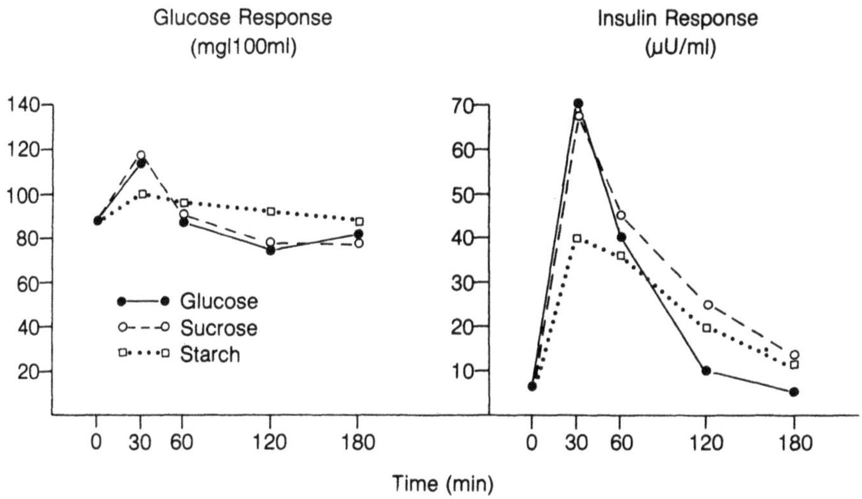

Fig. 5. Mean plasma glucose and insulin responses in 19 normal subjects to mixed-formula feedings containing 50 g of glucose, sucrose and starch (amylopectin).

b) In these experiments, the effect on plasma glucose and insulin responses of two forms of cooked starch was compared to that of glucose. Studies were carried out in 16 normal subjects and in 10 patients with chemical diabetes. Each patient consumed 50 g of glucose in the form of glucose, baked potato, and boiled rice, and the order of the three test meals was randomized. Because the dextrose was given in a 500 ml volume, the subjects consumed 500 ml of water along with each starch in order to eliminate volume as a variable. The test load was consumed in 15 minutes. Blood samples were drawn for measurement of plasma glucose and insulin before the meal, and at regular intervals for the next three hours.

The results in the subjects with normal glucose tolerance are illustrated in Figure 6. Mean plasma glucose levels in response to glucose and baked potato were identical, and significantly higher at 30 and 60 minutes than those observed after an equal amount of carbohydrate eaten as boiled rice (paired t-test, $p<0.001$). The mean plasma insulin response to glucose and baked potato were quite similar, differing only at the 30 min. interval. As in the case of the glucose response, the plasma insulin response to cooked rice was significantly lower than that following either glucose or baked potato at both the 30 and 60 min time interval.

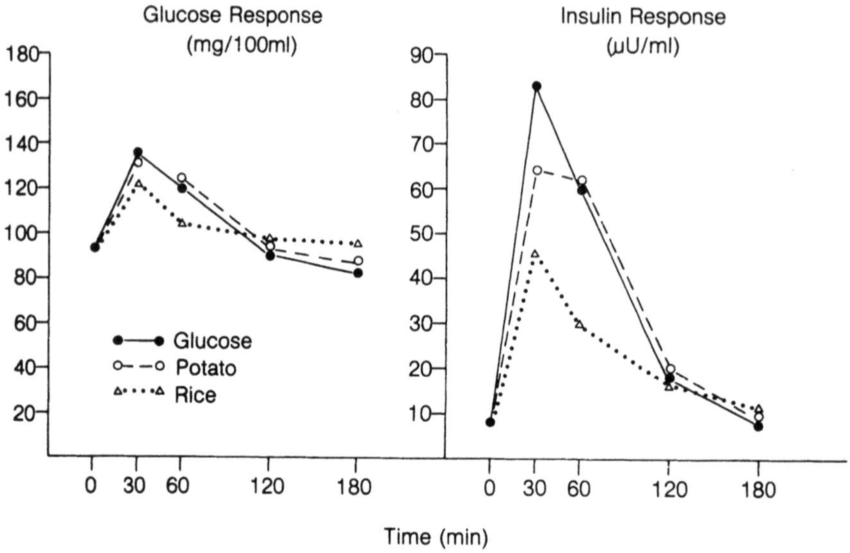

Fig. 6. Mean plasma glucose and insulin responses in 16 normal subjects following the ingestion of 50 g of glucose as glucose, baked potato and cooked rice.

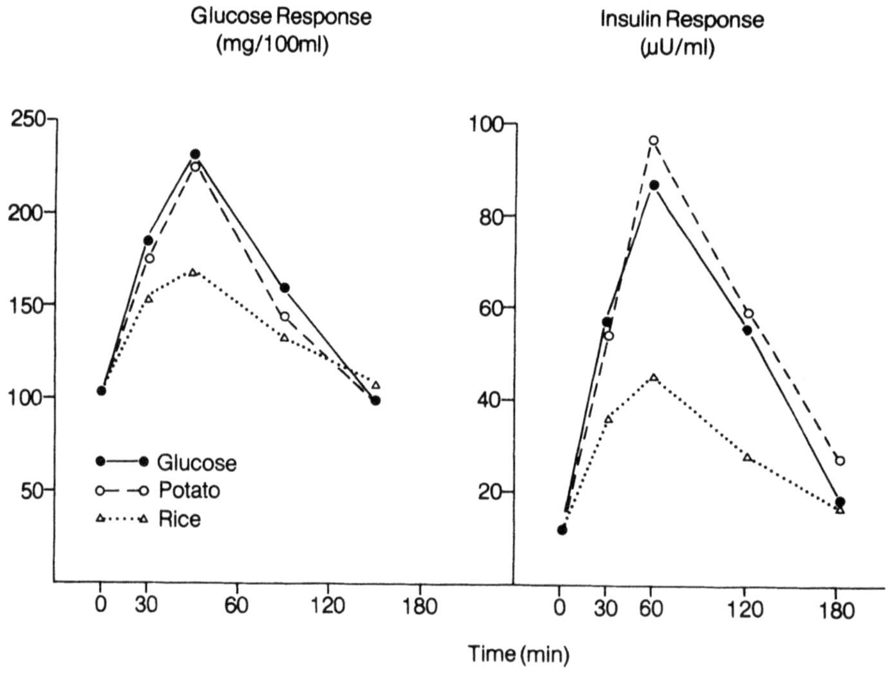

Fig. 7. Mean plasma glucose and insulin responses in 10 patients with chemical diabetes following the ingestion of 50 g of glucose as glucose, baked potato and cooked rice.

Qualitatively similar results were also seen following ingestion of the three carbohydrates in patients with chemical diabetes. However, as the results in Figure 7 clearly demonstrate, the magnitude of difference in the glucose and insulin responses to baked potato and glucose as compared to rice were accentuated in these subjects.

DISCUSSION

Several years ago, we suggested (1,9) that the basic defect in the majority of patients with endogenous hypertriglyceridemia was a loss of normal insulin sensitivity, leading to impaired glucose tolerance and a compensatory increase in insulin secretion. Glucose tolerance would be maintained at near normal levels as the result of elevated plasma insulin levels in such patients, but this would occur at the price of increased hepatic TG synthesis and secretion, and, eventually, hypertriglyceridemia. This combination of loss of normal insulin sensitivity, mild glucose intolerance, increased levels of circulating insulin, and hypertriglyceridemia is commonly seen in patients with chemical diabetes (Fig. 1).

If a large proportion of patients with chemical diabetes are hyperglycemic, hyperinsulinemic, and hypertriglyceridemic, certain approaches to dietary manipulation seem apparent. In the first place, significant numbers of such patients are overweight. Although not the focus of the current study, previous results (10) clearly indicate that weight loss will lead to an improvement in all three metabolic variables. However, the current results suggest that it is also possible to significantly modulate plasma glucose, insulin and TG responses with isocaloric diets. The data that have been presented demonstrate that plasma glucose and insulin responses, and fasting TG concentrations will all be reduced by lowering the relative proportion of carbohydrate in the diet (Fig. 4). Furthermore, plasma glucose and insulin responses can be reduced without changing the total carbohydrate intake by simply varying the manner of dietary carbohydrate ingestion. The results of the current study indicate that this can be achieved by at least two means. The data in Figs. 2, 3 and 5 suggest that the substitution of more complex carbohydrate for simple sugars will lead to lower plasma glucose and insulin responses. In addition, the data in Figs. 6 and 7 suggest that differences in the form of dietary starch can also modify plasma glucose and insulin responses. The observation that plasma glucose and insulin responses were lower after eating an identical amount of glucose as cooked rice as compared to baked potato was totally unexpected. An explanation for this disparate response is not certain, but is likely due to differences in gastric emptying time and physical availability of the starch to the hydrolytic enzymes. In any event, the observed differences emphatically underscore the potential benefit of this type of approach.

On the other hand, considerably more information is necessary before the information presented can serve as the basis for a dietary approach to patients with chemical diabetes. In the first place, the experiments described were all of short duration, and it is not clear that similar results would be seen over a longer time period. Secondly, the studies were carried out primarily on inpatients, under certain conditions in which control of dietary intake could be achieved. Whether similar results would obtain if subjects were studied as outpatients remains to be seen. Finally, all studies were carried out with formula feedings, and comparable results might not be seen if subjects were fed regular meals. All three issues must be dealt with before the practical implication of the experimental results can be truly evaluated. On the other hand, the striking metabolic changes that have been shown to result from manipulation of dietary carboydrate intake makes it essential that these additional studies be carried out.

REFERENCES

1. *Farquhar, J.W., et al.(1966). J. Clin. Invest. 45, 1648*
2. *Ginsberg, H., et al.(1976). J. Clin. Endocrinol. Metab. 42, 729*
3. *Crapo, P.A., et al.(1976). Diabetes 25, 741*
4. *Crapo, P.A., et al.(1977). Diabetes 26, 1178*
5. *Kadish, A.H., et al.(1968). Clin. Chem. 14, 116*
6. *Desbuquois, B. and Aurbach, G.D. (1971). J. Clin. Endocrinol. Metab. 33, 732*
7. *Kessler, G. and Lederer, H. (1976) in Automation in Analytic Chemistry Ed. L.T. Skeggs, Jr., New York, p. 341*
8. *Fajans, S.S. and Conn, J.W. (1959). Ann. N.Y. Acad. Sci. 82, 208*
9. *Reaven, G.M., et al.(1967). J. Clin. Invest. 45, 1756*
10. *Olefsky, J.M., et al.(1974). J. Clin. Invest. 53, 64*

This work was supported in part by grants from the National Institutes of Health, #HL 08506 and RR-70 from the Clinical Research Centers Branch, and from the Research Services of the Veterans Administration.

HIGH CARBOHYDRATE, HIGH FIBER DIETS FOR PATIENTS WITH DIABETES

J. W. Anderson*

Most dietary recommendations for patients with diabetes mellitus seem to be controversial. Traditional diets have been restricted in carbohydrate and generous in fat content. Some authorities (1,2) recommend low carbohydrate, high fat diets while others (3,4) suggest a liberalization of carbohydrate intake and a reduction in dietary fat. Unfortunately, these recommendations are empirical and not based on experimental data. I am unaware of any metabolic studies which demonstrate, in a convincing manner, that weight-maintaining diets (either low or high in carbohydrate) lead to reductions in average blood glucose values or insulin doses in lean individuals. For example, one careful study (5) demonstrated that conventional diets did not alter blood glucose concentrations of patients with diabetes fed weight-maintaining diets for 17-30 days on a metabolic ward (Figure 1). Because there was no conclusive data that dietary modifications altered blood glucose values or insulin doses in lean individuals, we began to evaluate high carbohydrate, high fiber (HCF) diets in 1974. For comparison, the average insulin doses of 12 lean men fed weight-maintaining control diets for eight days are presented in Figure 2. These control diets do not alter plasma glucose, cholesterol or triglyceride values or insulin does. In sharp contrast, when these men were placed on weight-maintaining HCF diets, insulin doses could be reduced promptly and significantly. On the HCF diets, fasting and postprandial plasma glucose values were significantly lower than values on the control diets. Our experience with HCF diets will be briefly reviewed.

METHODS

The composition of prototypical control, HCF and home maintenance diets are presented in Figure 3 (6). The control diet has 43% of energy as carbohydrate, 19% protein, 37% fat and 450 mg

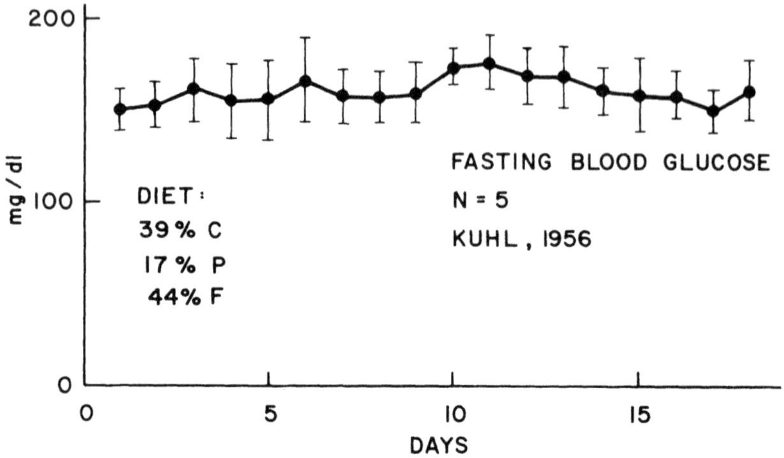

Fig. 1. Fasting blood glucose values on conventional diets (5).

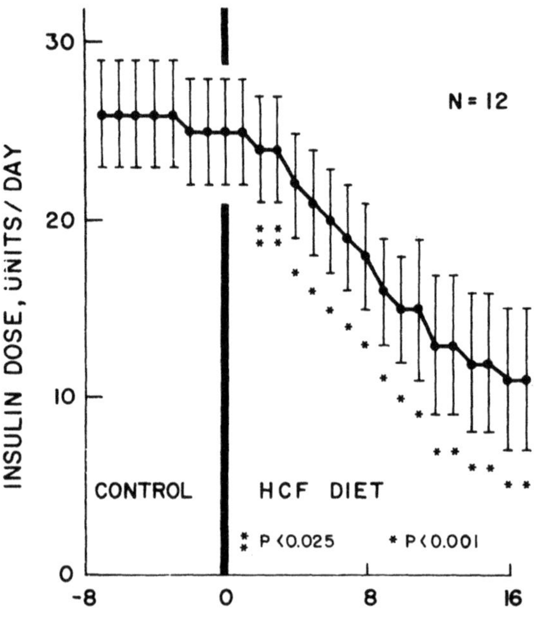

Fig. 2. Insulin doses on control and HCF diets.

cholesterol; it is similar to diets conventionally used to treat diabetes. The plant fiber content of the control diets (28 g/d) is 2-3 fold greater than the fiber content of conventional diabetic diets. HCF diets are high in carbohydrate (70%) and plant fiber (70-80 g/d) and very restricted in fat (11%) and cholesterol (45 mg/d). The diets used for home maintenance are also generous in carbohydrate (55-60%) and plant fiber (45-60 g/d) and limited in fat (21%) and cholesterol (<100 mg/d). Usually, patients are placed on the control diet for 6-11 days and fed weight-maintaining HCF diets for 12-21 days as demonstrated in Figure 4. Daily measurements of body weight, fasting glucose, cholesterol, triglycerides and urine glucose excretion are made. We have attempted to adjust the insulin dose to maintain a fasting plasma glucose value at approximately 150 mg/dl and urine glucose values less than 10 g/d throughout the study period.

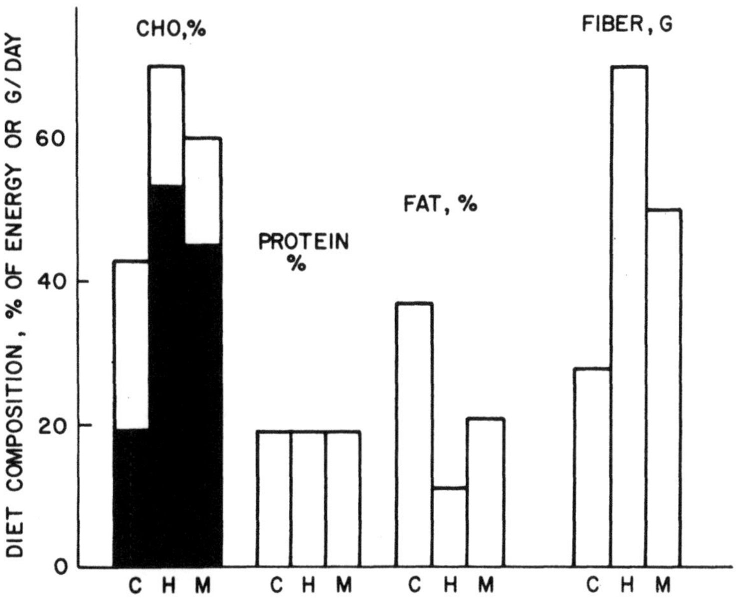

Fig. 3. Composition of control (C), HCF (H) and maintenance (M) diets.

RESULTS

The response of 6 representative patients to HCF diets are presented in Figures 4-6. There were no significant changes in body weights. Seventeen patients (11 lean, 6 obese) were receiving between 14 and 20 U/d of insulin on the control diets (Figure 7). Insulin therapy was discontinued in 16 of these patients on HCF diets. Insulin could be stopped within 7-10 days in patients who were well controlled on the control diet (5B) but was required for longer periods in patients who had fasting plasma glucose values above 200 mg/dl on the control diet (5C). For this group, insulin doses were reduced an average of 1 U/d and could be discontinued after an average of 14 days on HCF diets.

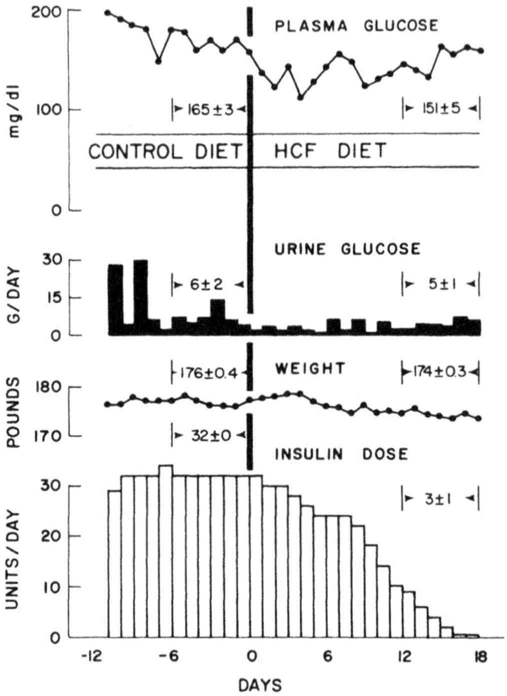

Fig. 4. Control and HCF diets.

Eleven lean men were receiving between 25 and 32 U/d of insulin on the control diets (Figure 7). The reductions in insulin doses on HCF diets demonstrated in Figure 2 and 6A are typical for this group. On the HCF diets average insulin doses could be reduced by 1 U/d while plasma glucose values fell significantly Thus, in one patient (6B) whose insulin dose was 32 U/d on the control diet, insulin could be discontinued after 33 days on the HCF diet. On the HCF diets, insulin therapy was stopped in 5 of these 11 men.

We have treated 5 lean men with the insulin-dependent (juvenile-onset) type of diabetes (Figure 7). On control diets their insulin doses averaged 44 U/d (40-55 U/d). On HCF diets, plasma glucose values were lower, urine glucose excretion was reduced, insulin reactions were less frequent and their insulin doses averaged 34 U/d (20-46 U/d).

Fasting serum cholesterol values have fallen in all patients treated with HCF diets (Figure 8). The average reduction was 52 mg/dl. Fasting serum triglycerides also decline in most patients on HCF diets and the average reduction was 30 mg/dl. Patients with hypertriglyceridemia show much greater reductions in triglyceride values on the HCF diets than do normotriglyceridemic individuals (7).

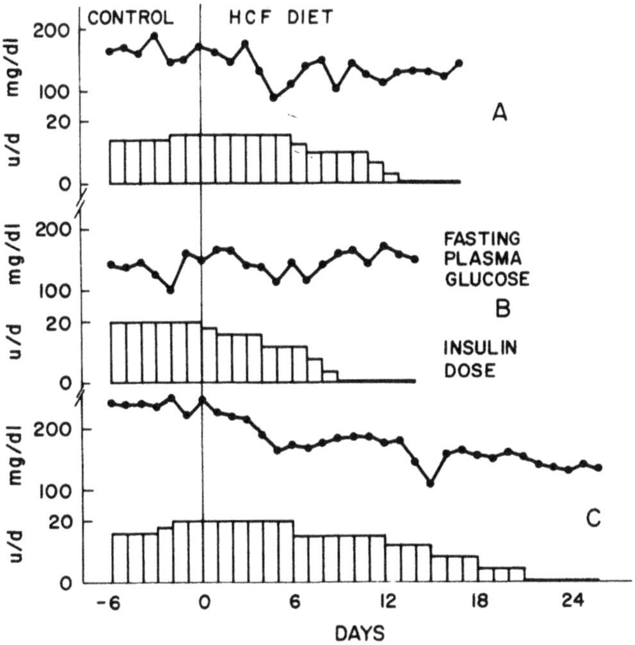

Fig. 5. Control and HCF diets.

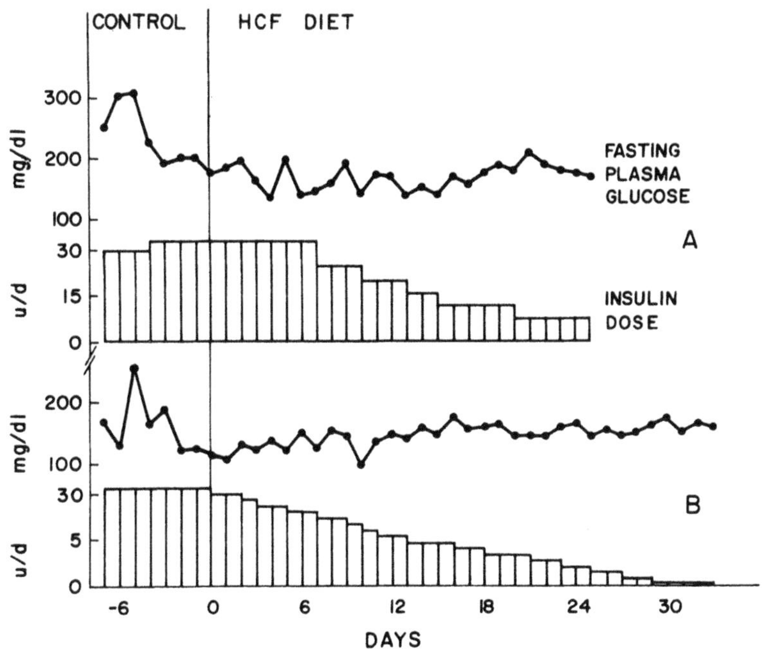

Fig. 6. Control and HCF diets.

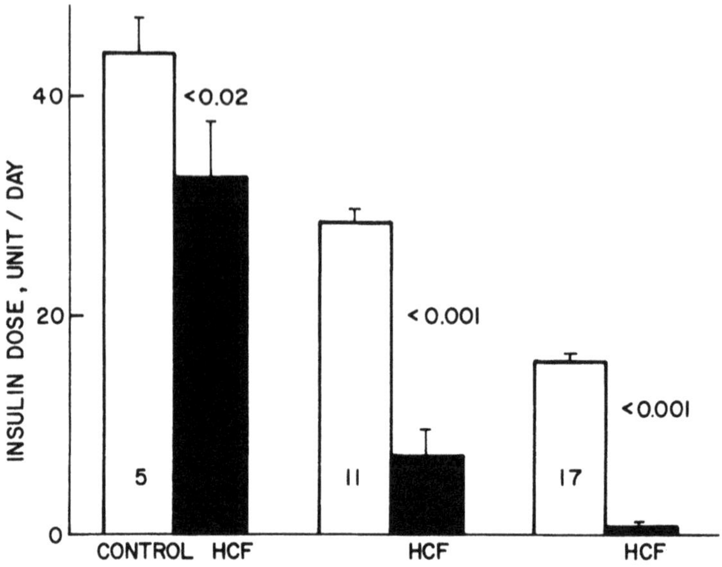

Fig. 7. Insulin doses on control and HCF diets.

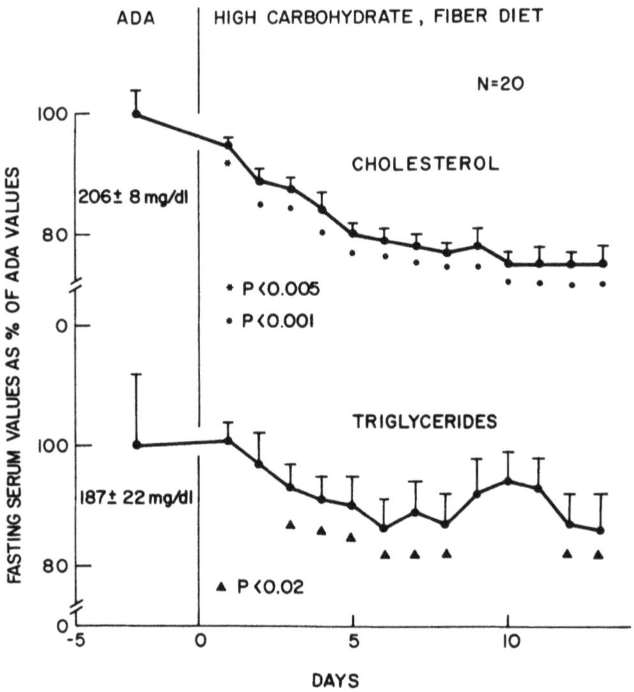

Fig. 8. Lipid responses to HCF diets.

Most patients who have a favorable response to an HCF diet in the hospital elect to follow a similar diet at home. In Figure 9 average insulin doses of 15 patients followed for an average of 16 months are summarized. On the control diets these men were receiving 15-55 U/d. On HCF diets insulin was discontinued in 11 men and on the maintenance diet, insulin was discontinued in one additional man. In sharp contrast, 9 patients who had favorable responses to the HCF diets (insulin was discontinued in 6) elected to resume a conventional diet (Figure 9). All patients had to resume insulin therapy and their current doses are slightly higher than on the control diet in the hospital. We have followed 10 patients on maintenance diets for a minimum of 6 months and an average of 20 months. These patients showed reductions in insulin doses and blood glucose and lipid values on HCF diets in the hospital and have sustained these improvements at home on maintenance diets (Figure 10). On the control diet all 10 were on insulin therapy, at home only two require insulin. Nevertheless, average fasting plasma glucose values at home are similar to values on HCF diets in the hospital. Serum cholesterol values have increased slightly at home but this is largely related to an increase in high-density lipoprotein cholesterol (Anderson, J.W. and Rees, D., unpublished). Despite the high carbohydrate content of these diets, serum triglyceride values have continued to decline at home.

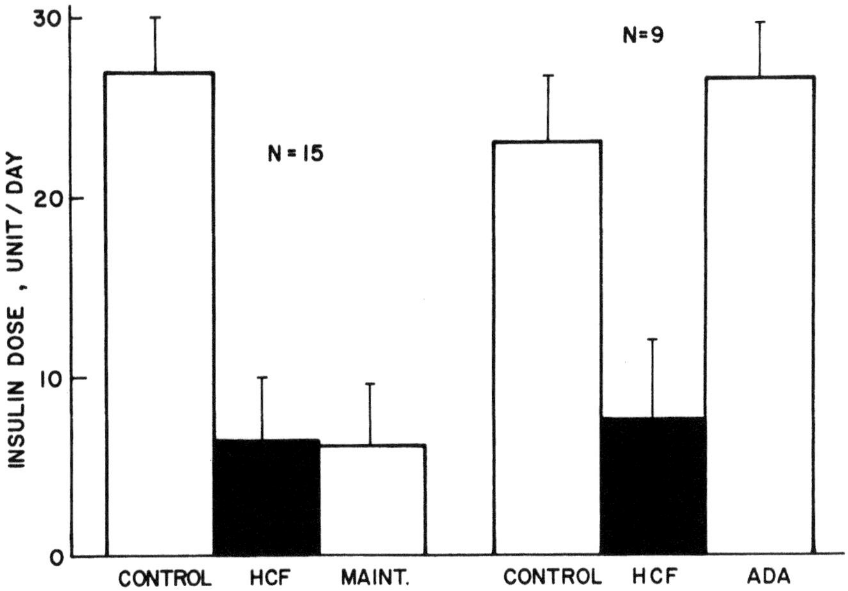

Fig. 9. Insulin doses on control, HCF, maintenance and conventional ADA diets.

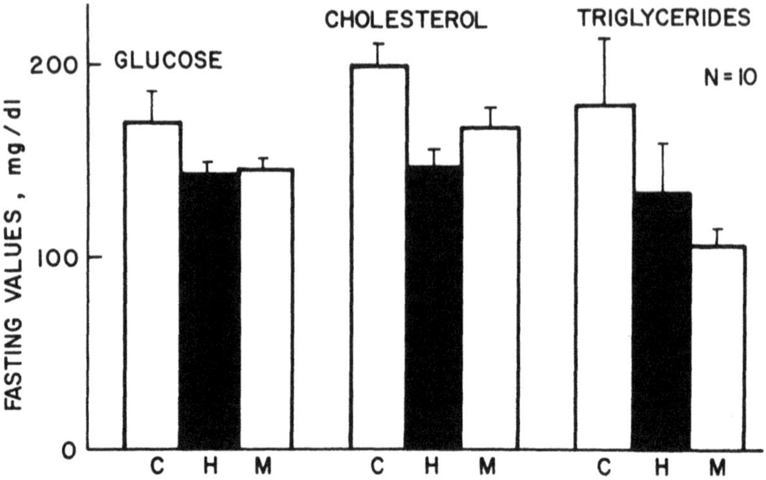

Fig. 10. Responses to control (C), HCF (H) and maintenance (M) diets.

DISCUSSION

Conventional diets have little impact on glucose or lipid metabolism of patients with diabetes. High carbohydrate, high fiber diets are accompanied by significant reductions in fasting blood glucose, cholesterol and triglyceride values and by lower insulin doses. The mechanisms responsible for these improvements in glucose and lipid metabolism have not been delineated. High carbohydrate, low fat diets are usually accompanied by improved glucose metabolism and by an apparent increase in sensitivity to insulin. We have examined the influence of control and HCF diets on insulin binding to monocytes (8). Improved glucose metabolism in insulin-treated or non-insulin treated patients on HCF diets was accompanied by increased binding of insulin by monocytes. Results from one representative patient is presented in Figure 11.

The effects of plant fiber on glucose metabolism in these patients is unclear. Plant fiber intake is accompanied by lower postprandial glucose values (9,10) and by decreased glycosuria in patients with diabetes (11). To examine the effects of plant fiber in our diets we have fed 8 patients with high carbohydrate (70%), low fiber (<25 g/d)diets. These patients have been matched by insulin dose and body weight with 8 patients fed standard HCF diets. The same protocol for reducing insulin doses was used for both groups of patients. The reduction in insulin dose in patients fed high carbohydrate, low fiber diets followed a similar pattern to that observed for patients fed the HCF diets (Figure 12). This suggests that the high carbohydrate and low fat content of HCF diets has a major role in the reduction in insulin doses on HCF diets. However, plant fiber may have an additive or syngergistic effect on glucose metabolism which was not detected by this comparison.

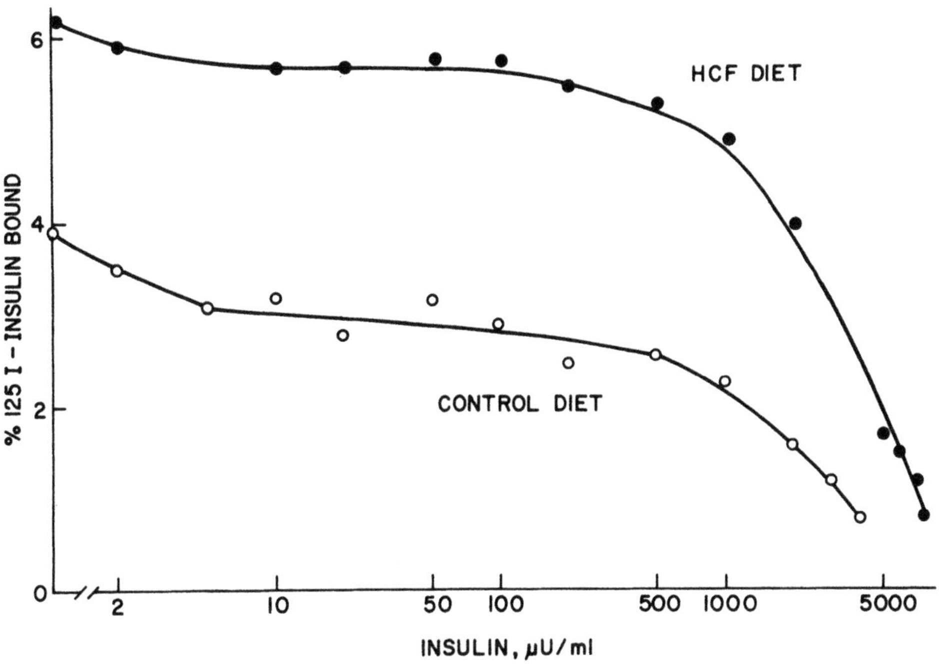

Fig. 11. Insulin binding to monocytes (5 x 10^6) on control and HCF diets.

Plant fibers have important roles in the absorption and metabolism of lipids (12). Water soluble plant fibers have distinct cholesterol-lowering effects. The reduction in serum cholesterol that we observed (Figure 8) on HCF diets is probably related to the soluble fiber content (∿20 g/d) of these diets as well as the restriction of saturated fats and cholesterol. Our studies (7, 13) suggest that a mixture of plant fibers lower fasting serum triglycerides in man and that the high fiber content of these HCF diets prevents the hypertriglyceridemia one would anticipate with 70% carbohydrate diets.

SUMMARY

Thirty-three insulin-treated men with diabetes were hospitalized on a metabolic ward and fed control diets (43% carbohydrate) for 6 to 11 days followed by high carbohydrate (70%), high fiber (HCF) diets for 12-35 days. Fasting blood glucose, cholesterol and

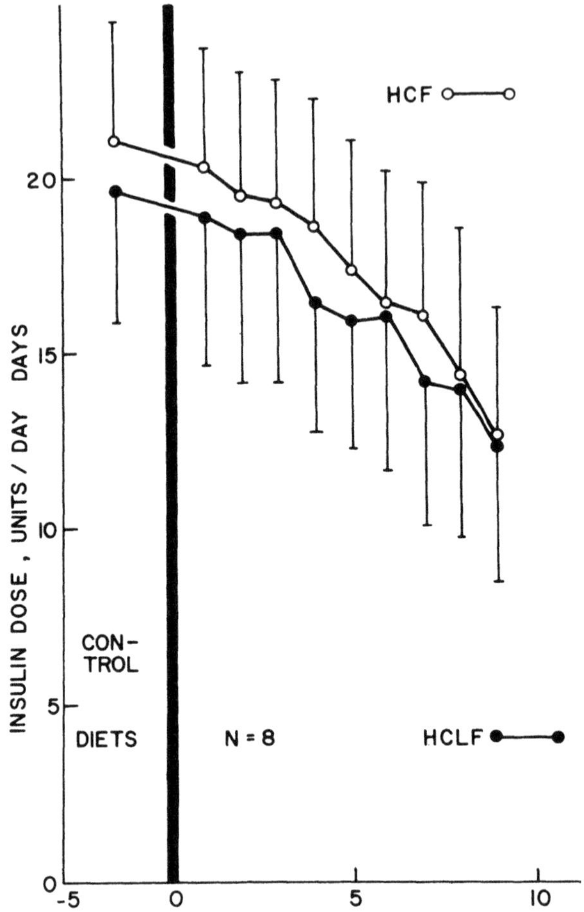

Fig. 12. Insulin doses on HCF and high carbohydrate, low fiber (HCLF) diets.

triglyceride values were significantly lower on HCF diets than on control diets despite significantly ($p<0.01$) lower insulin doses on the HCF diets. HCF diets were accompanied by increased insulin sensitivity and by binding of insulin by monocytes. Patients who responded well to the diet in the hospital have maintained comparable glucose, cholesterol and triglyceride values as well as lower insulin doses for an average of 20 months on maintenance diets (60% carbohydrate). The high carbohydrate and low fat content of these HCF diets seem to play the predominant role in the improved glucose metabolism of these patients whereas the high plant fiber content may be responsible for the reduction in serum cholesterol and triglyceride values. These studies suggest that HCF diets may have an important place in the management of patients with the maturity-onset type of diabetes.

REFERENCES

1. Perkins, J.R., et al. (1977). Diabetologia 13: 607
2. Wall, J. R., et al.(1973). Brit Med J, 1, 577
3. West, K.M. (1975). Nutr. Rev 33, 193
4. Bierman, E.L. and Nelson, R. (1975). World Rev Nutr Diet 22, 280
5. Kuhl, W.M. (1956). Metabolism 5, 953
6. Anderson, J.W., et al.(1978). Diabetes Care, 1
7. Anderson, J.W. (1978). Clin Res 26, 719A
8. Olefsky, J.M. and Reaven, G.M. (1974). J. Clin Invest 54, 1323
9. Jenkins, D.J.A., et al.(1976). Lancet 2, 172
10. Miranda, P.M. and Horwitz, D.L. (1978) Ann Intern Med, 88, 482.
11. Jenkins, D.J.A., et al.(1977). Lancet 2, 779
12. Anderson, J.W. and Chen, W. Am. J. Clin Nutr. In press.
13. Anderson, J.W. (1977) Cereal Foods World, 22, 12.

DIETARY FIBER AND DIABETIC THERAPY: A PROGRESSIVE EFFECT WITH TIME

D. J. A. Jenkins*, T. M. S. Wolever, R. Nineham,
S. Bacon, R. Smith, and T. D. R. Hockaday

Recent work has shown that fibre supplementation (1,5), especially of high carbohydrate diets (1,2), may reduce post-prandial glycemia (6), urinary glucose loss (3,4), and insulin requirement (1,2,3,4) in diabetics. The mechanism of action is uncertain but may follow slower absorption of nutrient (7) with more gradual post-prandial rises in glucose and amino acids. This, in turn would reduce the requirement for insulin to regulate nutrient concentration.

However, the reduction of urine glucose and insulin dosage produced by addition of a constant amount of fiber to a constant diet in diabetics is reported to be progressive (1,2). This suggests that the effect of fibre on carbohydrate metabolism may be related not only to the acute interaction of fiber and food in the gut but also to subsequent alterations in metabolism and alimentary structure and function. We have therefore measured the daily urinary glucose loss of diabetics for the first five days of fiber treatment and recorded the effect on insulin requirement and home urine glucose tests over 12 to 20 weeks.

METHODS

18 diabetics (11 men, 7 women, 45 $\pm$ 4yr, 107 $\pm$ 4% desirable weight (8), 14 taking insulin, 3 on oral agents and one treated by diet alone) were studied initially over 5-day control and 5-day guar periods either as out-patients (5 patients, 7 studies) or as in-patients on hospital metabolic ward diets (15 patients, 15 studies).

In metabolic ward studies, 14-25gm guar (mean 23gm) were added to the control menu in porridge, fruit juice, bread, soup, mashed potatoes, custards and chocolate mousse or latterly taken solely as guar crispbread (4). Apart from addition of guar, test and control diets were identical with the same menu repeated every 2 days.

Out-patients weighed and recorded their dietary intakes during the first 5-day period and repeated this 5 day menu during the second. They were provided with either weighed slices of guar and control bread and with tins of guar and control soup or with guar and control crispbread.

In metabolic ward and out-patient 5-day studies, complete 24-hr urine collections were made (7 a.m. - 7 p.m.) into 2-1 plastic bottles containing 10 ml concentrated HCl as preservative. The volumes were measured and the samples stored at -20° before being analysed for glucose (9).

Follow-up data are presented on 11 patients studied for 12-20 weeks after starting guar treatment. On average, they took 18 gm guar/day in crispbread form, although two patients also used processed guar. The results of home urine "Clinitest" (Ames), are the mean of 1 week of testing (pre-breakfast, pre-lunch, pre-dinner and pre-bed). They were obtained before starting guar treatment, and are compared with the values recorded while taking guar (9 patients). Similar data were obtained on changes in insulin dosage over 12 (9 patients) and 20 weeks (5 patients).

The results are expressed as means ± SEM and the significance given for differences between paired control and treatment values.

RESULTS

The mean urinary glucose loss during the last 3 days of the control period was 63 ± 13gm/24 hr. This figure, rather than the 5-day control mean, was chosen for comparison with reductions on guar to eliminate the carry-over effect of guar onto the first two days of the control which is seen in randomized trials (4). After beginning the guar diet the urinary glucose showed an overall 5-day reduction of 46 ± 9% ($P < 0.001$) (18 patients, 22 studies). (Fig. 1) Only one patient showed no reduction on guar. He was on a comparatively high dose of insulin at 76 U/day and his results lay more than 2 standard deviations from the group mean. After excluding him, recalculation of the data gave a mean control urinary glucose loss of 66 ± 14 g/day and an overall reduction on guar on 54 ± 6% ($P < 0.001$); (17 patients, 21 studies). On day 1 the reduction was 43 ± 6% ($P < 0.001$); day 2, 51 ± 9% ($P < 0.001$); day 3, 58 ± 6% ($P < 0.001$); day 4, 66 ± 6% ($P < 0.001$); and day 5, 52 ± 7% ($P < 0.001$) (Fig.2).

Follow-up of 9 patients for 12 weeks showed the progressive nature of the decrease in insulin requirements from 45 ± 5 to 36 ± 4 U/day ($P < 0.01$, Fig. 3). Insulin dosages were reduced when the

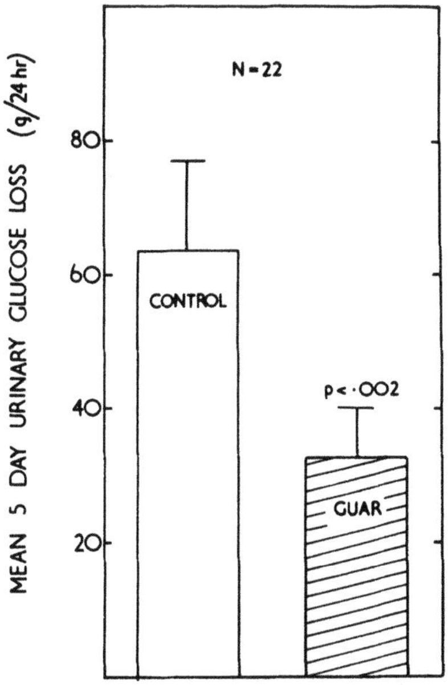

Fig. 1. Overall mean glucose loss in 18 diabetics (22 studies) over 5 days without (control) and with (test) guar supplementation.

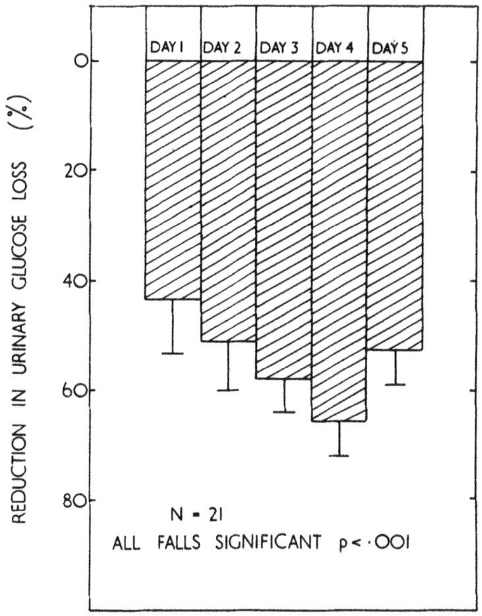

Fig. 2. Percentage reduction in urinary glucose loss of 17 diabetics (21 studies) during first 5 days on guar.

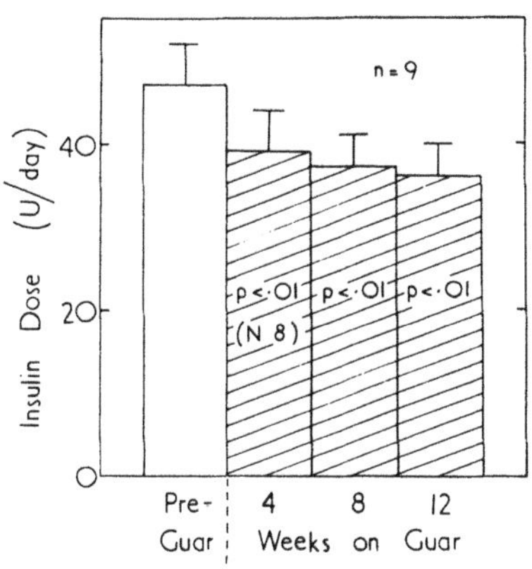

Fig. 3. Mean insulin dose of 9 diabetics before and during 12 weeks guar supplementation.

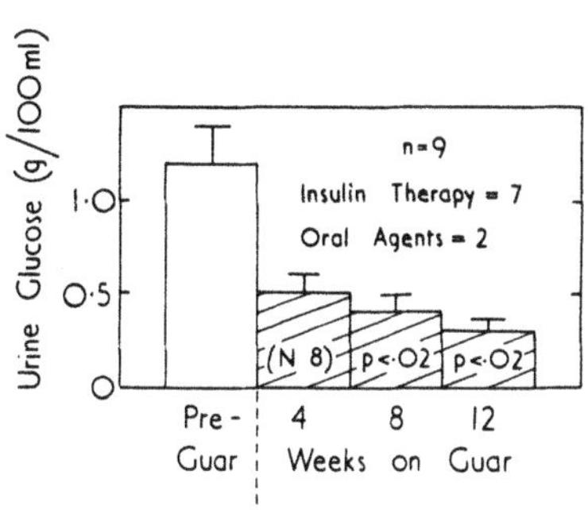

Fig. 4. Mean urinary glucose concentration on home testing of 9 diabetics before and during 12 weeks guar supplementation.

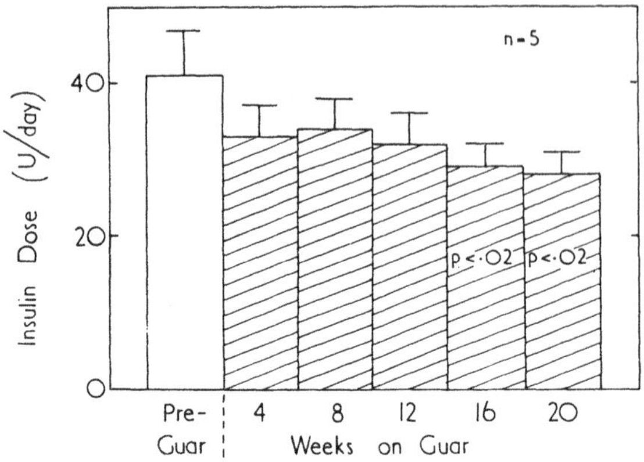

Fig. 5. Mean insulin dose of diabetics before and during 20 weeks of guar supplementation.

majority of the home urine tests over a 3-day period showed no glucose. In 9 patients (7 on insulin and 2 on oral agents) who had kept adequate urine testing charts throughout the day, the reduction in mean urinary glucose concentration was even more impressive (Fig. 4). Little further change was seen, however, in the insulin dosage (Fig. 5), and urinary glucose concentration of the 5 patients who were followed for the remainder of 20 weeks, although in this group the insulin reduction only reached statistical significance at 16 and 20 weeks.

DISCUSSION

These results further emphasize the observation that addition of fiber to the diet of some diabetics may reduce both the insulin requirement and the urinary glucose loss, but that the complete effect is not seen immediately and develops with time. The data indicate that in some diabetics the major change occurs during the first month of guar administration. Nevertheless, further reductions of small magnitude are seen for up to 12 weeks in urinary glucose concentration and insulin dose, while in the 5 patients followed for 20 weeks, the insulin reductions only became significant at 16 and 20 weeks.

Various types of dietary fiber have been shown to improve glucose tolerance in normal (10) and diabetic subjects (6) when added to test meals. It has also been shown that long-term administration of wheat bran to patients with diverticular disease improves glucose tolerance (11). Comparison of the effects of different types of fiber (7) suggests that the ability to increase the viscosity of gastrointestinal intraluminal contents is an important property in flattening the post-prandial glycemia. In part, this flattening may be related to slower mouth to caecum transit time and the slower absorption of carbohydrate (7). However, the acute gastrointestinal effects can only partly explain the metabolic changes induced by fiber.

Anderson and colleagues (1,2) showed the progressive effect of high fiber, high carbohydrate diets in allowing the sequential reduction of insulin dose in diabetics. Since food selection by the patient was not possible on the fixed metabolic ward diet, other adaptive changes must therefore have occurred which allowed insulin therapy to be withdrawn at a rate of approximately one unit per day, with no increase in fasting blood glucose.

Further evidence for a metabolic effect of dietary fiber is seen following 5 days guar administration. Here the reduction in urinary glucose output induced by guar remains for up to 3 days after guar has been removed from the diet (4).

This "carry-over" phenomenon not only shows that fiber has sustained metabolic effect but perhaps indicates that randomized cross-over studies may be inappropriate in this situation.

We conclude, therefore, that addition of certain types of fiber to the diet has both immediate and long-term effects. The latter may develop over days or weeks and may be useful therapeutically.

REFERENCES

1. *Kiehm, T.G., et al. (1976). Am. J. Clin. Nutr. 29, 895.*
2. *Anderson, J.W. and Ward, K. (1978). Diabetes Care 1, 77.*
3. *Jenkins, D.J.A., et al. (1977). Lancet 2, 779.*
4. *Jenkins, D.J.A., et al. (1978). Brit. Med. J. (in press).*
5. *Miranda, P.M. and Horwitz, D.L. (1978). Ann. Intern. Med. 88, 482.*
6. *Jenkins, D.J.A., et al. (1976). Lancet 2, 1972.*
7. *Jenkins, D.J.A., et al. (1978). Brit. Med. J. 1, 1392.*
8. *Diem, K. and Lentner, L. (1972). (Eds.) Documents Geigy: Scientific Tables, p. 712. Basle.*
9. *Werner, W., et al. (1970). Z. Analyt. Chem. 252*
10. *Jenkins, D.J.A., et al., (1977). Ann. Intern. Med. 86, 20.*
11. *Brodribb, A.J.M. and Humphreys, D.M. (1976). Brit. Med. J. 1, 420.*

TMSW and DN were supported by grants from the British Diabetic Association. We thank Mr. David Heath and Mr. Peter Lees for provision of guar crispbread and processed guar without which long term follow-up studies would not have been possible.

DISCUSSION

J. ANDERSON: *To eight individuals, we've fed 70% carbohydrate diets which were identical except that the fiber content was approximately 20 grams per day, a low fiber diet - almost as low as what the average American eats. With these low fiber diets, we saw a similar reduction in insulin dose. These eight individuals were matched, and we saw that the reduction in insulin dose was very similar in those patients fed low fiber diets as in those fed high fiber diets. In this type of examination, we cannot exclude an important effect of fiber, but it suggests that the major effect is related to the high carbohydrate and low fat content of our diet. We think that fiber plays the major role in preventing hypertriglyceridemia and perhaps in lowering the cholesterol. But, I think, with the type of fiber we use, its impact on glucose metabolism is less important than that of the nutrients.*

K.G.M.M. ALBERTI: *I think you've brought out a very important point there, that you've been using "fiber" and on that sort of global idea Jenkins and I have been looking specifically at guar and pectin because there the results are very striking. If you purely add guar, you do get an effect without changing any other part of the diet.*

J. TOBIN: *I thought, in your answer, you said that the triglyceride effects were due to the high fiber. In your eight low fiber patients, did their triglycerides also go down or up.*

J. ANDERSON: *No, they went up. That was a uniform phenomena. In eight out of eight, the triglycerides rose on the low fiber diet.*

J. TOBIN: *So, it's not a function of the complexity of the carbohydrates that protects?*

J. ANDERSON: *No.*

J. TOBIN: *The other question to Dr. Anderson and to Dr. Jenkins. Did you ever have the opportunity to measure the effect of gastric and gut hormones, like gastric inhibitory polypeptide, on the complex carboydrates? If not, were any studies on gastric motility done with high fiber diets?*

K.G.M.M. ALBERTI: *We found a very marked decrease in GIP secretion in both normal subjects and insulin dependent diabetics when we gave them a typical British breakfast of tomato soup, bread, butter and marmalade. But, the GIP went down very markedly with guar; it seemed to be a very important effect.*

J. ANDERSON: *A comment about the gastric emptying. Bread accelerates gastric emptying, but the soluble fibers, such as guar, seem to slow gastric emptying. Bran causes intestinal "hurry"; guar in the soluble fibers slow intestinal transit time.*

K.G.M.M. ALBERTI: *It's a very impresive effect. It's like eating glue, which is what it tastes like too. You would expect to get that sort of effect which you get with guar, but not with bran.*

J. BARBOSA: *Dr. Anderson, did you try high fiber, low carbohydrate diet?*

J. ANDERSON: *Yes, we have. We haven't done that extensively, but our limited experience shows that a high fiber diet of the mixed type of fiber we use has only a small impact on insulin doses. On our usual low carbohydrate diet, we see a reduction of a unit per day, roughly. We don't see that change on a standard carbohydrate, high fiber diet.*

K.G.M.M. ALBERTI: *Actually, in the British studies with a low carbohydrate diet, we found that guar decreases postprandial glycemia, smoothing out the curve. But, I don't know about long term effects.*

J. BARBOSA: *Our group reported last year about potato, rice and corn breakfast in both normals and chemical diabetics. We found marked differences between these types of complex carbohydrates and differences were even more marked for chemical diabetics, just like Dr. Reaven's data. Corn raised plasma glucose and plasma insulin more than both potato and rice. I wonder how many other factors influence these differences, even the age of the potato, because there is some breakdown of complex carbohydrates as the potato ages, and even the preparation of food - how long it is cooked. For instance, we used corn meal, but I think you used corn in a different form. So, there must be a multitude of factors. Therefore, these studies must be very, very strictly controlled to arrive at conclusions.*

R. CAMERINI-DAVALOS: *Dr. Anderson, have you tried to decrease the amount of insulin in your patients without any change in the diet?*

J. ANDERSON: *Yes, we have. We treated people with conventional diets for up to two weeks, and we've never been able to achieve greater than a 15% reduction in insulin dose.*

R. CAMERINI-DAVALOS: *And the blood sugar went up?*

J. ANDERSON: *Yes, the insulin reduction was accompanied by a rise in the blood sugar. In contrast with the HCT (high carbohydrate fiber) diet, the minimum we've reduced insulin is 15%, but this was accompanied by a reduction in blood sugar.*

R. CAMERINI-DAVALOS: *In one of our hospitals in New York, 70% of the patients are Puerto Ricans. If you prescribe a high protein diet for them, they comment "I cannot do it, I don't have the money for it." So, 70% of their diet is comprised of rice. We have great difficulty in controlling them. We bring them to the hospital and put them on a diet with carbohydrate and protein. Subsequently, we achieve what we call "good control". Upon returning home, they follow your diet, high in carbohydrates, high in rice, and the control is terrible. Why? If your data is correct what is wrong with those patients? Have you any suggestions?*

J. ANDERSON: *We had to do a careful dietary analysis of what they actually eat. I think they would probably get a fair amount of fat. I don't know whether they deep fry many things, but probably the fat content of their diet is moderately high. Also, they're probably eating refined carbohydrates, such as white rice and probably potatos without skins. When they do eat potatos, they are french fried potatos. I think the fat and the refined carbohydrate makes up a large component of their diet, whereas we provide essentially no refined carbohydrate. All of our foods are unrefined, like our forefathers ate.*

H. LEBOVITZ: *I have several questions for Dr. Anderson. I have had similar experiences as Dr. Camerini. In North Carolina, we likewise have a relatively high indigent population of patients who eat a very high carbohydrate diet. This precipitates very significant adult onset or insulin-independent diabets. We've been able to effectively control a significant number of these patients, who are not on insulin, by cutting the carbohydrate content down to 45%. The difference is that, with the 45% carbohydrate diet, we eliminate all of the simple sugars, so that we're now talking about the kind of complex carbohydrates to which Dr. Reaven referred. I wonder whether it may not be just total carbohydrate, but the percentage of the kinds of carbohydrates. Are the types of carbohydrate in your control period different?*

J. ANDERSON: *No. Basically, they're similar.*

H. LEBOVITZ: *So basically you're using exactly the same kinds of carbohydrates?*

J. ANDERSON: *Similar, yes. Obviously, our control diet is 43% carbohydrate. If that amounts to 210 grams of carbohydrate a day, that would be roughly 110 grams of simply carbohydrate and 100 grams of complex, and that's a breakdown fairly similar to diabetic diets that I've analyzed - roughly, half-complex, half-simple carbohydrate. What we do is, in essence, to add complex carbohydrate to that, and retain the simple carbohydrate.*

K.G.M.M. ALBERTI: *I think one of the very important points about you and Dr. Camerini's problems and ours with our Indian and Pakistani population, is not so much the fact they eat a lot of rice, but that they're eating too many total calories, and our biggest problem is maintaining body weight. If one got them on some type of isocaloric diet, which could maintain body weight in the normal range, perhaps many of these problems would disappear along with very irregular eating patterns which, on an insulin-independent diabetic, even with high carbohydrate, or plenty of guar in his diet, is going to play havoc with control.*

H. LEBOVITZ: *I was interested, secondly, in your insulin-binding studies. I'm not sure how to interpret them. These patients were on insulin initially, is that right, when the initial binding study was done?*

J. ANDERSON: *That's right.*

H. LEBOVITZ: *Well, then that really invalidates the significance of the differences.*

J. ANDERSON: *We studied eight people. Four were on insulin, four were not; four were chemical diabetics, two on sulfonylureas. We see similar results in people who were chemical diabetics on diets without sulfonylureas and on chemical diabetes treated with sulfonylureas. I think that does play a role, but it's difficult to interpret.*

H. LEBOVITZ: *The last question concerns again our experience with diet. It's very easy to lower the fasting blood sugar in people put on a modest carbohydrate diet. Do you have, say, sampling every two hours, or postprandial sampling to conclude that you really have achieved what you want? Insulin dosage is a very subjective matter, and whether the fasting sample is a valid way to measure it is questionable.*

J. ANDERSON: *Routinely we measure glucose excretion, which is an index, at least, in people with fasting blood sugars of 200. We have also routinely measured 3:00 p.m. plasma glucose. Then, on selected days, we made measurements throughout the day. We find that the fasting sugar is a fairly reasonable predictor of postprandial values on these diets.*

R. CLEMENTS: *Dr. Reaven, to follow up on Dr. Barbosa's comment, you showed a very impressive difference between feeding potato and boiled rice to your patients. Did you feed them the water in which you boiled the rice? Or, if you didn't, how much glucose and disaccharides do you discard?*

G. M. REAVEN: *Well, we didn't drain it. We fed it as we would have fed any baked potato or boiled rice. I wasn't aware that there was that much content of disaccharide in rice.*

R. CLEMENTS: *The only reason I bring it up is because we ran into this same problem with apple preparations, where we got a significantly lower glycemic excursion feeding boiled apple to a patient. However, if we fed them the juice in which it was boiled, we found no difference between the boiled and the raw.*

G. M. REAVEN: *That's probably not quite comparable.*

J. ANDERSON: *Apples are simple two-thirds carboydrate.*

R. CLEMENTS: *I'm just wondering how much you can leech out of something like rice?*

K.G.M.M. ALBERTI: *This is definitely a culinary sort of problem, because some people will boil rice in a large volume of water, drain the water away, and the rice then becomes somewhat white and frothy. Others will boil rice in a small, fixed amount of water and eat it when all the water is absorbed. It depends on whether you use that horrible package stuff or do it properly.*

G. M. REAVEN: *I'd like to make a few more comments. I think that one can show a moderate increase in insulin sensitivity by feeding a high carbohydrate diet, but I believe that the binding data are very controversial. In our, Jesse Roth's, and a group in Arhaus' hands, there's no question that feeding a high carbohydrate diet led to a decrease in insulin binding. Again, the results were comparable, that a few days of high carbohydrate diet led to a decrease in binding, due to a decrease in affinity. After a week or so, the decrease was due to a decrease in the number of receptors. Now, I'm surprised at your data, and I think they may well be explained by the fact that perhaps half of your patients were ones who were on insulin. Therefore, I think that there is some support for the notion that high carbohydrate is going to lead to some improvement in sensitivity. I'm not so sure about the binding, and I'd be very careful on that, because I believe many of us right now agree that's not the case. I think also, along with Dr. Camerini, that it would be more persuasive if you took patients at random and assign them at the same insulin level. If they came in on dose X, you put some on your diet, and decreased the insulin, some you kept on the control diet and tried to decrease the insulin, thereby demonstrating that there really was a difference. Many of us realize that "insulin requirement" is a vague term. Often, it is a function of what the doctor is giving the patient more than what the patient must take.*

G. GERRITSEN: *Two simplistic questions. One is for Dr. Reaven. Have you done metabolic balance studies, so that you know that the absorption of glucose from rice and from potato are similar?*

G. M. REAVEN: *We have not. The difference is not so much the biochemistry of these compounds, but the fact, as with guar, that you have a whole series of physical and mechanical GI factors taking place, which just slow down entry, rather than gross malabsorption.*

G. GERRITSEN: *The other question is for Dr. Anderson. On your high fiber diets, do you see a weight reduction in these individuals?*

J. ANDERSON: *We have fed weight-maintaining diets by design. On outpatients, we've seen weight reductions. We think these are good diets for weight reduction, because although they have a high satiety value; weights were maintained as constant as possible.*

DIETARY *MYO*-INOSITOL AND DIABETIC NEUROPATHY

R. S. Clements, Jr.*

A marked decrease in motor nerve conduction velocities can be demonstrated within days following the spontaneous development of hyperglycemia in man (1,2) or following the induction of experimental diabetes in the rat (3). When insulin therapy is instituted, this abnormality is promptly restored towards normal in both man and rodent. The rapidity of such fluctuations in peripheral nerve function has led to speculation that the neuropathy associated with early diabetes may be the consequence of acute biochemical alterations within the nerve which result from exposure of this tissue to elevated ambient glucose concentrations.

A disorder of neural *myo*-inositol metabolism has been proposed as one biochemical mechanism that could be responsible for these reversible functional abnormalities of the diabetic nerve. *Myo*-inositol is a six-carbon, cyclic polyhydric alcohol which is present within the nerve in a concentration roughly 50-times that of plasma. This extraordinary gradient has been speculated to play an important role in nerve function since it may facilitate the incorporation of *myo*-inositol into the phosphoinositides of the axolemmal membrane (4,5) that accompanies nerve impulse conduction and synaptic transmission.

The free *myo*-inositol concentration of the rat sciatic nerve is significantly decreased within weeks following the induction of streptozotocin diabetes (3,6). When the nerve free *myo*-inositol content is restored to normal by oral *myo*-inositol supplementation, the functional defect in motor nerve conduction velocity is obviated despite the persistence of elevated polyol pathway intermediates in this tissue (3). Since we previously observed that the human diabetic excretes excessive amounts of *myo*-inositol in his urine despite rigid control of his blood glucose concentration, we speculated that (as in the rat) abnormalities in neural *myo*-inositol metabolism could play a role in the pathogenesis of acute diabetic neuropathy (7). To test this hypothesis, we have studied the effect of variations in dietary *myo*-inositol intake upon peripheral nerve function in patients with distal symmetrical diabetic neuropathy.

METHODS

Following their provision of fully-informed consent, twenty patients with symptomatic diabetic polyneuropathy were studied at the Clinical Research Center of the University of Alabama. This group contained six women and 14 men whose average age was 42 years. They had been known to be diabetic for an average of 9 years, and had noted symptoms of neuropathy for an average of 17 months prior to entrance into this study. All patients complained of pain and numbness of the lower extremities and manifested bilateral stocking hypesthesia as well as absent Achilles reflexes.

Following measurement of baseline diurnal plasma glucose and *myo*-inositol concentrations, 24-hour urinary *myo*-inositol excretion, and nerve conduction velocities, the patients were randomized to groups which ingested diets with either a low or a high *myo*-inositol content for a period of 16 weeks. Biochemical analyses and nerve conduction velocity determinations were repeated after 1, 2, 4, 8, and 16 weeks on the diet. Subsequently, the patients were crossed-over to the alternative diet and the studies described above were repeated.

Plasma glucose was determined enzymatically and dietary, urinary, and plasma *myo*-inositol was quantified by gas-liquid chromatography as previously described (7). Repeat nerve conduction velocities were always performed in the same extremity in a given patient. Each determination was repeated 10 times, the values corrected to a skin temperature of 35°C, and the mean value utilized for subsequent analysis (8).

RESULTS

As shown in Table 1, the *myo*-inositol content of the low diet was reduced by 30% and that of the high diet was increased by 10% when compared with that of the control diet. Plasma *myo*-inositol concentrations fell by 16% on the low and rose by 31% on the high-*myo*-inositol diet when similarly compared. Urinary *myo*-inositol excretion decreased by 20% on the low diet and more than tripled on the high-*myo*-inositol diet. The diurnal plasma glucose concentrations were similar on all of the diets, although they tended to decrease slightly on the low and to increase slighly on the high-*myo*-inositol diet.

Table 1

PLASMA GLUCOSE AND *MYO*-INOSITOL (MI) CONCENTRATIONS AND URINARY *MYO*-INOSITOL EXCRETION WHILE PATIENTS WERE INGESTING DIETS WITH VARIOUS *MYO*-INOSITOL CONTENTS

Diet	Dietary MI Intake (mM/day)	Diurnal Plasma MI Concentration (mM)	Urinary MI Excretion (mM/day)	Diurnal Plasma Glucose Concentration (mM)
Control	3.45 ± 0.44	0.038 ± 0.004	0.15 ± 0.05	8.64 ± 1.72
Low MI	2.43 ± 0.36	0.032 ± 0.002	0.12 ± 0.06	7.66 ± 0.87
High MI	7.13 ± 1.50*+	0.046 ± 0.003+	0.50 ± 0.17	9.31 ± 1.45

*p versus control diet < 0.05
+ p versus low-MI diet < 0.05

All nerve conduction velocities were profoundly decreased in the neuropathic diabetics (Table 2). When the nerve conduction velocities were analyzed as groups, the values observed on the low- and the high- *myo*-inositol diets did not differ significantly from each other or from the values observed while the patients were ingesting the control diet. However, when each patient served as his own control, analysis of paired differences revealed that both motor nerve conduction velocities fell significantly while the patients were ingesting the low-*myo*-inositol diet and both of the sensory nerve conduction velocities rose substantially while they were ingesting the high-*myo*-inositol diet (Figure 1).

DISCUSSION

These studies indicate that variations in the dietary intake of *myo*-inositol can be utilized to manipulate the diurnal plasma *myo*-inositol concentration and the urinary *myo*-inositol excretion in patients with diabetic neuropathy. Furthermore, they suggest that increased dietary *myo*-inositol intake may have a salutory effect upon sensory nerve function in the "well-controlled" neuropathic diabetic. Conversely, a decrease in the dietary intake of *myo*-inositol appeared to further impair the motor nerve conduction velocities in this group of patients.

Table 2

NERVE CONDUCTION VELOCITIES IN NORMAL SUBJECTS AND IN NEUROPATHIC DIABETICS ON CONTROL, LOW-AND HIGH-*MYO*-INOSITOL (MI) DIETS

	Nerve Conduction Velocity (m/sec)			
	Median Motor	Median Sensory	Peroneal Motor	Sural Sensory
Normal Subjects (n = 16)	63.1 ±0.5	46.4 ±0.7	55.9 ±0.9	45.7 ±0.6
Diabetic Patients (n = 20)				
Control Diet	51.7 ±0.8	41.9 ±1.8	40.7 ±1.1	33.3 ±1.6
Low-MI Diets	52.1 ±0.5	41.5 ±1.4	41.3 ±0.8	33.9 ±1.2
High-MI Diets	52.4 ±0.5	42.6 ±1.3	41.2 ±0.7	36.1 ±1.1

The explanation for the disparate effects of variations in dietary *myo*-inositol intake upon the function of the motor and sensory nerves of the neuropathic diabetic is not clear. However, the speculation that the sensory nerves are exquisitely sensitive to the slight decrease in diurnal plasma *myo*-inositol concentrations observed in this group of patients (38.0 μM versus 50.0 μM in non-diabetic control subjects),whereas the motor nerves may only be affected by more substantial losses of *myo*-inositol could offer a possible explanation. Such an hypothesis would account for the impairment of motor nerve function observed on the low-*myo*-inositol diet as well as the improvement in sensory nerve conduction velocities observed on the high-*myo*-inositol diet. In addition, it could provide an explanation for the rapid improvement in motor nerve conduction velocities (without parallel improvement in sensory nerve function) that has been observed following the initiation of insulin treatment and the concomitant termination of excessive urinary *myo*-inositol excretion in the uncontrolled diabetic (1,2,7).

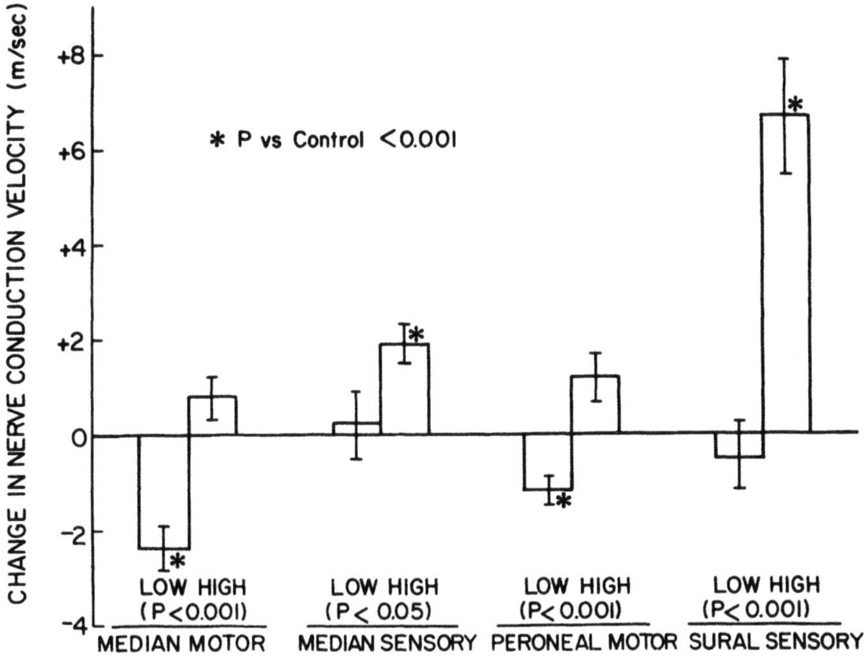

Fig. 1. Changes in nerve conduction velocity in twenty neuropathic diabetics on low-and high- myo-inositol diets. The asterisks refer to statistically significant differences from the control determinations (P values all < 0.001). The P values resulting from comparison of the changes observed on the low and high diets are given in parenthesis.

Recently two reports have appeared which support the aforementioned speculations. It has been observed that in the mildly diabetic rat (mean plasma glucose 17.2 mM), oral *myo*-inositol supplementation has little influence upon motor nerve conduction velocities (9). This observation is consistent with a lack of effect of a slightly decreased total body *myo*-inositol pool size upon motor nerve function. In contrast, the salutory effect of oral *myo*-inositol supplementation upon motor nerve conduction velocities in severely diabetic rats (mean plasma glucose 30.4 mM) may reflect the severity of the decrease in the *myo*-inositol pool of these animals prior to treatment (3). In agreement with the present study, it has recently been reported that the oral administration of 3.0 grams per day of *myo*-inositol had no effect upon the mean motor nerve conduction velocities of a group of sixty treated human diabetics (10).

In sum, the currently available data suggest that slight depletion of the body pool of *myo*-inositol (as is observed in the treated human diabetic and the mildly diabetic rat) may impair sensory nerve function. More profound losses of *myo*-inositol (such as are seen with decreased dietary *myo*-inositol intake and with severe hyperglycemia in both man and rodent) may be required before an effect upon motor nerve function can be detected. The possibility that oral *myo*-inositol supplementation will prove to be of value in the treatment of established diabetic neuropathy or in the modification of the natural history of nerve dysfunction in diabetic patients without symptoms of neuropathy must await the results of further investigations.

REFERENCES

1. *Gregerson, G. (1968). Diabetologia 4, 273*
2. *Ward, J.D., et al.(1971). Lancet 1, 428*
3. *Greene, D.A., et al.(1975). J. Clin. Invest. 55,1326*
4. *Hawthorne, J.N. and Kai, M. (1970) in Handbook of Neurochemistry, Lajtha, A. ed., Plenum Press, New York, p. 491*
5. *Gould, R.M. (1976). Brain Res. 117, 168*
6. *Palmano, K.P., et al.(1977). Biochem. J. 167,229*
7. *Clements, R.S. and Reynertson, R. (1977). Diabetes 26, 215*
8. *Oh, S.J., et al.(1978). Ann. Neurol. 4, 369*
9. *Jefferys, J.G.R., et al.(1978). J. Neurol. Neurosurg. Psych. 41, 333*
10. *Gregerson, G., et al.(1977). Diabetologia 13, 397*

This research was supported by grants from the Veterans Administration, the Diabetes Trust Fund, the Juvenile Diabetes Foundation and Grants RR-32 and AM-21065 from the National Institutes of Health.

DISCUSSION

J. BARBOSA: *We have done some oral myoinositol tests, and we essentially confirmed all of Dr. Clements' findings. But, since we have so many diabetic kidney recipients around, and since the kidney was possibly one of the main sites for the metabolism of myoinositol, we also obtained oral myoinositol intolerance tests in patients who had received their kidneys about two to three years prior. Their control was as poor as any other patient's but their creatinine clearance was normal. To our great surprise, the oral myoinositol in these kidney recipients was normal. We could think of only two explanations, but we have not tested these hypotheses. One is that the patients were on prednisone, which could possibly change the myoinositol absorption. The other possibility is that, in the diabetics who had diabetes for 10 to 15 years, there might be a lesion in the kidney responsible, at least in part, for myoinositol intolerance, a lesion which was not present in the transplanted kidneys. I would be interested in Dr. Clements' comments on this.*

R. CLEMENTS: *The kidney is the major organ for the disposal of myoinositol, both by excretion and, as it turns out in the rat and in man, by oxidation. The normal human kidney makes about two grams of myoinositol a day, so we make four grams of myoinositol per day in our kidneys when we're fasting. The total turnover of myoinositol in normal human subjects is about nine grams a day. Our dietary intake makes only about 10% of the total turnover of myoinositol. However, if we look at myoinositol turnover in the patient who is a recipient of a kidney, it is decreased to about 4, 4½ grams per day, implying that the kidney does contribute a significant amount of myoinositol to the total circulating myoinositol pool. The speculations that Dr. Barbosa mentioned are quite reasonable ones. That is, the lesion kidney may not yet have lost the capacity to oxidize myoinositol. In addition, the fact that the patient is now uninephric may be responsible for less myoinositol input into the system, which in turn may account for the normalization of the oral myoinositol tolerance.*

K.G.M.M. ALBERTI: *Two questions for information: First, do capillary cells metabolize myoinositol at all? Secondly, what are the foods which are particularly rich in myoinositol?*

R. CLEMENTS: *With regard to the capillary metabolism of myoinositol, it is not understood and has not been well studied. The capillary does contain concentrations of about 10 times that of plasma, or the aorta does, at least. However, it does not seem to actively concentrate the material. I don't know if Dr. Freinkel has been able to get much of any tissue to actively concentrate the material. Even the pancreatic islet won't actively concentrate it either in our hands or in the hands of Dr. Paul Lacy. With regard to the foods that are high in myoinositol, grain foods are extraordinarily high; fruits, particularly canteloupe and cherries, are high. Fish are low. White breads are low, and whole grain breads are high. We use a simple exchange list, and go heavy on either the low or high foods to try to maintain the various diets.*

M. VRANIC: *You have shown that tolerance for myoinositol is abnormal in diabetes. How does that correlate to the abnormal glucose tolerance test? How does it correlate with severity of diabetes? Could this be used as an index of early diabetes?*

R. CLEMENTS: *This was our hope years ago, and once we found that the oral myoinositol tolerance could completely be normalized by careful control of the hyperglycemia, we became aware that it was secondary to the hyperglycemia, rather than a primary genetic abnormality. We haven't looked at this in a broad range of patients with varying degrees of abnormal carbohydrate tolerance, however.*

N. FREINKEL: *More than a decade ago, we tried to see whether concentration gradients could be established in vitro. We were unable to establish this to any meaningful degree. We felt that might be because the exit flux so preponderated over the influx, that we had an artificial situation. So, we went on to an in vivo turnover, to see where the concentration gradients and specific activity equilibrium could be achieved, and that was also very, very slow. Equilibrium was not achieved over any rapid interval. The problem then arises that, if one can't establish intracellular concentration gradient, then, theoretically, therapeutic efficacy would require elevating plasma levels to a point where diffusion per se restored intracellular concentration of the myoinositol to a putative normal level. Since that is so slow to achieve with isotope exchange experiments, one would be very hard put to understand what is achieved with feeding regimes which affect relatively minor changes in circulating myoinositol levels.*

R. CLEMENTS: *I think that's a very valid point. We increase plasma myoinositol concentrations by only about 20% in these individuals. But, interestingly enough, the diurnal plasma myoinositol concentration in diabetics on high myoinositol diet was very similar to that of our control subjects on a normal diet. If there is competitive inhibition for transport, this should not have any marked effect on intracellular concentration.*

EFFECT OF INSULIN TREATMENT ON THE MESANGIAL STRUCTURE OF KK MICE

W. Oppermann*, H. Wehner, A.S. Reddi
and R.A. Camerini-Davalos

In previous communications, we described specific glomerular changes in genetically diabetic KK mice (1-4). These changes include an increase in mesangial matrix and thickening of the glomerular basement membrane. Increase in the mesangium was found as early as two months of age, which gradually progressed with aging (3-4). Similar findings were described by other investigators.

The highly predictable, spontaneous occurrence of glomerular lesions in the KK strain motivated us to attempt to delay, ameliorate or even prevent the formation of these findings. A protective effect without significant alterations in the fasting blood sugar or serum IRI levels or in body weight was demonstated by treatment with Pyridinolcarbamate (PDC), an antibradykinin agent (5,6). Other studies revealed that the early control of hyperglycemia by glyburide, a sulfonylurea compound, delays the progression of glomerulosclerosis in these mice (7).

In the present investigation, we report the effect of insulin treatment on the mesangial structure in KK mice. For this purpose, the number of mesangial cells, mesangial area and also total glomerular area in insulin and saline treated mice were quantitated. In addition, the quantification of epithelial and endothelial cells was performed. This method defines the severity of glomerulosclerosis especially in very young mice in a more accurate and quantitative manner.

MATERIAL AND METHODS

The KK mice used in this study have been inbred in our laboratory for 12 years. They were fed the Old Guilford mouse laboratory chow ad libitum.

Lente Pork insulin (Squibb & Sons Lab ., Princeton, N.J.) was diluted (0.1 m/1 2.5 U) in 0.9% saline containing 1% albumin. 25 U/kg were injected subcutaneously into the nuchal area once a day for 7 days a week in KK mice of both sexes. An equal number of saline injected KK mice served as controls. All mice were weighed weekly. The animals were treated from 20 days of age until they were sacrificed at 40 and 100 days of age.

Blood was collected from the orbital sinuses of mice fasted for 18 hr. into capillary tubes. Twenty microliters of whole blood was mixed with 1% NaF in a unopette (B.D. Co., Rutherford, N.J.) for sugar determination by the ferricyanide method of Hoffman on the Technicon Autoanalyzer.

The mice were sacrificed by cervical dislocation, the kidneys were excised, weighed, and a portion of the kidney was fixed in 10% neutral formalin. Morphometric analyses were performed as described previously (8). All measurements were done in a blind fashion.

RESULTS

Table 1 contains general information on KK mice studied. The body weight and kidney weight remained similar in mice of both age groups treated with insulin or saline. The fasting blood

TABLE 1

	TREATMENT	AGE IN DAYS 40	100
Body Weight (g)	Saline	20.9 ± 0.6 (9)	27.1 ± 0.7 (11)
	Insulin	21.4 ± 0.4 (9)	26.8 ± 0.3 (9)
Blood Sugar (mg/dl)	Saline	96.0 ± 4.0 (9)	110 ± 3.0 (11)
	Insulin	88.0 ± 5.0 (9)	99.0 ± 6.0 (9)
Kidney Weight (g)	Saline	0.225 ± 0.011 (9)	0.303 ± 0.011 (11)
	Insulin	0.228 ± 0.010 (9)	0.322 ± 0.010 (9)

General information on KK mice. Values are means ± S.E. numbers in parentheses represent number of animals.

sugars showed a lower tendency in insulin treated KK mice in both age groups, although the means fall short of statistical significance.

Table 2 illustrates data from the morphometric analysis of glomeruli in KK mice treated only for 20 days (age of mice 40 days). Although a decreasing tendency in the number of epithelial, endothelial and mesangial cells was found in insulin treated mice, the differences were not statistically significant.

TABLE 2

	SALINE (n = 9)	INSULIN (n = 5)
Epithelial Cells	12.0 ± 0.5	10.1 ± 0.8
Endothelial Cells	15.0 ± 0.8	13.2 ± 0.8
Mesangial Cells	13.5 ± 1.1	11.0 ± 0.2
Total Glomerular Cells	40.2 ± 2.0	34.3 ± 1.6
% Epithelial Cells	30.2 ± 1.1	29.1 ± 1.4
% Endothelial Cells	36.6 ± 0.5	38.3 ± 1.3
% Mesangial Cells	33.0 ± 1.0	37.7* ± 1.1

* $P < 0.05$
Morphometric studies of glomeruli in KK mice treated from 20 to 40 days of age. Values are means ±.S.E.

Table 3 summarizes the glomerular and mesangial areas in mice treated with saline or insulin for 20 days. The total, as well as the percent, mesangial areas were significantly lower in insulin treated mice ($p < 0.02$). Total glomerular area was not different between the two groups of mice.

The results of the morphometric analysis of kidneys of KK mice treated either with insulin or saline for 80 days (age of mice 100 days) are shown in Tables 4 and 5. No significant differences in various cell types were found between saline and insulin treated mice (Table 4). Similar results were observed with regard to the glomerular and mesangial areas (Table 5).

TABLE 3

	SALINE (n = 9)	INSULIN (n = 5)
Glomerular Area ($\mu 2$)	4550.0 ± 102.7	4145.3 ± 130.7
Mesangial Area (μ^2)	609.6 ± 29.1	445.0 ± 32.4*
% Mesangial Area	13.0 ± 0.5	10.8 ± 0.6**

* $P < 0.02$; ** $P < 0.05$

Glomerular and mesangial areas in KK mice treated from 20 to 40 days of age. Values shown are means ±.S.E.

TABLE 4

	SALINE (n - 14)	INSULIN (n = 9)
Epithelial Cells	12.0 ± 1.0	13.2 ± 1.0
Endothelial Cells	15.4 ± 0.3	15.8 ± 0.8
Mesangial Cells	13.2 ± 1.0	11.2 ± 0.5
Total Glomerular Cells	40.4 ± 1.9	40.2 ± 1.3
% Epithelial Cells	30.0 ± 1.5	32.8 ± 2.0
% Endothelial Cells	38.1 ± 1.0	38.8 ± 1.3
% Mesangial Cells	32.5 ± 1.3	28.5 ± 1.0

Morphometric studies of glomeruli in KK mice treated from 20 to 100 days of age. Values are means ± S.E.

TABLE 5

	SALINE (n = 14)	INSULIN (n = 9)
Glomerular Area (u^2)	5038.0 ± 137.0	5323.8 ± 145.1
Mesangial Area (u^2)	643.0 ± 39.0	690.1 ± 46.4
% Mesangial Area	12.9 ± 0.7	12.9 ± 0.7

Glomerular and mesangial areas in KK mice treated from 20 to 100 days of age.

DISCUSSION

A smaller absolute number ($p<0.02$) and percentage of mesangial area was observed in 40 day-old KK mice after treatment with the medium acting Lente Pork insulin (LPI) for 20 days (Table 3). We could demonstrate, therefore, by morphometric studies that the treatment with LPI over a short period exerts a protective effect on the development of glomerular changes in genetically diabetic mice with spontaneously occurring glomerulosclerosis.

In the long term experiment, no significant difference was observed between KK mice, injected with insulin or saline for 80 days (sacrificed at 100 days) (Table 5). This finding appears to be in disagreement with our previous communications, in which we described a delay in the progression and severity of glomerular lesions in KK mice by long term treatment with pyridinolcarbamate or glyburide (5-7).

The treatment studies of KK mice with monocomponent insulin (MC insulin) and immunologically active insulin (depot insulin) offer some explanation (8). The protective influence of the MC insulin versus the ineffectiveness of the depot insulin on the progression of glomerular changes in these experiments indicate that improvement in carbohydrate metabolism without concurrent antibody formation is responsible for the prevention of glomerulosclerosis.

The data presented by us support these observations. It can be assumed that the demonstrated protective effect on the development of glomerulosclerosis in our KK mice, treated with insulin for 20 days, was also at least over part of the experimental period associated with lowered blood sugars (although not statistically significant) without concurrent antibody formation. The delay in the progression and severity of glomerular changes in KK mice treated with pyridinolcarbamate (5,6) or glyburide (7) can similarly be explained by the absence of insulin antibodies. Antibody formation to the depot insulin (Lente Pork insulin), on the other hand, appears to be responsible for the lack of protective effect on the development of glomerular changes in KK mice treated for 80 days. This would explain why some diabetic patients develop severe microvascular complications despite long term insulin therapy.

REFERENCES

1. *Treser, G., et al (1965). Glomerular lesions in a strain of genetically diabetic mice. Proc. Soc. Exp. Biol. Med. 129, 820.*
2. *Camerini-Davalos, R.A. (1970). Studies of vascular and other lesions in KK mice. Diabetologia 6, 324*
3. *Ehrenreich, T., et al (1973). In "Vascular and Neurological Changes in Early Diabetes" (R.A. Camerini-Davalos and H.S. Cole, eds.), pp. 271-280. Academic Press, New York.*
4. *Oppermann, W., et al (1973). In "Vascular and Neurological Changes in Early Diabetes" (R. A. Camerini-Davalos and H.S. Cole, eds.) pp. 281-290 Academic Press, New York*
5. *Oppermann, W., et al (1976). Attempts to delay the progression of inherited vasculopathy. Ann. N.Y. Aca. Sci., 275, 348-362.*
6. *Reddi, A.S., et al (1977). Diabetic Microangiopathy in KK Mice II. Suppression of Glomerulosclerosis by Pyridinolcarbamate Exp. Mol-Pathol. 26, 325.*
7. *Reddi, A.S., et al (1978). Diabetic microangiopathy in KK mice. III. Effect of prolonged glyburide treatment on glomerulosclerosis. Exp. Mol. Pathol. 29, 92.*
8. *Wehner, H., et al (1978). Influence of short-term insulin therapy on the mesangial structure in young KK mice. Nephron 22, 460.*

INSULIN TREATMENT FOR ADULT ONSET DIABETES: A REPORT OF THE UNIVERSITY GROUP DIABETES PROGRAM

T. E. Prout*

The University Group Diabetes Program was a long-term prospective clinical trial designed to evaluate the effects of various hypoglycemic agents on the vascular complications of patients with asymptomatic adult-onset non-insulin dependent diabetes. Among patients enrolled in this study, insulin used either in fixed dose or in variable doses in an attempt to normalize blood glucose was no better than diet alone in prolonging life or in preventing macrovascular or microvascular complications (1). The purpose of this paper is to explore the implications of this finding and to comment on other interpretations of the data.

The follow-up status of the patients in the report consists of 619 individuals, or approximately 200 patients in each of three treatment groups. All patients were available for follow -up over a period of nine years, and 460 patients (74%) were followed for 11 or more years. This is by far the largest group of patients studied prospectively in a clinical trial for this long a period of time.

The mean fasting blood glucose values for a cohort of patients followed for approximately nine years is shown in Fig. 1. The standard error of the mean for glucose values in each treatment group at standard times is approximately 7.3 mgs.%. The mean dose of insulin needed for patients in the variable insulin group increased from 10 units per patient per day at baseline to 47 units at the close of the study. Fifteen patients in this group were on two injections of insulin per day, and hypoglycemia was diagnosed in 80 patients in the variable insulin group. These observations can be compared to those of the insulin standard group in which the mean dose of insulin was 15 units throughout the study, and the hypoglycemic episodes reported were 22. This effect at control resulted in fasting blood glucose values of less than 150 mg./dl. more than 75% of the time in 65% of the variable insulin group compared to 40% in the patients treated with diet alone. Equally important, the blood glucose was more than 150 mg./dl. only 7% of the time for the variable insulin group as compared to 23% in the diet alone group. This degree of difference in glucose control would be expected to indicate whether insulin therapy as it is now used is effective in preventing degenerative complications in these patients over that achieved by diet alone.

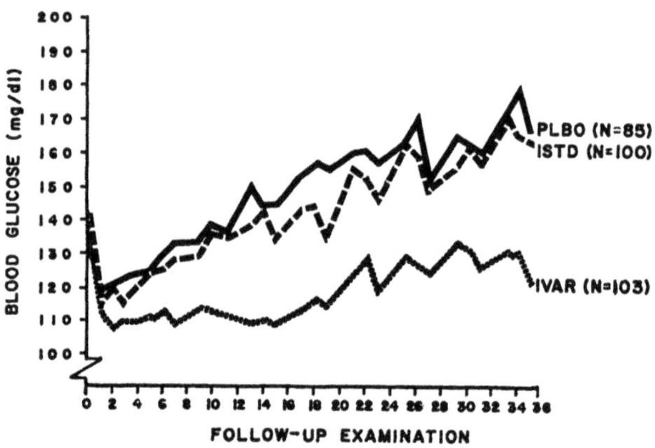

Fig. 1. Mean fasting blood glucose for cohort followed for 35 examinations.

In contrast to the differences in glucose control, there were no significant differences in mortality rates among these treatment groups. Death due to cardiovascular causes were 14.1%, 12.9%, and 14.2% in patients treated with diet alone, insulin standard, and variable insulin respectively. Similarly, death from all causes in these groups were 26.3%, 22.9% and 24.0%.

As regards non-fatal events, there were no significant differences among treatment groups in EKG abnormalities, angina, hypertension, fundus abnormalities, urine protein, or arterial calcification as shown in Table 1. The percentage of patients with an elevation of serum creatinine above 1.5 mg./dl. was 16.3% for patients treated with diet alone, 8.3% for insulin standard patients, and 9.1% for variable insulin patients. The p value for these treatment differences was 0.03 and 0.06 for insulin standard and insulin variable respectively.

Table 1

INSULIN ANALOGS WITH MODIFICATIONS AT THE N- AND C-TERMINAL AMINO ACID RESIDUES OF THE A CHAIN[a]

Insulin Analog	(S=sheep) (P=pig)	IU/mg MC	GO	DGT	RIA	% of Natural Insulin RB
Des(tetrapeptide A^{1-4})	(S)	0				0.03 (LM)
Des(tetrapeptide A^{1-4})	(P)	0				
Deamino-A^{1}	(S)	7-10				
[Sarcosine^{1}-A]	(S)	20			9	
[L-Alanine^{1}-A]	(S)	7.5-9	2.3	3		10 (FC)
[D-Alanine^{1}-A]	(S)	10.5-12	23	24		100 (FC)
[Isoasparagine^{21}-A]	(S)	21			16	
[D-Asparagine^{21}-A]	(S)	8			4	
[Arginine^{21}-A]	(S)	10.5-12	9.5		8.5-12	40 (FC); 18 (LM)
[Asparaginamide^{21}-A]	(S)	17			4	68 (LM)
[Sarcosine^{1}-, Isoasparagine^{21}-A]	(S)	15			7	

[a] MC, mouse convulsion assay; GO, glucose oxidation assay in isolated fat cells; DGT, 2-deoxy-D-glucose transport assay; RIA, radioimmunoassay; RB, receptor binding; LM, liver membranes; FC, fat cells.

Although serum creatinine may be a sensitive marker for the microvasculopathy in patients with diabetes, these differences were not borne out by similar findings in the microvascular pathology seen in the fundus. The changes in the eye have been watched with particular interest because of the ease and accuracy with which changes in the fundi can be photographed and quantitated. If treatment differences were to be seen under the conditions of this study, they should be found in relation to pathologic changes with a high rate of occurrence. Thus, in spite of the fact that fundus abnormalities occurred at a rate of approximately 4% per year, no treatment differences were found. This suggests that we will need to understand the pathogenesis of macro-and microvascular changes better before we are able to apply more meaningful therapeutic measures to the treatment of patients with adult-onset diabetes to prevent these complications.

These results have reignited the debate as to the effectiveness of present methods of insulin usage in adult-onset, non-ketone prone diabetic patients. As one reviews the possible reasons for failure to detect the influence of insulin in this group, a number of possibilities must be considered. Among these must be listed the possibility that the blood glucose level found in these patients is not an independent factor in the pathogenesis of vascular disease. Weight reduction through caloric control has been shown to be an effective way to control all of the metabolic abnormalities in the diabetic patient and to improve the effectiveness of endogenous insulin. For this reason dietary management deserves greater emphasis in these patients than it has recently received.

On the other hand, attempts to find a different conclusion in these data through re-analysis is hazardous. It will be recognized that the inclusion of patients into groups into which they were randomized is conservative, as noted by Cornfield (2) and "dilutes whatever treatment effects, beneficial or adverse, are present. The comparison based on patients with good adherence only is generally considered unsafe because the original comparability provided by randomization may be impaired". When subgroup analysis is needed, patients should be reviewed by degree of adherence. When the percentage of patients in each treatment group who took all or some of the prescribed medications 75% or more of the time are compared, no evidence of treatment effect is shown.

Other attempts have been made to analyze these data after serious manipulations of the composition of the treatment groups (3). The authors of this critique have made the unproven assumption that all patients who died within the first year must be eliminated from analysis. This is justified by the authors by stating that "only subjects with the life expectancy of five years were supposed to be recruited into the study". Although the physicians could not be infallible, the selected patients had an overall rate of survival above that expected. In any event, there is no justification for removing patients from analysis who died during the first year. An analysis by adherence by treatment group is also an accepted way of subgroup analysis for the problem of dropouts.

Having eliminated the individuals who died during the first year, the authors decided arbitrarily to eliminate all patients over 70 who did not die, but the total number of patients 70 years or older in the study was only 5.5% at baseline. Further elimination of patients with diastolic blood pressures equal to or greater than 110 suggests that there is no need to study the effect of insulin therapy in anyone but healthy young people. Elimination of patients with FBS at baseline greater than 150 mg./dl. (or greater than 200 mg./dl.) implies that insulin therapy should not be tested in severe diabetics and leads to the conclusion that variable insulin reduces mortality in patients with fasting blood sugars at baseline that are less than 150 mg.%.

Legitimate differences of opinion undoubtedly exist concerning the way data should be analyzed. It is essential, however, that these differences of opinion be subjected to peer review and to competent scientific scrutiny. The controversies concerning the UGDP findings and their clinical significance cannot be resolved except by careful analysis of data that are presented in referred scientific publications.

REFERENCES

1. *UGDP: (1978) JAMA 240, 37.*
2. *Cornfield, J. (1971) JAMA 217, 1676.*
3. *Kilo, C. et al. (1979) in Treatment of Early Diabetes. ed. R. Camerini-Davalos and B. Hanover, Plenum, New York,*

REFUTING THE UGDP CONCLUSION THAT INSULIN TREATMENT DOES NOT PREVENT VASCULAR COMPLICATIONS IN DIABETES

C. Kilo, J. R. Williamson*, S. C. Choi, and
J. P. Miller

If the "late" complications of diabetes are indeed the direct and/or indirect consequences of insulin deficiency, we would anticipate that therapeutic measures which effectively normalize blood glucose levels should reduce the frequency and severity of cardiovascular complications associated with diabetes. Therapeutic measures which substantially reduce blood glucose levels but fall short of achieving euglycemia might also be expected to reduce cardiovascular complications if the relationship between the two is linear, but not necessarily if the relationship is more complex.

Indeed, Pirart (1) has suggested that such factors might account for the discrepancy in his findings of a strong association between diabetic neuropathy, retinopathy and nephropathy with the duration and severity of hyperglycemia, whereas macrovascular disease correlated better with age of the diabetic and with duration of diabetes, but not with severity of hyperglycemia or degree of control achieved. Thus neuropathy and microangiopathy may be more directly related to hyperglycemia whereas the pathogenesis of macroangiopathy may be much more complex (multifactorial).

In contrast to Pirart's observations, UGDP investigators (2) recently reported that insulin treatment which significantly lowered blood glucose levels (achieving values close to normoglycemia) did not reduce the frequency of macro- or microangiopathy in mild, asymptomatic maturity-onset diabetics. Because of several questions regarding the UGDP approach to data analysis, we have examined patient data recently released by the UGDP coordinating center, in an effort to determine whether their inability to demonstrate an association between cardiovascular disease and control of hyperglycemia might be related to their method of analysis or to other unrecognized discrepancies in the data.

MATERIALS AND METHODS

The data based utilized for our analysis was comprised of computer printout sheets of patient data provided by the UGDP Coordinating Center in Baltimore, Maryland. It should be noted that the patient information released by the UGDP did not include ECG data or history of heart disease (use of digitalis, hospitalization for heart disease, or angina pectoris). Since the objective of the UGDP study was to assess the long term effects of hypoglycemic therapy on cardiovascular complications in patients with asymptomatic adult-onset diabetes, we eliminated from our analysis all subjects who:

1) died or dropped out in the first year of the program (before any significant beneficial effect of therapy might be anticipated) and,

2) were unavailable for follow-up for 4 consecutive quarterly examinations (1 year) and/or changed medication for the same period of time.

RESULTS AND DISCUSSION

Of the approximately 619 subjects recruited into the three treatment groups under analysis (Placebo = PLBO, Insulin Standard = ISTD, and Insulin Variable = IVAR)*, 25 (4%) died or dropped out in the first year of the program. An additional 39% of all subjects were unavailable for follow-up and/or were on medication not originally assigned for 4 consecutive scheduled visits or longer. In fact, these subjects, whom we designated drop outs or medication changes (DO·MC), were on medication different from that originally assigned or missed their scheduled examinations, an average of 23 $\pm$ 12 quarters (or 5.75 years) compared to 2.5 $\pm$ 3 quarters for the remaining subjects. Thus, in our opinion, 43% of all subjects recruited into these treatment groups should have been excluded from analyses designed to assess effects of insulin treatment on vascular complications.

When we looked at the mean fasting blood glucose values of the remaining subjects for the duration of the study, we found that they were only 16 mg% lower for the IVAR group than for the PLBO group (Table 1). Note that the standard deviations are quite large which indicates that blood glucose values were much higher than the mean of 119 mg% in many individuals.

*PLBO treatment consisted of dietary control and administration of an inactive pill or capsule. ISTD consisted of administration of a fixed dose of insulin which was proportional to body weight and therefore was varied only when there was significant weight change; and IVAR treatment consisted of insulin injection, the quantity of which was adjusted in an effort to normalize blood glucose levels. See UGDP publications (2) for further details.

Table 1. Mean Fasting Blood Glucose Values in Subjects Who did not Drop Out or Change Medication

	MEAN $\pm$ SD
PLBO	135 $\pm$ 56 (mg%)
ISTD	132 $\pm$ 55
IVAR	119 $\pm$ 40

In this regard, it should be noted that most subjects in the IVAR group received only a single daily injection of Lente (intermediate acting) insulin. Thus, even if the UGDP conclusion that insulin treatment is ineffective in prevention of vascular complications in diabetics is correct, the conclusion would apply only to that treatment schedule. A number of recent publications (1,3,5) as well as preliminary data from studies of our own indicate that much better control can be achieved by use of multiple injections of regular insulin, or two daily injections of properly balanced mixtures of regular and intermediate acting insulin, one given in the morning before breakfast and the other before the evening meal. The risk of significant hypoglycemic reactions with these regimens is much less than when improved control is attempted by increasing the amount of intermediate acting insulin given in a singly daily injection, the approach utilized by UGDP investigators.

When we examined baseline characteristics of the remaining subjects (DO·MC subjects) who subsequently died of cardiovascular causes, we found that a disproportionate number (14 of 17 = 82%) of IVAR subjects, compared to placebo subjects (5 of 17 = 29%) were age 70 or over, had diastolic blood pressure (DBP) equal to or greater than 110 mmHg and/or had fasting blood glucose (FBS) values equal to or greater than 150 mg% at the time they entered the study. Thus, they were at much higher risk of dying of cardiovascular causes at the start of the study than were placebo subjects. This same tendency was evident in a previous UGDP publication dealing with effects of tolbutamide (6), in which disproportionate numbers of subjects in the IVAR group (compared to the placebo group) who died of cardiovascular causes, were over age 70 and/or had sum glucose tolerance test values in excess of 1100 mg% at baseline. Therefore, we also excluded from analysis those subjects whose baseline parameters equaled or exceeded any one of these values (age $\geq$ 70, FBS $\geq$ 150 mg%, or DBP$\geq$110 mmHg) in order to render all groups comparable at baseline in terms of age, diastolic blood pressure, and severity of diabetes. 48.5% of all IVAR subjects, compared to 34% of all placebo subjects who did not change medication or drop out according to the above criteria, were at increased risk in terms of these variables. Cardiovascular deaths were 4 times as frequent in the remaining placebo subjects

(Figure 1) as in IVAR subjects ($\chi^2 = 5.76$, $P<0.025$). If subjects with baseline FBS values up to 200 mg% were included, cardiovascular deaths were still twice as frequent in the placebo as in the IVAR group. Thus, when the data is examined in this manner, it is clear that the IVAR treatment schedule was indeed efficacious in reducing the frequency of cardiovascular deaths in mild, adult-onset diabetics.

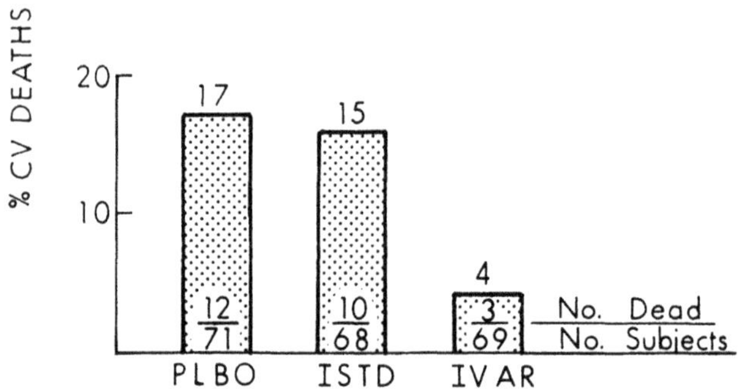

Fig. 1. % CV Deaths in Reminaing Subjects (-DO.MC) With Baseline FBS<150, DBP<110, or Age<70.

In light of the fact that use of multiple insulin injection techniques (as described above) would undoubtedly permit much better control in the vast majority of diabetics who are receiving a single daily injection of insulin, we would suggest that excess cardiovascular deaths (as well as non-fatal complications) in diabetics can be greatly reduced by use of therapeutic measures presently available to virtually all diabetics and their physicians.

These preliminary findings clearly indicate that UGDP investigators were in error in concluding that insulin is ineffective in prevention of diabetic vascular complications. These findings, together with recent FDA audit documentation of numerous discrepancies in baseline cardiovascular risk factors and causes of death reported by UGDP investigators, attest to the urgent need for an in depth reassessment of the entire UGDP study, including validation of the data base, consideration of alternate approaches to data analysis such as those we employed, and retraction of inappropriate and/or erroneous conclusions.

REFERENCES

1. *Pirart, J. (1978). Diabetes Care 1, Part I 168, Part II 252.*
2. *University Group Diabetes Program, (1978). JAMA 240, 37.*
3. *Johnsson, S. (1960). Diabetes 9, 1.*

4. Peterson, C.M., et al. (1977). Ann. Int. Med. 86, 425.
5. Danowski, T.S. and Sunder, J.H. (1978). Diabetes Care 1, 27.
6. University Group Diabetes Program (1970). Diabetes 19, (Suppl. 2), 789.

DISCUSSION

Invited Discussant: M. P. COHEN - *We have found that glomeruli from streptozotocin-diabetic rats are larger, and contain and produce more basement membrane (GBM) than do glomeruli from non-diabetic animals. These changes are prevented if insulin is administered throughout the duration of the diabetes.*

Renal cortex was obtained from kidneys of male white rats; diabetic animals were sacrificed 4-6 weeks after injection of streptozotocin, and non-injected litter mates served as controls. Some groups of diabetic rats received insulin (2-5 units/kg/day) beginning the day after induction of diabetes and continued until the time of sacrifice. Glomeruli were isolated by sequential sieving through a series of stainless steel meshes. The number of glomeruli obtained with this technique reflects that proportion of all glomeruli with a diameter between the 63-149 μm limits of the sieving system. This indirectly allows determination of glomerular size, confirmed by micrometric measurement. For isolation of GBM, glomeruli were suspended in cold buffered saline containing proteolytic inhibitors and ultrasonically disrupted. The basement membranes were collected by rapid low-speed centrifugation, washed with the above buffer, lyophilized, and subjected to appropriate analytical procedures such as total protein determination, agarose gel chromatography and SDS-gel electrophoresis following reduction and/or denaturation, and amino acid analysis after hydrolysis in 6N HCl.

Comparable numbers of glomeruli isolated from normal, diabetic, and insulin treated diabetic animals were incubated with ^{14}C-lysine, following which the GBM and cell sap were analyzed for ^{14}C-protein, and for OH-^{14}C-lysine after acid hydrolysis. In other experiments, the 17,000 x g supernatant prepared after homogenization of isolated glomeruli from these groups of rats was used as enzyme source and incubated with underhydroxylated, ^{14}C-lysine-rich protocollagen substrate. Lysyl protocollagen hydroxylase activity was determined from the formation of labeled OH-lysine, measured in acid hydrolysates.

Streptozotocin diabetic animals were markedly hyperglycemic and exhibited stunted *growth at the time of sacrifice. Since mean glomerular diameter is proportional to body weight (Grant, et al., 1975. Eur. J. Biochem 54: 531), this consideration is necessary when comparing glomerular or GBM yields between experimental groups. Glomerular yields were significantly greater in diabetic preparations (Table). Although this finding could in part represent a decrease in the non-glomerular mass of diabetic rats, it is also consistent with an increased mean glomerular diameter in diabetic kidneys, an interpretation confirmed by micrometry. The yield of GBM was also significantly greater in diabetic preparations, and calculation of the amount of GBM protein per glomerulus demonstrated that this finding actually represented GBM accumulation rather than the (unlikely) possibility that diabetic samples have more glomeruli.*

Glomerular and Basement Membrane Yield in Normal and Diabetic Rats

	Non-Diabetic(7)	Diabetic(5)
Body Wt. (gm)	348 ± 23	236 ±13*
Blood glucose (mg/dl)	<140	414 ±12*
No. glomeruli/gm cortex/gm wt	70.4 ± 21.0	170.0±41.7*
Basement membrane/gm cortex/gm wt (10^{-8} gm protein)	7.95 ± 1.44	23.66±3.91*
Basement membrane/glomerulus/gm wt (10^{-12} gm protein)	3.53 ± .64	7.22±1.70*

Values represent mean ± SEM of results obtained with pooled renal cortical tissue from 9-30 animals in each experiment; no. of experiments in parenthesis.
** p <.05 compared to non-diabetic values*

These increases in glomerular size and basement membrane appear to result at least in part from increased GBM synthesis. Glomeruli isolated from streptozotocin-diabetic rats and incubated with ^{14}C-lysine synthesize more protein (non-dialyzable ^{14}C), collagen (OH-^{14}C-lysine in non-dialyzable protein), and basement membrane (^{14}C and OH-^{14}C-lysine in membrane protein) than do glomeruli from non-diabetic animals. When these animals were treated with insulin throughout the duration of diabetes, however, all of these in vitro parameters of glomerular protein, collagen, and basement membrane synthesis were partially or completely normalized. Lysyl hydroxylase activity, a parameter of basement membrane biosynthesis, was also significantly increased in homogenates of isolated glomeruli obtained from streptozotocin-diabetic rats. Furthermore, when glomerular homogenates from streptozotocin-diabetic rats which were treated with insulin throughout the duration of diabetes were used as enzyme source, lysyl hydroxylase activity did not differ from that of non-diabetic preparations.

Molecular sieve chromatography of reduced and denatured GBM from both normal and diabetic animals revealed several major absorbance peaks, including one at the void voluem. Elution profiles of normal and diabetic samples were similar, with neither the presence nor absence of any specific peak noted in the diabetic preparations. Reference to a calibration curve, obtained with reduced and denatured proteins of known molecular weight (i.e., collagen β and α chains, procollagen, bovine serum albumin and trypsin) indicated that these components had apparent molecular weights ranging from about 30,000 to 300,000 daltons. Each of the peaks identified on agarose gel analysis of normal and diabetic GBM is probably heterogeneous and it was not surprising that the chromatographic patterns were similar. Nevertheless, SDS-polyacrylamide gel electrophoresis of both normal and diabetic GBM revealed several components which, on the basis of migration coefficients, were identical in both preparations.

The findings that biosynthetic parameters of GBM production are elevated in experimental diabetes, and are normalized with continuous insulin therapy, support the hypothesis that the duration and degree of hyperglycemia (and/or other metabolic abnormalities of diabetes) substantially contribute to the development of diabetic nephropathy. Evidence that these biochemical changes are of pathologic significance is provided with the demonstration of increased glomerular size and increased GBM in rats with experimental diabetes. Glomerular expansion, in part resulting from excess deposition of solid material and in part due to a compensatory hypertropy of functioning open glomeruli, as well as accumulation of basement membrane are early hallmarks of human diabetic nephropathy (Gundersen H.J.G. and Osterby, R. 1977. Diabetologia 13:43). These changes occur despite loss of protein and fat in other tissues, findings that agree with results from other studies which have shown that protein synthesis paradoxically increases in diabetic kidneys (Cohen, M.P. and Vogt, C.A. 1975. Horm. Metab. Res. 7:338). Diabetic GBM, although quantitatively increased, appears qualitatively similar to that of normal, suggesting that it is a general increase in protein (and collagen) synthesis which contributes to the accumulation of GBM in diabetes. Restoration of normal renal protein synthesis with amelioration of the insulin deficient state would also diminish the rate of GBM synthesis, and, in turn, allay the development or progression of diabetic microangiopathy.

(Supported in part by NIH Grant No. RR-5384-11, the American Diabetes Association, the National Kidney Foundation, Affiliated Internists Corporation, and the Juvenile Diabetes Foundation.)

T. PROUT: *I'm surprisingly delighted with the Williamson analysis, and it is my delight now to have an adversary who, in fact is reputable and who has given a method by which an analysis is made, which is contrary perhaps to what we have, but whose methods of analysis are clear, unequivocal, and about which we can do battle on a scientific basis. The other delight is, of course, that if this is true, it's where our gut feelings are. That there is improvement of the pathologic changes of diabetes as a result of intense insulin treatment. It's what we all hoped to come from the UGDP. I think this raises an important philosophical question.*

For the most part, one is safest in doing analysis simply on the basis of how the randomization was done, and then looking at it from the point of view of adherence. It's the way that we, in UGDP, have looked at adherence. Two or three methods here will illustrate minor differences, if you will, that have been seen. In the first, we see that all patients are analyzed for cardiovascular death and cancer, and there are few differences. Then, when we look at all medications that were taken, 75-100% of the same, again the figure is, in fact, about one-half. Again, we see very little variation in our analysis of cardiovascular, cancer or all causes. When you take some medication all of the time now to find 75-100% of the time, one begins to see some differences in cardiovascular death, and perhaps this is where the argument is beginning to take some form. I think that one has to be very careful when one makes subgroup analyses like this, and the idea of excluding patients, who did not get blood sugars better than 150 mg percent, does not appeal to me.

J. R. WILLIAMSON: *There were several things I didn't say in the presentation. I was a little uneasy about the 150 mg percent as a cutoff, because I know many of you would feel that that's a fairly low blood glucose level, and we're excluding most of the diabetics. I would just add, if we raised the level to 200 mg percent, we still see a twofold difference in the mortality. That is, cardiovascular deaths were still twice as frequent in the placebo group as in the IVAR group.*

G. M. REAVEN: *This is a question for both Dr. Prout and Dr. Williamson. One of the things that has struck me about the study is that so many of the patients were not terribly hyperglycemic. I think one of the reasons for the relatively good control data, in terms of placebo versus insulin variable, is because a lot of the people already began underneath those levels. I wonder, if you had a chance to look at that the other way around? Suppose you had taken patients who were quite hyperglycemic, glucoses above 200 or above 250, where one has more room to really improve things.*

J. R. WILLIAMSON: *We have not done that, but it is important. I'd like to also see what happened to that 15% of patients with retinopathy, who came into the study and who were well controlled. That would be a very interesting group, and I hope to have that very soon.*

A. S. REDDI: *Dr. Cohen, Dr. Biswinger was unable to show any increase in collagen synthesis. On the other hand, Michael Grand and yourself have been able to show an increase in collagen synthesis in streptozotocin diabetic rats. Would you like to comment on that?*

M. COHEN: *The best explanation probably has to do with technical differences. The animals used for those experiments had very little data provided, in terms of what their blood glucoses were and how long they were diabetic. The basement membrane, by virtue of its amino acid analysis, did not seem to be a particularly pure preparation, and there were a number of other technical difficulties, which might help explain the differences that we found.*

J. TOBIN: *I'm a little confused about the animal studies. If I got Dr. Cohen's presentation correctly, she treated the streptozotocin diabetic rats with two units per kilo of insulin and got some reduction of blood sugar, but not completely back to normal. Dr. Oppermann I think your slide said 25 units per kilo in the mice, and without really much of a change in the blood sugar, if I understood that. Ten mg% difference, but I'm not sure if that was significant. Could you comment on that?*

W. OPPERMANN: *All I can say is that those were our observations. We're dealing with the mouse and the rat, and they are different. Maybe that's part of the explanation.*

S. FAJANS: *The question of achievement of control by insulin variable in the UGDP was brought up. It is my recollection that, in the insulin variable group, only 49% of the subjects actually came in the classification of good control. Is this correct?*

T. PROUT: *I don't recall, but I think in the insulin group it was 64.5%.*

J. R. WILLIAMSON: *I would like also to say I accept the graciousness with which Thad (Prout) accepts our challenge of the UGDP data. I hope our differences remain philosophical rather than personal.*

NEW SYNTHETIC INSULINS

P. G. Katsoyannis*

Modification of the insulin molecule may alter its biological profile, either by altering its binding ability to the receptor or by altering the "message region" of the molecule so that the insulin analog-receptor complex cannot initiate the biological response in the same fashion as the natural hormone-receptor complex.

It is therefore obvious that a broad spectrum of inulin analogs must be synthesized and biochemically evaluated in terms of biological and immunological activity and receptor binding ability, in order to be able to draw meaningful conclusions regarding the functional areas of the insulin molecule. The availability of efficient methods, both for the synthesis of the insulin chains and their combination to produce the active hormone in highly purified form, make the synthesis of a variety of insulin analogs a readily attainable task. In our laboratory, we have chemically synthesized thus far some forty new insulins and the synthesis, at will, of any new insulin is only a matter of time.

MODIFICATIONS AT THE AMINO AND CARBOXYL TERMINAL REGIONS OF THE A CHAIN

Table 1 shows some of the analogs we have synthesized, with modifications at the terminal regions of the A chain. Removal of the N-terminal tetrapeptide sequence from the A chain [des(Tetrapeptide A^{1-4}) insulins] (1) leads to total inactivation, whereas replacement of the α-amino group of the A^1 glycine with hydrogen [Deamino A^1 insulin] (2) results in ca@65% inactivation. Methylation of the α-amino group of the A^1 glycine, a modification that increases the basic character of that residue (pK_2 of A^1 glycine 9.6 and of A^1 sarcosine 10.0), results

@approximately

([Sarcosine^1-A]insulin) (3) in a very small decrease in the biological activity and a more pronounced decrease of the immunoreactivity of insulin. Substitution of the A^1 glycine with L- and D-alanine ([L-Alanine^1-A] and [D-Alanine^1-A] insulins)(4) results in analogs which, in the in vitro assays, have relative potencies of ca 10% and 100%, respectively, of that of insulin. It is interesting to note that the relatively binding affinities and the relative in vitro biological potencies of these analogs are the same. A similar situation regarding relative binding affinity and biological activity was encountered with all other analogs which we have tested. Our data demonstrate the importance of the A^1 amino acid residue to the biological activity of insulin and are in agreement with data from other laboratories, pointing to the suggestion that the A^1 glycine is one of the amino acid residues involved in receptor binding, and that the insulin binding site and the site responsible for activating cellular processes may reside on the same region of the molecule.

The X-ray structure of insulin reveals that the B chain folds itself within the insulin molecule in a way that the A^{21} asparagine and the B^{22} arginine are brought in such juxtaposition as to insure salt bridge formation between the α-carboxyl group of A^{21} asparagine and the guanidium group of the B^{22} arginine. This structural arrangement appears to stabilize the tertiary structure of insulin. Since [Isoasparagine^{21}-A] insulin (5), where the A^{21} asparagine is replaced with isoasparagine which has a free β-carboxyl group, has similar biological behavior to the natural hormone, it is concluded that the α- and β-carboxyl moieties of the A^{21} residue are nearly equivalent in the formation of the A^{21}-B^{22} salt bridge. On the other hand, in [D-Asparagine^{21}-A] (6) insulin the α-carboxyl moiety of the A^{21} D-amino acid residue is less favorably disposed for A^{21}-B^{22} salt bridge formation as Courtauld atomic models of that region reveal, an event that probably causes distortion in the tertiary structure and hence a decrease in the biological activity of the hormone.

In the [Arginine^{21}-A] insulin (7), the A^{21} arginine still retains the A^{21}-B^{22}salt bridge capability. Yet this analog is only 50% as active as the natural hormone. This implies that other factors, perhaps steric hindrance, come into play which involve the side chain of the A^{21} amino acid residue. The high biological activity of [Asparaginamide^{21}-A] insulin (8), where the A^{21} asparagine has both its α- and β-carboxyl groups as amides, and hence cannot form a salt bridge with the B^{22} arginine, may suggest that a salt-bridge stabilization involving A^{21}-B^{22} residues is not essential for activity.

As was the case with the [Sarcosine^1-A] insulin, the [Sarcosine^1-, Isosaparagine^{21}-A^5] analog exhibits a slightly lower biological activity, but a significantly lower immunological activity, as compared to the natural hormone. This suggests that the change in the relative positive charge at the N-terminus of the A chain is responsible for the considerable decrease in the immunoreactivity of these analogs.

Several more analogs, however, must be prepared before the observed differential effect on biological activity and immunoreactivity of insulin is ascribed primarily to changes in the basicity of the N-terminus of the A chain.

Table 1

PERCENT OF PATIENTS WITH NEW NON-FATAL EVENT

	PLBO	ISTD	IVAR
Abnormal EKG	20.0	16.7	17.6
Angina	19.6	15.5	16.6
Hypertension	50.0	54.7	55.6
Abnormal Fundi	43.3	45.3	43.2
Urine Protein	4.2	2.1	5.8
Creatinine	16.3	8.3*	9.1**
Calcification	29.6	28.8	28.4

P value = * 0.03 ** 0.06

See original paper (1) for definitions of the non-fatal events shown. PLBO = Diet + Placebo. ISTD = Insulin Standard. IVAR = Insulin Variable.

MODIFICATIONS OF THE INTRA-AND INTER-CHAIN DISULFIDE BRIDGES

Table 2 shows the analogs with modifications in the disulfide bridges of insulin. The [Alanine^{6,11}A] insulin (9) which differs from the parent molecule in that the A^6 and A^{11} cysteine residues have been replaced with alanine residues and hence lacks an intra-chain disulfide bridge, has a potency 8-10% of that of the natural hormone. Furthermore, the [Homocysteine^{6,11}-A] insulin (10) which because of the presence of homocysteine instead of cysteine at positions A^6 and A^{11} has an enlarged (22-membered) intrachain cyclic system, possesses a potency ca 30% of that of the natural hormone. This demonstrates that the intrachain disulfide system does not participate functionally in the mechanism of action of insulin. This finding is in agreement with X-ray structure which indicates that the intrachain bridge is completely buried and is part of the hydrophobic core in the interior of the insulin molecule. On the other hand, [Homocysteine^{7,20}-A] insulin (11), in which the cysteine residues at positions A^{7} and A^{20} have been replaced with homocysteine residues and hence the interchain cyclic system has been enlarged by two carbon atoms, is biologically inactive. This indicates that the biological activity of insulin depends critically on a particular geometry conferred on the molecule by the proper placement of its individual chains.

Table 2

INSULIN ANALOGS WITH MODIFICATIONS IN THE INTRA- AND INTER-CHAIN DISULFIDE BRIDGES[a]

Insulin Analog (Sheep)	IU/mg		
	MC	GO	RIA
[Alanine^{6,11}-A] (no intrachain -S-S-)	2-2.5	-	2-2.5
[Homocysteine^{6,11}-A] (enlarged intrachain -S-S-)	7-8	-	7-8
[Homocysteine^{7,20}-A] (enlarged interchain -S-S-)	0	-	2

[a] MC, mouse convulsion assay; GO, glucose oxidation assay in isolated fat cells; RIA, radioimmunoassay.

MODIFICATIONS IN THE INTERIOR OF THE A CHAIN

Analogs in this category are shown in Table 3. Substitution of the A^{2} isoleucine, which is buried and is part of the hydrophobic interior of the molecule, with norleucine causes a dramatic decrease of the biological activity of insulin. The [Norleucine^{2}-A] insulin analog (8) shows, by circular dichroism measurements, a change in its secondary structure and fails to dimerize as it happens with the natural hormone. Indeed, the X-ray model of insulin shows that the A chain is folded upon itself so that the A^{19}tyrosine, which is on the surface of the molecule, is in van der Waals contact with the A^{2} isoleucine, and in agreement with our data, this interaction contributes to the stability of the structure of insulin. Modifications at the A^{19} position also demonstrate the importance of the A^{19} tyrosine to the biological activity of insulin. Substitution of the L-tyrosine with the D-isomer, [D-Tyrosine^{19}-A] insulin (8), or inversion of the location of the A^{19} tyrosine with A^{18} asparagine, as is the case with [Tyrosine^{18}-, Asparagine^{19}-, Arginine^{21}-A] insulin (8), leads to total inactivation. Even replacement of A^{19} tyrosine with phenylalanine, as is the case in [Phenylalanine^{19}-A] insulin (8) leads to 50% decrease in the biological activity. The importance of the A^2 and A^{19} residues is further demonstrated by the fact that substitution of the weakly interacting hydrophobic residues A^2 isoleucine and A^{19} tyrosine with the strongly interacting polar residues α,γ-diaminobutyric acid and glutamic acid residues, respectively ([Diaminobutyric acid^2-, Glutamic acid^{19}-A] insulin) (12), leads to total inactivation.

The A^5 glutamine, an invariant amino acid residue in insulin sequences from various species, is on the surface of the molecule and has no known structural role. Substitution of this hydrophilic residue, however, either with the hydrophilic threonine or with the hydrophobic leucine, affords the [Threonine^5-A] and [Leucine^5-A] insulins (8), respectively, which exhibit only 30% of the biological activity of insulin. The relative binding affinity of one of these analogs, which was measured, is the same as the relative biological activity. It is tempting to speculate that the A^5 glutamine is in the receptor-binding region of insulin.

MODIFICATIONS AT THE AMINO AND CARBOXYL TERMINAL REGIONS OF THE B CHAIN

The X-ray model of insulin shows that in the B chain the residues B^{20}-B^{23} form a U-turn within the insulin molecule so that the carboxyl terminal segment of the B chain is folded back and lies in antiparallel fashion against the central segment of that chain. In this configuration the B^{27}-B^{30} sequence is not involved in stabilizing interactions and does not appear to be important to the structure and hence the activity of insulin. Similarly, the X-ray model indicates that the N-terminal segment of the B chain is on the surface of the insulin molecule as an extended chain and is folded across in an antiparallel fashion to the central portion of the A chain. In this configuration, the sequence B^1-B^3 does not appear to be involved in stabilizing interactions that affect the structure and hence the activity of the insulin. However, the B^4 glutamine and particularly the B^5 histidine appear to be involved in interactions (with A^{11} and A^7 cysteines, respectively) of importance to the structure and activity of the hormone. Our synthetic analogs, shown in Table 4, verified all these predictions of the X-ray model. The des (Tripeptide B^{28-30}) insulin (13) is fully active, indicating that the C-terminal tripeptide sequence of the B chain is not important to the biological activity of insulin. Subsequent elimination of amino acid residues from the C-terminal region of the B chain, however, is accompanied by a gradual decline of the potency of the hormone. Des (Tetrapeptide B^{27-30}) insulin (14) is ca 55% as active as insulin and des (Pentapeptide B^{26-30})insulin (15) is only ca 35% as active as the natural hormone. Amidation of the carboxyl terminus of the truncated B chain moieties of the latter two insulin analogs results in a slight increase of their potencies. [Des (Tetrapeptide B^{27-30}), Tyrosinamide^{26}-B] insulin (8) is ca 68% and [des (Pentapeptide B^{26-30}), Phenylalaninamide^{25}-B] insulin (8) is ca 42% as active as the natural hormone.

Table 3

INSULIN ANALOGS WITH MODIFICATIONS IN THE INTERIOR OF THE A CHAIN[a]

Insulin Analog (Sheep)	IU/mg			% of Natural Insulin
	MC	GO	RIA	RB
[Norleucine^{2}-A]	1	0.25	2-3	0.6
[Diaminobutyric acid^{2}-, Glutamic acid^{19}-A]	0		0	
[Threonine^{5}-A]	6.5-7.5		5.3	
[Leucine^{5}-A]	6-9		8-10	30
[Phenylalanine^{19}-A]	11-12.5		9.6	
[D-Tyrosine^{19}-A]			0.22	1.4
[Tyrosine^{18}-, Asparagine^{19}-, Arginine^{21}-A]	0		0.35	

[a] MC, mouse convulsion assay; GO, glucose oxidation assay in isolated fat cells; RIA, radioimmunoassay; RB, receptor binding in liver membranes.

The three dimensional structure of insulin indicates that the amino acid residues B^{12} valine, B^{16} tyrosine, B^{24} phenylalanine, B^{25} phenylalanine and B^{26} tyrosine, which constitute the hydrophobic core of the molecule, are the points of contact between insulin monomers in the formation of the insulin dimer. It is speculated that these same amino acid residues are members of the binding region of the hormone and hence the binding of insulin monomer to the receptor is similar to the formation of the insulin dimer from two monomers. As was mentioned earlier, however, the amino acid residues A^{1} glycine, A^{5} glutamine, A^{19} tyrosine and A^{21} asparagine, which are not involved in the dimerization of insulin, do contribute to the binding of insulin to the receptor.

It is tempting to speculate that the gradual decline in the biological activity observed as amino acid residues are eliminated from the C-terminus of the B chain is due to the proximity of a polar group (the carboxyl group of the newly formed C-terminal residue) to the hydrophobic core of the molecule with consequent deleterious conformational changes.

It has been shown, in other laboratories, that des (B^1) and des (Dipeptide B^{1-2})insulins are fully active and des (Tripeptide B^{1-3}) insulin is ca 70% as active as the natural hormone. This indicates that the first three amino acid residues at the N-terminus of the B chain are not important to the biological activity of the hormone. Since the synthetic des (Tetrapeptide B^{1-4}) insulin (16) possesses ca 54% of the biological activity of insulin, it appears that the B^4 glutamine, as is the case with the B^1 phenylalanine, B^2 valine and B^3 asparagine, is not involved directly in the expression of the biological activity of insulin. There is a dramatic decrease, however, in the biological activity of insulin when the B^5 histidine is also eliminated. Thus the des (Pentapeptide B^{1-5}) insulin (16) is ca 5% as active as the natural hormone. This, of course, demonstrates the crucial role of the B^5 histidine, an invariant amino acid residue in all insulin species, to the biological activity of insulin, and supports the prediction of the X-ray model that this residue is involved in intramolecular interactions of structural importance.

Table 4

INSULIN ANALOGS WITH MODIFICATIONS AT THE N- AND C-TERMINAL REGIONS OF THE B CHAIN[a]

Insulin Analog	(H=human) (B=bovine)	IU/mg MC	IU/mg GO	IU/mg RIA	% of Natural Insulin RB
Des[tripeptide B^{28-30}]	(B)	25			
Des[tripeptide B^{28-30}]	(H)	17-20			80
Des[tetrapeptide B^{27-30}]	(H)	11-15		7	
Des[pentapeptide B^{26-30}]	(H)	8.5-9		11	
[Des(tetrapeptide B^{27-30}), Tyrosinamide^{26}-B]	(H)	17		10.8	
[Des(pentapeptide B^{26-30}), Phenylalaninamide^{25}-B]	(H)	10.5		14	
Des(tetrapeptide B^{1-4})	(H)	13		7.6	
Des(pentapeptide B^{1-5})	(H)		1.2	3.7	

[a] MC, mouse convulsion assay; GO, glucose oxidation assay in isolated fat cells; RB, receptor binding in liver membranes; RIA, radioimmunoassay.

MODIFICATION IN THE INTERIOR OF THE B CHAIN

Analogs in this category are shown in Table 5. Substitution of the B^{22} arginine with lysine results in the [Lysine^{22}-B] insulin (17) which was found to possess a potency ca 56% of that of the natural hormone. The high biological activity of this analog may indicate that the presence of a positive ion at B^{22} with a concomitant establishment of a salt bridge with the A^{21} carboxylate group contributes greatly to the degree of hormonal activity. The fact that guinea pig insulin, which has aspartic acid at B^{22}, is endowed with considerable biological activity (2.14 IU/mg) does not contradict this speculation. Indeed, even in guinea pig insulin, there is an interaction between B^{22} and A^{21} (although considerably weaker than in the case of B^{22} arginine or lysine insulins) that contributes to the stabilization of the structure of insulin. Since, however, [Asparaginamide^{21}-A] insulin, which cannot form an A^{21}-B^{22} salt bridge, is highly active, the importance of this ionic bridge is at present in doubt.

Substitution of the hydrophilic serine at B^9, which is on the surface of the insulin molecule, with the hydrophobic leucine, results in the [Leucine^9-B] insulin (18) which possesses a potency ca 55% of that of the natural hormone. We attribute the partial loss of activity of this analog to the perturbing influence that the bulky hydrophobic side chain of leucine may have in the aqueous environment on the interactions of that region or to steric effects that this bulky side chain may generate during hormone-receptor interactions.

The considerable biological activity (ca 45% of that of the natural hormone) of [Leucine^{10}-B] insulin (19), where the B^{10} histidine is substituted with leucine, demonstrates that the B^{10} histidine, in contrast to the B^5 histidine, is not involved directly in the biological activity of the hormone. The decreased biological activity of the [Leucine^{10}-B] insulin as compared with the natural hormone might be due, as was the case with the [Leucine^9-B insulin], to the perturbing effects on the structure of that region of the molecule which may be produced by the substitution of a polar by a non-polar amino acid residue.

The B^{12} valine is a member of the hydrophobic core of the insulin molecule, which is the contact region of the monomer in the formation of the insulin dimer. It is speculated that this region is also part

Table 5

INSULIN ANALOGS WITH MODIFICATIONS IN THE INTERIOR OF THE B CHAIN[a]

Insulin Analog (Human)	IU/mg MC	GO	RIA	% of Natural Insulin RB
[Lysine^{22}-B]	13-14		8.1	
[Leucine^9-B]	13-14		11-12	30
[Leucine^{10}-B]	10-11		9	
[Asparagine^{12}-B]		ca 0.01	5	< 0.1

[a] MC, mouse convulsion assay; GO, glucose oxidation assay in isolated fat cells; RIA, radioimmunoassay; RB, receptor binding in liver membranes.

of the contact area between the insulin monomer and the receptor. Substitution of the hydrophobic B^{12} valine with the hydrophilic residue asparagine affords the [Asparagine^{12}-B] insulin (8) which possesses only trace of biological activity. I believe this finding is the first evidence that supports the involvement of the hydrophobic core of insulin in the biological activity of the hormone.

In conclusion, a considerable amount of information has been already accumulated regarding the contribution of various structural features of insulin to the expression of the biological profile of this protein. Our own data and those obtained in other laboratories have shown that changes in the biological activity of insulin are related to changes in its binding affinity to the receptor and suggest that the binding site and the site responsible for activating cellular processes may reside in the same region of the insulin molecule. This region includes the amino acid residues A^1 Gly, A^5 Gln, A^{19} Tyr, A^{21} Asn, B^{12} Val, B^{16} Tyr, B^{24} Phe, B^{25} Phe and perhaps B^{26} Tyr. However, the possibility cannot be excluded that the structural features involved in insulin binding to the receptor and in the expression of biological activity, apparently overlapping, may be dissociated. The recent finding that hagfish insulin has about 23% receptor binding affinity, but only 4.6% ability to activate lipogenesis, as compared to pig insulin, is consistent with this speculation. There is already good evidence that discrete regions of activity and binding are present in the glucagon and ACTH molecules. Should this be the case with insulin, it might be feasible to synthesize insulin analogs with more favorable characteristics than the natural hormone in respect to potency, immunoreactivity or duration of action.

I believe that the availability of several more insulin analogs will facilitate the solution of this problem.

REFERENCES

1. *Katsoyannis, P.G. and Zalut, C. (1972). Biochemistry 11, 3065*
2. *Katsoyannis, P.G. and Zalut, C. (1972). Biochemistry 11, 1128*
3. *Okada, Y. and Katsoyannis, P.G. (1975). J. Amer. Chem. Soc. 97, 4366*
4. *Cosmators, A., et al. (1978). J. Biol. Chem. 253, 6586*
5. *Cosmatos, A., et al. (1976). Biochemistry, 15, 4076*
6. *Cosmatos, A., et al. (1975). J. Chem. Soc. Perkin I, p. 2157*
7. *Ferderigos, N., et al. (1978). Int. J. Peptide Protein Res. (in press)*
8. *Unpublished data from this laboratory*
9. *Katsoyannis, P.G., et al. (1973). Biochemistry 12, 2516*
10. *Cosmatos, A. and Katsoyannis, P.G. (1973). J. Biol. Chem. 248, 7304*

11. *Cosmatos, A. and Katsoyannis, P.G. (1975). J. Biol. Chem. 350, 5315*
12. *Ferderigos, N. and Katsoyannis, P.G. (1977). J. Chem. Soc. Perkin I p. 1299*
13. *Katsoyannis, P.G., et al. (1971). Biochemistry 10, 3884*
14. *Katsoyannis, P.G., et al. (1973). J. Amer. Chem. Soc. 95, 6427*
15. *Katsoyannis, P.G., et al. (1974). J. Chem. Soc. Perkin I, p. 1311*
16. *Schwartz, G. and Katsoyannis, P.G. (1978). Biochemistry, 17, 4550*
17. *Katsoyannis, P.G., et al. (1975). J. Chem. Soc. Perkin I, p. 464*
18. *Schwartz, G. and Katsoyannis, P.G. (1976). Biochemistry, 15, 4071*
19. *Schwartz, G. and Katsoyannis, P.G. (1977). J. Chem. Research (S), 220; J. Chem. Research (M), 2453*

I am indebted to my co-workers, Drs. G. Schwartz, A. Cosmatos, N. Ferderigos, Y. Okada, C. Zalut, J. Ginos, K. Cheng, and G.T. Burke, who have contributed at various time intervals to this work. This research was supported by the National Institute for Arthritis, Metabolism and Digestive Diseases, USPHS (AM 12927).

DIFFERENTIAL RESPONSE OF INSULIN-DEPENDENT DIABETICS TO INFUSIONS OF BOVINE AND HIGHLY-PURIFIED PORCINE INSULINS: A PRELIMINARY REPORT

K.G.M.M. Alberti*, R. Nosadini, G. Noy
and A.B. Kurtz

Highly purified and single peak porcine insulins have been available now for nearly eight years. More recently single peak bovine insulin has been introduced and highly purified bovine insulins are on the point of being commercially available. The reason for the introduction of these purer insulins, apart from pharmaceutical desirability, has rested mainly on the discovery of anti-insulin antibodies in the serum of nearly all diabetic patients treated with traditional insulin preparations (1). It was originally thought that this antigenicity of the older bovine insulins was due to the structural differences between bovine and human insulin or to abnormal metabolism of the injected insulin. It is now clear, however, that the antigenicity is greater in impure insulin preparations. The a-component is particularly antigenic while antibodies to proinsulin and insulin derivatives are also found (2). In addition Bloom and his coworkers (1976) have shown that patients treated with conventional bovine insulin preparations have significant antibody titres against other pancreatic hormones such as pancreatic polypeptide, glucagon and VIP.

Since the introduction of the highly purified porcine insulins many studies have been published showing the lower immunogenicity of the new insulins both in patients treated only with these insulins and in those changed from conventional to highly purified porcine insulin (see Alberti and Nattrass (3) for review). In addition a fall in antibody titres has been reported in patients changed to highly purified porcine insulin from conventional porcine insulin (4) confirming that species difference alone is not responsible.

The main argument now is whether, despite the lower immunogenicity of the new insulins there is any real advantage to their use. Already there is concern that converting all patients to porcine insulins will lead to a world shortage of insulin from this species although the advent of the highly purified bovine insulins may help to avoid this problem. Certainly there is clear indication that patients require less of the new insulins than of the older insulins (4,5) although this decreased requirement is restricted mainly to those patients previously on a high dose of bovine insulin (6). Also massive insulin resistance, insulin allergy and insulin lipoatrophy are rarely seen with the new insulins.

There is still much dispute, however, with regard to the clinical significance of insulin antibodies. This is obviously central to the question of whether all patients should be changed to the new insulins. It has been suggested that the presence of antibodies may decrease the effectiveness of the residual insulin secretion which is found during the first years of treatment of insulin dependent diabetes, although this depends on the relative avidity of the antibodies to endogenous and exogenous insulins (7). It has also been shown that insulin antibodies may cross the placenta (8) (Kurtz and Stowers, unpublished data), and that they may be involved in, or contribute to, the development of diabetic microangiopathy (7).

The most important consideration, however, is whether the presence of insulin antibodies has any influence on diabetic control. It has been strongly suggested by Dixon et al (9) amongst others that the presence of antibodies improves control by providing a buffer against sudden changes in free insulin. Others have suggested the contrary: that a decrease in insulin antibodies leads to improved glycaemic regulation (10,11). This latter is an appealing concept but in none of these studies were proper control groups included. Indeed in perhaps the only published study with adequate controls (12) no difference in control could be shown when patients were changed from conventional to highly purified insulin although numbers were small and all patients were so called "brittle" diabetics. Thus there is as yet little information about the precise effects of the new insulins and of antibodies on hour to hour regulation of blood glucose levels.

It is worth reconsidering the aims of insulin therapy. In normal man insulin is secreted in response to meals with onset of action within minutes of ingestion and the peak effect occurs after 45 to 60 minutes. If the aim of therapy in diabetes is to normalise metabolism then insulin regimens should be designed to mimic the natural response. Unfortunately, insulin absorption from subcutaneous sites is slow, even for rapid acting insulins with onset of action at about 1 hour and peak effects at 2 1/2 to 6 hours.

It is possible, indeed probable, that high titres of circulating antibodies will delay the onset of action and prolong the duration of the peak effect and further dissociate the actual pattern of insulin response from the desired profile. This is indeed suggested by the work of Munksgaard Rasmussen et al (13) who showed that patients with high antibody and total serum insulin levels tended to have more severe late hypoglycaemic reactions. Little data is available, however, either on this or on exact effects of different types of insulin on the early response to insulin injection.

We have therefore made a preliminary study of patients treated with either conventional bovine insulins (n = 5), and patients treated with highly purified porcine insulin (n = 3) of whom two had been treated with bovine insulin until two years before study.

METHOD

The protocol was as follows. Patients fasted overnight and were then connected to the "artificial pancreas" (glucose-controlled-insulin-infusion system, Biostator, Life Science Instruments, Ulm, West Germany) via a superficial venous cannula through which blood was withdrawn continuously; a return cannula for infusion of insulin and glucose by the Biostator was inserted in an antecubital vein.

Once the level of plasma glucose was established, the Biostator was programmed to (a) infuse insulin at a rate of 0.01 units/kg/hr. and (b) maintain constant glycaemia at 10-20 mg/100 ml below the admission value. Frequent intermittent blood samples were taken for measurement of metabolites, glucagon, growth hormone, free insulin and insulin binding (total antibody titre) (14). The insulin infusion was continued for 2 hours and the experiment continued for a further 2 hours. Each patient was studied on at least two occasions: on one, bovine soluble insulin (Wellcome) was infused and on the other, porcine Actrapid MC (Novo) insulin was used. At least one week separated studies and the two insulins were used in random order. If initial blood glucose and ketone body levels did not match on the two occasions a third infusion was performed, and the studies discarded if a good match was not achieved on this occasion.

The principle of the method is shown in Fig. 1. This shows in the upper part that blood glucose concentrations were closely matched on the two occasions. Below, the amount of glucose infused per minute is shown. The rate of glucose infused in the first 30 minutes of the study gives an indication of the rate of response to a particular insulin infusion. The amount of glucose infused after cessation of the insulin infusion indicates any residual insulin effect which might be expected if biologically

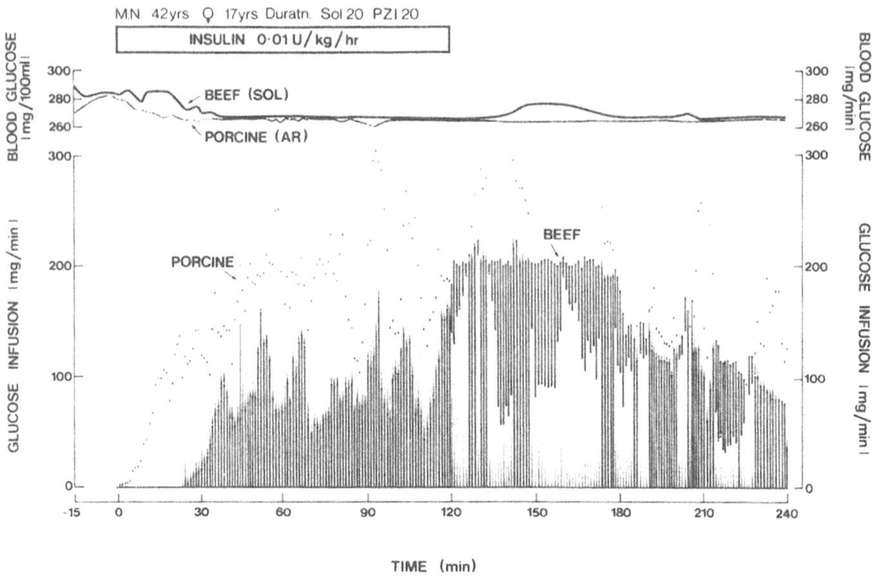

Fig. 1. Insulin-glucose clamp in diabetic patient given either soluble (bovine) or Actrapid MC (porcine) insulin.

Amounts of infused glucose required to maintain constant glycaemia are shown as single bars each representing glucose infused in one minute.

Solid bars - during bovine insulin infusion. Faint *bars - during porcine insulin infusion.*

active insulin was released from antibodies. The total amount of glucose infused gives an indication of the total sensitivity of the system.

RESULTS AND DISCUSSION

Fig. 1 shows clearly that for one subject normally receiving 40 units/day of bovine insulin more glucose was infused during the early part of the insulin infusion when porcine insulin was given than with bovine insulin. In this case the difference was maintained for the whole of the insulin infusion the difference disappearing only after stopping the insulin. In the other subjects normally treated with bovine insulin the same results were found only for the early part of the infusion. Total glucose infused varied widely between subjects, and there was no consistent difference between the two insulin infusions. There was, however, a highly significant difference in the amount of glucose infused in the first 30 minutes. Thus, all five subjects normally treated with bovine insulin received more glucose in the first 30 minutes of the porcine insulin infusion than during the same period of the bovine infusion. The same was true for the two patients treated with porcine insulin who had previously received bovine insulin, the only exception being the one subject studied to date who has never received beef insulin. This is shown in Fig. 2 where glucose infused in the first 30 minutes is expressed as % total glucose infused during the four hours.

Differences were also found in responsiveness of ketone bodies to the insulin infusions (Fig. 3). Thus patients normally receiving porcine insulin showed a more rapid fall in ketone body concentration when infused with beef insulin than those patients who were normally treated with beef insulin.

There is thus a greater early response of beef-insulin treated patients to pork than to bovine insulin. This could not be accounted for on the basis of differential antibody binding of beef and pork insulin, which has been described previously (14), or on total insulin antibodies in that some patients had virtually no circulating antibodies and only two had clear evidence of differential binding of pork and beef insulin. Free insulin levels did, however, show a difference in the five beef-insulin treated patients. The increase in free insulin levels above basal was greater in these subjects when given porcine than beef insulin, although total insulin levels did not vary. Similarly there was a strong correlation ($P<0.01$) between free insulin levels and the amount of glucose infused in the first hour.

It is obviously important that the beef insulin treated patients showed a more rapid response to porcine than to bovine insulin. It also appears that switching to porcine from beef insulin, even for two years, does not remove this differential effect. This has clear therapeutic implications although confirmation is required.

Antibodies, as measured by us, do not explain the observed effects so other explanations must be sought. Others have described two populations of anti-insulin antibodies (16): a high affinity group with low capacity and long half life of association/dissociation, and a second low affinity group with a shorter half life and bigger capacity. It is possible that we were missing change in one or other population. It should also be remembered that our comparison is between a conventional bovine and a highly-purified porcine insulin. Some properties of the insulin suspension could be responsible for the lower free insulin levels found with bovine insulin infusion, earlier observations

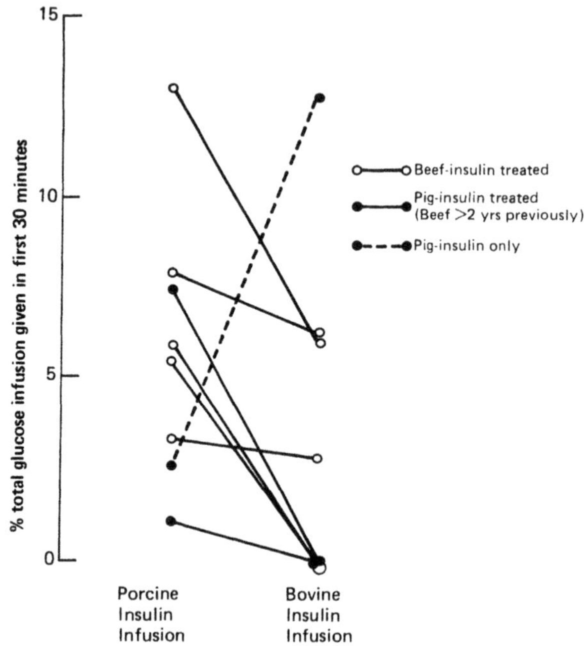

Fig. 2. Glucose infused during first 30 minutes of porcine or bovine insulin infusion. Results are expressed as % total glucose infused during 4 hours. Each pair of joined circles represents one subject.

having shown differences in half life between high molecular weight and single component radioactive insulins in the rat (15). Differential binding of insulin to fixed tissue proteins could be responsible as may differences in the effects of the two insulins at the insulin receptors. A final possibility is that different amounts of insulin were infused but a consistent error of this kind is unlikely.

None of the explanations offered seems entirely satisfactory. Obviously more studies will be needed to substantiate these findings, and comparisons are also necessary between highly purified beef and highly purified porcine insulin. More patients who have never been treated with beef insulin are also required. Nonetheless the finding remains of potential clinical importance as the first demonstration of a clear difference in metabolic effect and rate of response between the old and the new insulins.

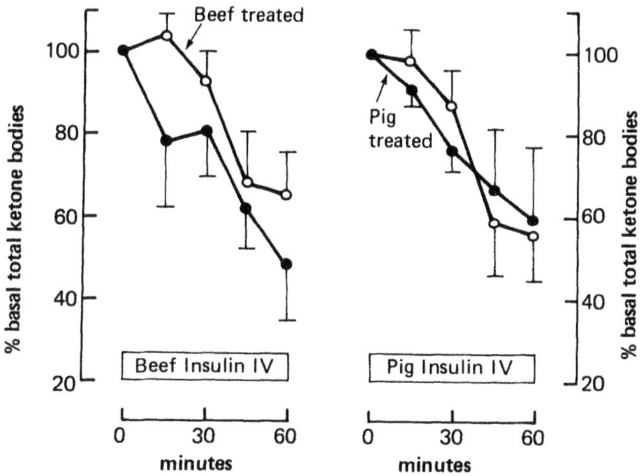

Fig. 3. Effect of prior treatment with pig or beef insulin or ketone body response to insulin infusion. Results are expressed as % initial (basal) blood ketone body infusion. n = 5 for soluble (bovine) insulin treated subjects; n = 3 for Actrapid MC (porcine) insulin treated subjects.

REFERENCES

1. Deckert, T. (1964). Insulin antibodies. Copenhagen: Munksgaard
2. Schichtkrull, J., et al.(1974). Horm. Metabl. Res., 5 (Suppl.), 134
3. Alberti, K.G.M.M. & Nattrass, M. (1978). Diabetologia, 15, 77
4. Andreani, D. (1973). Excerpta Medica Int. Congr. Ser., 316, 68
5. Oakley, N.W. (1976). Lancet, i, 994
6. Bloom, S.R., et al.(1976). Diabetologia, 12, 381
7. Anderson, O.O. & Egeberg, J. (1978). Acta Paediatr. Scand. Suppl., 270, 63
8. Persson, B. (1975). Isr. J. Med. Sci., 11, 609
9. Dixon, K., et al.(1975). Q.J. Med., 176, 543
10. Lavaux, J.P., et al.(1973). Excerpta Medica Int. Congr. Ser., 316, 40
11. Asplin, C.M., et al.(1978). Diabetologia, 14, 99
12. Yue, D.K. & Turtle, J.R. (1975). Diabetes, 24, 625
13. Munksgaard Rasmussen, S., et al (1975). Diabetologia, 11, 151
14. Kurtz, A.B., et al.(1978). Diabetologia, 15, 19
15. Goldman, J., et al.(1978). Diabetes, 27, 653
16. Antoniades, H.N. (1976). Endocrinology, 99, 481

DISCUSSION

E. PFEIFFER: *Dr. Katsoyannis, when do you think we will have human-like insulin made available for clinical therapy? And, Dr. Alberti, you selected .01 units of insulin per kilo per hour. This means by calculation 10-12 milliunits per minute, and the blood glucose came up to 280 mg percent. This 10 milliunits per minute is the basal value which is needed when the patient is well regulated. But, you were in the range of 280 mg percent, which is too high. Really, I cannot explain it.*

P.G. KATSOYANNIS: *Dr. Pfeiffer, I think the time to have available human insulin for clinical trials was ten years ago. They could have made the insulin ten years ago. The procedures are here, but who is going to make it?*

E. PFEIFFER: *CIBA already made it, as far as I know.*

P. G. KATSOYANNIS: *That's what I said, the technology is here. I said it should have been available ten years ago.*

K.G.M.M. ALBERTI: *Dr. Pfeiffer, first, all patients were not at 280. Each patient was matched so that the two admissions were at the same level. That happened to be the one I used as a demonstration. Two or three of the patients were at relatively normal glycemic levels, between 80 and 130. In fact, there was no correlation between the amount of glucose infused and the starting dose, looking at just the eight patients. The reason we chose .01 of a unit/kg/hour was because we did studies with a whole range of concentrations, and we didn't want to get to a level where we infused more than needed. All I can say is, with that dose, we got these very clear differences in requirement to maintain the blood glucose at whatever level it started.*

T. PROUT: *A number of years ago, we injected triple purified pork insulin back into the pig, and were surprised to find that it developed antibodies. This raised a disquieting double point that either when we crystallized insulin or we do things with it, we fold it or double it, or do something that has the animal see it as a foreign protein. I don't know if that is even theoretically possible, Dr. Katsoyannis. The possibility is, of course, that this is going to carry over into human insulin. George (Alberti), one would guess that you have higher free insulin in those first weeks and, as the antibody becomes saturated and the pork antibody gets lit up, that it begins to increase its binding and decrease its free insulin.*

P. G. KATSOYANNIS: *I think you mentioned that you have crystallized your insulin.*

T. PROUT: *Yes.*

P. G. KATSOYANNIS: *The crystalline insulin is like a crystalline protein and it doesn't do very much in regard to homogeneity. We have used crystalline insulin, which we crystallized ten times, and then put on isometric focusing. Then, a computer is needed to count the balance, several of them, 7 or 8. So, when we now say we use pure insulin, we have to mention what criteria. In my experience, the only way to get pure insulin is by isometric focusing.*

K.G.M.M. ALBERTI: *I think, in fact, Dr. Deckert published similar studies by injecting insulin into humans and showing an antigenicity or showing some form of antibody formation.*

T. DECKERT: *I wonder why people are asking for human insulin, because we can give highly purified soluble porcine insulin to human beings without raising antibodies. We can do it with human insulin also. However, the problem of antibody formation arises when we have to give patients retarded insulin preparations, the zinc insulin or protamine insulin. Then, we cannot avoid antibody formation. So, the problem is not human insulin or porcine insulin, but the preparation of long-acting insulin preparations. I think I agree fully with you. The problem is whether we can achieve better control with the highly purified insulin preparations, since we cannot mimic the normal insulin peak after meals because the normal insulin peak is half an hour after the meal.*

G. M. REAVEN: *Alberti, I get the impression that this beneficial effect is very short-lived, such as a half an hour during a two-hour infusion. It rather stuns me, in terms of thinking of mechanisms. Out of curiosity, would you try to correlate this in any way with insulin binding, taking, for example, the monocytes just before you start your infusion?*

K.G.M.M. ALBERTI: *I think that is an important point. Yes, there is this clear distinction which is reproduceable, if you repeat the experiment. Simplistically, when you start your infusion with a porcine insulin, much less of it is being bound. When you begin with a bovine insulin, more is being bound, but then you're starting to see it being released again and you may get some degree of saturation. We haven't yet done the studies which you suggest, which are very much on the cards, to look at actual monocyte binding in these patients.*

R. CAMERINI-DAVALOS: *I would like to go back to Dr. Deckert's comment. You made a statement that, in giving purified insulin, pork insulin, we don't need to worry at all about antibodies for life. If that is the case, am I right in thinking that the only problem we are facing now is the manner in which we will deliver this soluble, short-acting insulin? Dr. Katsoyannis, I'm a little bit confused. If it's true that we have the possibility of manufacturing the ideal insulin today, what do you look for tomorrow?*

T. DECKERT: *If we used highly purified, soluble insulin, subcutaneously, in our treatment, then we can avoid the formation of insulin antibodies. We have shown this in studies over half a year. However, the patient will no longer accept these insulin injections three times a day. Therefore, we had to change to these long-acting insulin preparations, but with long-acting insulin preparations, also made of highly purified porcine insulin, insulin antibody formation cannot be totally avoided, but it can be very much reduced.*

R. CAMERINI-DAVALOS: *So, we're still aiming at producing human insulin?*

T. DECKERT: *Well, I have done studies with soluble human insulin, given to humans for three months or so in psychiatric patients. These patients were given very high doses of human insulin. But, this insulin was not highly purified and, therefore, some of these patients developed insulin antibodies against these human insulin preparations. Therefore, we will repeat this experiment with the highly purified human insulin, but I think the results will come out the same as with the highly purified porcine insulin.*

R. CAMERINI-DAVALOS: *If we have the ideal insulin, all we need is a better way to inject it; or, if we do not have the ideal insulin, then we must look for that as well.*

K.G.M.M. ALBERTI: *I think what Dr. Deckert suggests is that even if you took highly purified human insulin and complexed it with zinc protamine, etc., you would still get an antigenic response. The antibody titers which you get with the highly purified pork insulins are impressively low. I'm particularly interested in seeing whether we'll get the same effect with a highly purified beef insulin, which will be available shortly.*

P. G. KATSOYANNIS: *Dr. Camerini, as protein chemists, we look for an insulin which is degraded at a much lower rate than human insulin which, in turn, will have a longer duration of action, disposing of all the additives, protamines, zincs and everything else. I'm looking for an insulin molecule which can be injected and which will remain for two days without requiring anything else. I'm looking for an insulin molecule which is less antigenic than the natural hormone.*

K.G.M.M. ALBERTI: *I would argue quite quickly with one of the things you said. I'm not looking - and I would discourage you from doing so - for an insulin with a very prolonged action. That's fine in the subcutaneous tissues and non-antigenic insulin there, but once it's in the circulation, you want snappy action and you want to try to mimic the insulin mealtime response.*

T. PROUT: *Just a comment on Dr. Deckert's observation. Lockwood and I showed also that given crystalline porcine insulin for 42 weeks there was no antibody formation. We had a patient who was very resistant to beef insulin, whom we changed over to crystalline pork, about 1956. I followed her for about ten years on regular insulin, three times a day, without any significant development of porcine antibodies.*

N. FREINKEL: *The physiological desideratum, is somewhere in between. I think we need both; to mimic basal insulinization, you need something that's going to give you a sustained flow of insulin action. The puzzle in the acute phase is an ad hoc response to alimentation, so really both would be desirable. If one had a non-modified, long-acting insulin to provide that and to supplement with the acute, that would obviously be the most physiological replication.*

S. PODOLSKY: *I have a clinical question. One of the advantages of the single component is that, as no other, it is not associated with lipoatrophy. There have even been reports that injecting single component insulin into the site of lipatrophy has been associated with filling up of these areas. I wonder if this has held up? I've not been impressed with this reversal of pre-existing lipoatrophy.*

K.G.M.M. ALBERTI: *My feeling is that there is a very strong point there - that it does work. However, if you use beef insulin in many patients, ordinary beef insulin, you get the things to fill up too. This has certainly been reported by one or two people. We, in fact, use the highly purified insulin.*

DELAY OF CARBOHYDRATE ABSORPTION BY INHIBITORS OF INTESTINAL α-GLUCOSIDASES

W. Puls* and H.P. Krause

The therapeutic value of a suitable diet as an aid to the treatment of metabolic disease is just as undeniable as the blood pressure lowering effect of a low salt diet in the therapy of hypertension. Since the introduction of saluretics into the modern hypertension therapy, the very strict low salt diet, which is only rarely accepted by the patients, can be eased or even almost completely dispensed with, since these saluretics reliably and very effectively increase the excretion of sodium in the urine.

Another example for the substitution of a diet is the surgical treatment of obesity by jejuno-ileostomy (1,2,3). The shortening of the small intestine reduces the digestive and absorptive capacity for proteins, fat and carbohydrates. The nutrient remains undigested in the small intestine for a longer period of time, passes less rapidly into the body and is excreted partially undigested in the feces. The reduction of gross overweight is achieved in most patients without prescribing a reduction diet. However, due to the high and also life-endangering side effects, the jejuno-ileostomy is only reserved for a very limited number of patients (4) and should not be considered a substitute for diet therapy in carbohydrate-dependent metabolic disease.

For pathophysiological reasons the alimentary carbohydrates are of major interest in patients with diabetes mellitus, obesity and hyperlipoproteinemia type IV. In diabetics they cause hyperglycemia,in obese people hyperinsulinemia and in patients with a familial hypertriglyceridemia an increase in the VLDL synthesis. Furthermore, the carbohydrates make up approximately 45% of the calories and are the most important source of energy in our diet. Thus particular attention should be directed to alimentary carbohydrates which are rapidly hydrolyzed to monosaccharides and absorbed from the intestine. A delayed absorption of carbohydrates as achieved by strict dieting can be obtained using inhibitors of intestinal α-glucosidases.

In loading tests with starch the postprandial increment of blood glucose and serum insulin are dose-dependently reduced in animals and man by the amylase inhibitors BAY d 7791 and BAY e 4609 (5,6). The same effects were achieved in sucrose loading tests by administration of TRIS (Tris-(hydroxymethyl)-aminomethane) as a competitively acting sucrase inhibitor (7).

RESULTS

In loading tests on rats with sucrose + starch the inhibitors were without effect on postprandial blood glucose increment, when given singly (Fig. 1). Only after combination of both the amylase and the sucrase inhibitor a marked reduction in blood glucose increment occurred.

As our diet very often contains startch as well as sucrose, a combination of an amylase inhibitor with a sucrase inhibitor is necessary or we must find a new glucosidase inhibitor which delays the digestion of both carbohydrates to absorbable monosaccharides. These demands are fulfilled by the glucosidase inhibitor BAY g 5421 (8).

When rats are given 0.6 mg BAY g 5421 plus 500 mg sucrose/rat, then significantly more undigested sucrose is found in the small intestines of these animals after 15, 30 and 60 minutes than in the control animals without an inhibitor (Fig. 2).

The blood glucose increment in rats is dose-dependently reduced in sucrose loading tests (Fig. 3). The oral ED_{50} is 1.1 mg BAY gm5421/kg rat. In loading tests with starch the inhibitor is of the same order of potency. The ED_{50} is 1.5 mg. BAY gm5421/kg rat. This fact was somewhat surprising because in vitro BAY gm5421 inhibits pancreatic α-amylase very slightly, compared with the amylase inhibitor BAY e 4609. The mechanism by which the digestion of starch is inhibited by BAY gm5421 has not, as yet, been fully established.

In healthy volunteers, the ED_{50} in loading tests with 43 g sucrose plus 67gm starch is approximately 80 mg BAY g 5421/person when measured against the reduction of the capillary blood glucose increase, and 60 mg BAY gm5421 when measured against the reduced postprandial insulin increase (9).

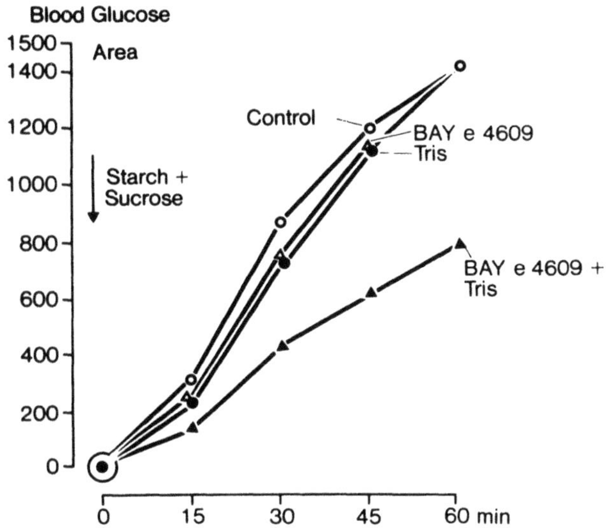

Fig. 1. Reduction of postprandial blood glucose increment in rats by administration of BAY e 4609 + Tris in loading with sucrose + starch.

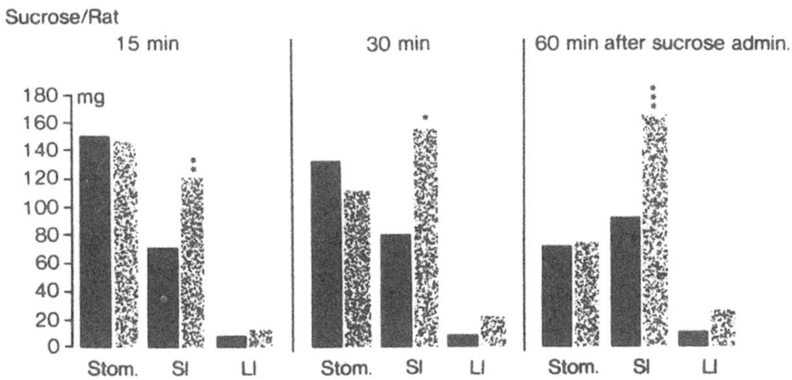

*Fig. 2. Gl sucrose content of rats 15,30 and 60 min after administration of 500 mg sucrose ■ + 0.6 mg. Bay g 5421 ▒ /rat. Stom. = Stomach, SI = Small intestine, LI = Large intestine *P 0.05, **P 0.01, ***P 0.001.*

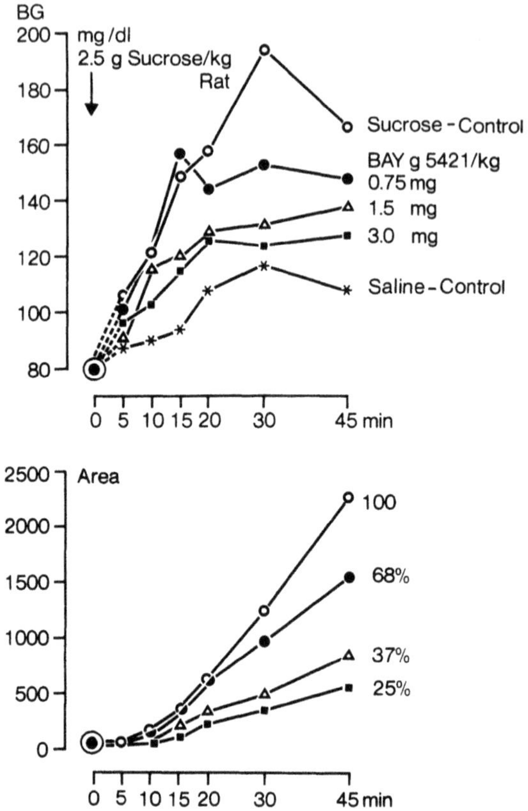

Fig. 3. Blood glucose concentrations (mg/dl, upper part) and 'area under the curve' (lower part) of rats in sucrose loadings tests ± BAY g 5421

From these results, one can conclude that the postprandial hyperglycemia in diabetic patients and the postprandial hyperinsulinemia in obese patients are reduced by this inhibitor. First results in clinical trials with insulin dependent diabetics confirm this conclusion (10).

Subacute doses of the inhibitor in a feed containing sucrose and starch caused a dose-dependent reduction in body weight-gain of genetically obese and hyperinsulinemic rats (Fig. 4). In higher concentrations the inhibitor even caused a loss in weight. Feed consumption is dose-dependently reduced.

After feeding rats with the inhibitor for 42 days, the lipid content of the carcasses of these rats was significantly reduced and the protein content after 37.5 mg BAY g 5421/100 gm feed was significantly increased.

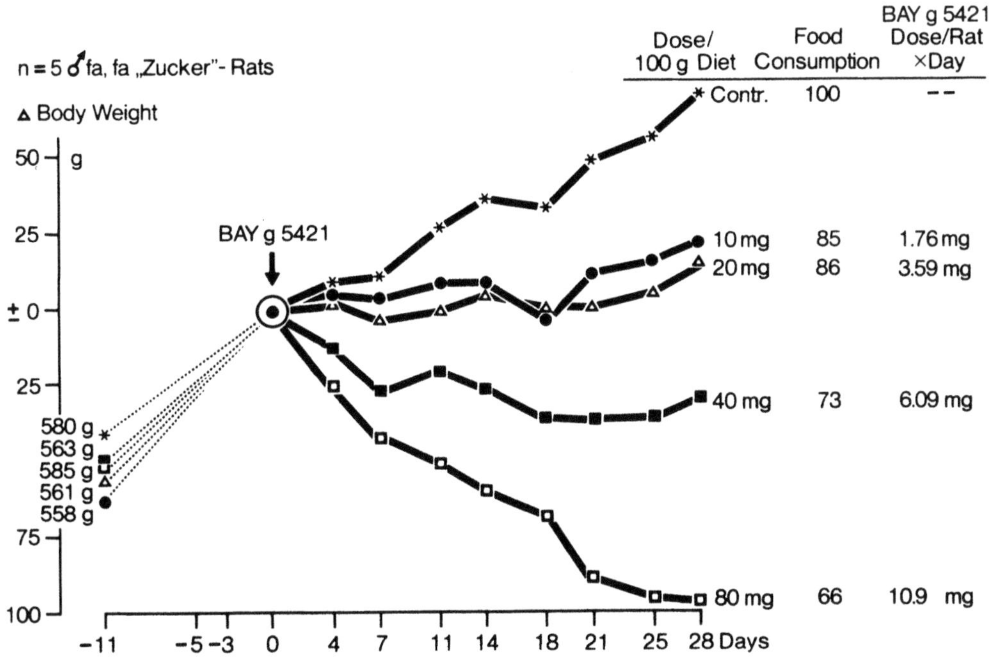

Fig. 4. Effect of BAY 5 5421 on body weight gain and food intake of genetically obese "Zucker"-rats

The biosynthesis of VLD-lipoproteins can be greatly increased in animal and man by a diet rich in carbohydrates and low in fat. After offering a fat free diet for three days to genetically hypertriglyceridemic rats, the serum triglyceride concentrations increased from approximately 500 mg to more than 3000 mg/dl due to an increased biosynthesis of VLDL (Fig. 5). The triglyceride concentration did not increase but rather, when compared with the initial value, decreased after 20 mg BAY gm 5241/100 gm feed.

CONCLUSIONS:

(a) The glucosidase inhibitor, BAY g 5241, caused a dose-dependent delay in the digestion of starch and sucrose in the small intestines of rats. It also reduced the postprandial increment of blood glucose and serum insulin dose-dependently in animal and man.

(b) In feeding experiments the intake of feed, the body weight-gain and the total lipid content in the carcasses of genetically obese "Zucker"-rats were dose-dependently reduced by BAY g 5421. The VLDL increase in the serum of genetically hypertriglyceridemic "Zucker"-rats was inhibited completely by BAY g 5421.

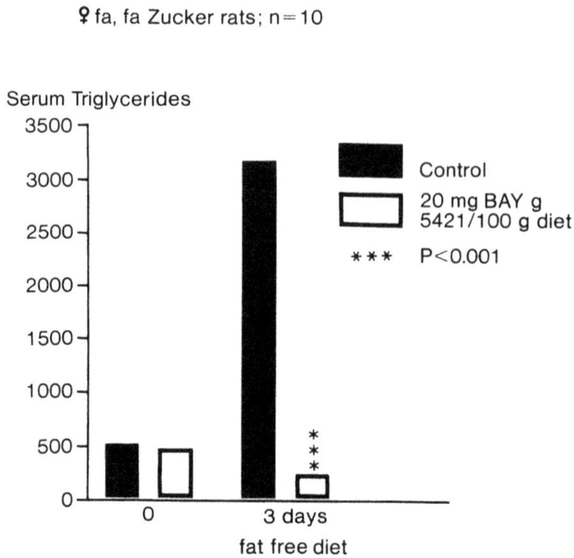

Fig. 5. Serum triglyceride concentrations before and three days after offering genetically obese "Zucker"-rats a fat free diet ± BAY g 5421

(c) From these results one can assume that metabolic disorders in carbohydrate dependent metabolic diseases can be effectively controlled by delaying carbohydrate digestion in the small intestines.

REFERENCES

1. *Iber, F.L. & Cooper, M. (1977). Am. J. Nutr. 30, 4*
2. *Quaade, F. (1977). Am. J. Clin. Nutr. 30, 16*
3. *Husemann, G. (1973). Dtsch. med. Wschr. 98, 2343*
4. *Gries, F.A., et al.in Adipositas. Pathophysiologie, Klinik und Therapie. Springer Verlag, Berlin.*
5. *Puls, W. & Keup, U. (1973). Diabetologia 9, 97*
6. *Puls, W. & Keup, U. (1975). Recent Advances in Obesity Research: I. Proceedings of the 1st International Congress on Obesity. Howard, A. ed., Newman Publishing LTD, London*
7. *Puls, W. & Keup, U. (1975). Metabolism 24, 93*
8. *Schmidt, D.D., et al.(1977). Naturwissenschaften 64, 535*
9. *Puls, W., et al.(1977). Naturwissenschaften 64, 536*
10. *Jaeger, H., et al. 84. Tagg. Dt. Ges. Inn. Medizin in Wiesbaden, 2 , Abstr. 394*
11. *Sachse, G. & Willms, B. (1979) (submitted for publication)*

INHIBITION OF POLYOL PATHWAY ACTIVITY IN DIABETIC AND GALACTOSEMIC RATS BY THE ALDOSE REDUCTASE INHIBITOR CP-45,634

M.J. Peterson*, R. Sarges, C.E. Aldinger
and D.P. MacDonald

Studies in animal models and man suggest that conversion of glucose to sorbitol via the polyol pathway may be causative in the pathogenesis of diabetic cataracts and peripheral neuropathy (1-3). Elevated levels of sorbitol have in fact been detected in both the lens (2) and the peripheral nerves (3) of diabetic man. The NADPH-linked conversion of glucose to sorbitol is catalyzed by the enzyme aldose reductase which also catalyzes the conversion of other sugar aldehydes to their respective sugar alcohols (e.g., galactose to galactitol). Although aldose reductase has low substrate affinities (K_m = 70 and 20 mM for glucose and galactose), conditions such as diabetes or galactosemia lead to elevated flux through the polyol pathway and tissue accumulation of sorbitol and galactitol, respectively. In either case, such elevations in sugar alcohols are thought to be responsible for the cataractous process in lens and depressed nerve conduction velocity in peripheral nerves (1). In support of this, inhibitors of aldose reductase have been shown to delay cataract formation in both diabetic (4) and galactosemic (5) rodents and to delay depressions in motor nerve conduction velocity in galactosemic rats (6). These findings, taken together with the observations that aldose reductase is present in other tissues in which diabetic complications occur (e.g., retina and aorta) (1-7), suggest that aldose reductase inhibitors may be of value in the treatment of some of these complications. This report describes studies undertaken in diabetic and galactosemic rats with a novel and highly potent aldose reductase inhibitor, CP-45,634 (d-6-fluoro-spiro[chroman-4,4'-imidazolidine]-2',5'-dione).

MATERIALS AND METHODS

Male rats (200-250 grams) were of the Charles River strain and were fed ad libitum (Laboratory Rat Pellets or Ground Rat Chow, Ralston Purina Company, St. Louis, Mo.). Rats were made diabetic by an intravenous injection of streptozotocin (85 mg/kg in a 0.01M solution of citrate buffer). Galactosemia was produced by placing rats on a 30% galactose diet. Galactose was mixed with Ground Rat Chow in a Hobart Model A-200 mixer. Aldose reductase was partially purified (75% ammonium sulfate fraction) from frozen calf lens (Pel Freeze Biologicals, Inc., Rogers, Ark.) by the method of Hayman and Kinoshita (8). Enzymatic activity was also determined by the method of Hayman and Kinoshita (8). For whole cell in vitro studies, sciatic nerves were quickly removed from normal anesthetized rats (pentobarbital, 60 mg/kg, intraperitoneally) and incubated for two hours at 37°C in Krebs-Ringer bicarbonate buffer containing 4% Bovine Serum Albumin and 50 mM glucose.

Sorbitol was assayed enzymatically using sheep liver sorbitol dehydrogenase (Boehringer Mannheim, New York) by a modification of the method of Clements et al (9). The assay was carried out in diethanolamine buffer (100 mM) containing 10 mM $MgCl_2$ and 5 mM EDTA. Galactitol was assayed chromatographically with a Tracor MT-220 gas chromatograph by the procedure of Hayman, et al (10). Glucose was measured with a ferricyanide reduction method using an autoanalyzer. Extraction of sciatic nerves and lenses for sorbitol determinations was done in an ice cold 8% perchloric acid, 40% ethanol (v/v) solution. Nerves and lenses removed from anesthetized rats (and nerves from incubation media) were homogenized in 1.0 ml of the extraction fluid. The homogenates were centrifuged at 37,000 x g and the supernatants neutralized with 3M K_2CO_3 in a 0.5 M triethanolamine solution. The neutralized extracts were again centrifuged and the supernatants assayed for sorbitol. For extraction of lenses for galactitol determinations, lenses were initially homogenized in 1 ml of ice cold water. The homogenates were centrifuged at 4000 x g and the supernatants were treated with 0.1 ml of 3% (w/v) $ZnSO_4$ and heated at 50°C for 10 minutes. The solutions were then neutralized by the addition of 0.1 ml Ba $(OH)_2$, the concentration of which was approximately 3.3% (w/v). The resultant suspensions were centrifuged and 0.1 ml of the supernatants were lyophilized overnight. The trimethylsilyl ethers were prepared by the method of Sweeley, et al (11).

Lenticular opacities in galactosemic rats were determined by placing 5 μl of Homatropine Hydrobromide (Alcon Laboratories, Fort Worth, Tex.) in each eye followed by examination with a flashlight in a darkened room. As an index of the severity of the opacity, the area of the lens involved was used. Areas of involvement were designated as < 20%, 20% to < 50% and 50% to > 50%. These correspond to Stages 1-A, 1-B, and 1-C through 5, respectively, as described by Sippel (12).

RESULTS

CP-45,634 was found to be a highly potent inhibitor of partially purified aldose reductase, with an IC_{50} (concentration of inhibitor required to produce a 50% inhibition of the enzyme) of approximately 5×10^{-7} M. Kinetic analysis showed the inhibition to be uncompetitive in nature (Figure 1).

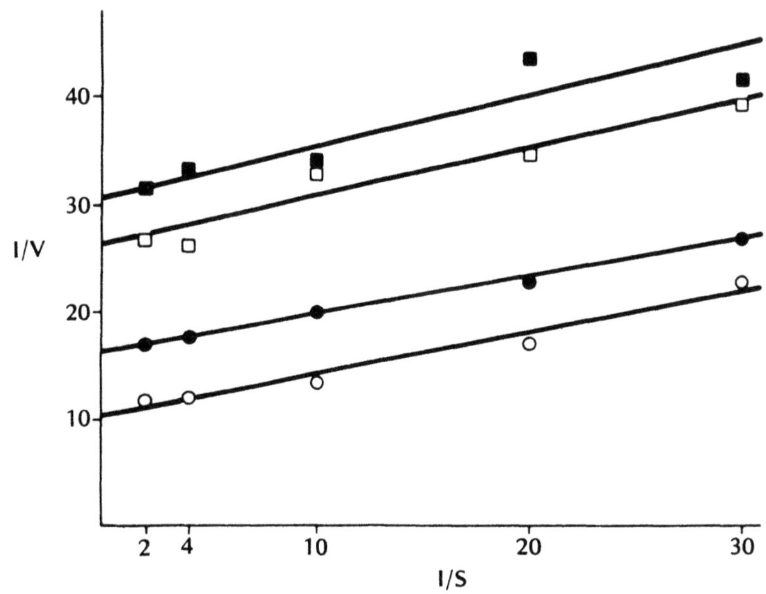

Fig. 1. Effect of CP-45,634 on the Lineweaver-Burke plot of enzyme activity with glyceraldehyde as substrate. The ordinate represents the reciprocal of initial velocity expressed as the change in optical density per 15 minutes. The abscissa represents the reciprocal of glyceraldehyde concentrations ranging between 0.033 and 0.5 mM. The open circles represent the uninhibited enzyme; the closed circles, open squares and closed squares represent enzyme inhibited by CP-45,634 at 2.5×10^{-7}, 5.0×10^{-7} and 7.5×10^{-7}M, respectively.

In isolated sciatic nerves incubated in the presence of high (50 mM) glucose concentrations, CP-45,634 essentially eliminated sorbitol accumulation at 1 x 10^{-5} M and produced a 50% decrease at 1 x 10^{-6} M (Table 1).

Table 1

INHIBITION OF SORBITOL ACCUMULATION[a] IN ISOLATED RAT SCIATIC NERVES INCUBATED IN THE PRESENCE OF 50 mM GLUCOSE

	% Inhibition	
In Vitro Concentration (M)	1 x 10^{-5}	1 x 10^{-6}
CP-45,634	92	51

[a]In control incubations, sorbitol rises from approximately 50-100 nmoles/gm tissue to 400 nmoles/gm tissue in 2 hours.

In order to determine if the in vitro activity of CP-45,634 would translate to in vivo models, initial studies employed a streptozotocinized rat model in which sorbitol accumulation in sciatic nerves was measured 27 hours after the induction of diabetes. In Table 2, the effects of CP-45,634 are shown. CT-45,634 produced substantial inhibition of sorbitol accumulation at oral doses as low as 0.25 mg/kg, t.i.d. It should also be noted that CP-45,634 did not produce depressions in blood glucose, an activity which would be expected to cause depressions in sorbitol levels.

To determine the ability of CP-45,634 to reduce already elevated sorbitol levels, rats with streptozotocin-induced diabetes of 2 weeks duration were treated orally with CP-45,634 for 7 days (Table 3). Sorbitol measurements were carried out in both the sciatic nerve and lens. At the end of the 2 week untreated period (i.e. Day #1, Table 3) a control group (Control Group 1) was sacrificed for baseline sorbitol determinations and the remaining two groups received either CP-45,634 (2.5 mg/kg, b.i.d.) or water (Control Group 2). After 7 days, sciatic nerve and lens sorbitol levels in the control group had risen above baseline values. After 7 days of treatment with CP-45,634 substantial depressions of sorbitol levels were observed in both the sciatic nerve (92%) and lens (90%).

Table 2

EFFECT OF CP-45,634 ON BLOOD GLUCOSE AND ON SORBITOL ACCUMULATION[a] IN SCIATIC NERVES OF DIABETIC RATS

Streptozotocin was administered at 85 mg/kg, intravenously, at 0 hour. Compound was administered orally at 4,7 and 24 hours. Values are means ± SEM; n = 5.

		Time (Hours)				
	Compound and Dose	4	6	24	27	% Inhibition
Experiment 1	Control					
	Blood Glucose (mg%)	171 ± 9	117 ± 14	371 ± 15	327 ± 12	---
	Nerve Sorbitol (n moles/gm)	–	–	–	413 ± 20	---
	CP-45,634 (0.25 mg/kg)					
	Blood Glucose (mg%)	199 ± 25	150 ± 19	382 ± 10	337 ± 7	---
	Nerve Sorbitol (n moles/gm)	–	–	–	220 ± 19	47

		Time (Hours)				
	Compound and Dose	4	6	24	27	% Inhibition
Experiment 2	Control					
	Blood Glucose (mg%)	231 ± 11	196 ± 23	367 ± 15	382 ± 11	---
	Nerve Sorbitol (n moles/gm)	–	–	–	614 ± 78	---
	CP-45,634 (0.75 mg/kg)					
	Blood Glucose (mg%)	265 ± 27	212 ± 35	402 ± 8	378 ± 5	---
	Nerve Sorbitol (n moles/gm)	–	–	–	136 ± 10	78

[a]In normal rats, sorbitol levels are approximately 50-100 nmoles/gm tissue.

As an index of efficacy, the effect of CP-45,634 on cataract development in galactosemic rats was determined. This model was chosen since rats fed a diet rich in galactose begin to develop cataracts within a few days as compared to a few months in diabetic rats. The reason for this difference is due to a more rapid accumulation of polyol in galactosemia. Prior to the efficacy study, the ability of CP-45,634 to prevent galactitol formation in lenses of acutely galactosemic rats was determined (Table 4). Lens galactitol levels rose from essentially undetectable levels to over 30 μmoles/gm in rats fed a 30% galactose diet for 7 days. In rats receiving CP-45,634 in the diet in addition to galactose, galactitol accumulation was inhibited by over 95% at dose levels approximating 10 and 20 mg/kg.

Table 3

EFFECT OF CP-45,634 ON SORBITOL LEVELS IN THE SCIATIC NERVE AND LENS OF CHRONICALLY DIABETIC RATS

Streptozotocin was administered at 85 mg/kg, intravenously. Rats remained untreated for 2 weeks. Control Group 1 was sacrificed at the end of the 2 week period. CP-45,634 was then administered to a group at an oral dose of 2.5 mg/kg (b.i.d.) and a second control group (Control Group 2) received water. Treatment was continued for 7 days. Rats received their a.m. dose on day 8, and were sacrificed 3 hours post-dose. Values are means ± SEM; n = 6 for control groups; n = 5 for the CP-45,634 treated group.

	Treatment Day	1	4	8
Blood	Control Group 1	456 + 8	–	–
Glucose	Control Group 2	429 + 20	461 + 18	426 + 11
(mg%)	CP-45,634	441 + 11	444 + 25	419 + 16
Sciatic Nerve	Control Group 1	1,161 + 99	–	–
Sorbitol	Control Group 2	–	–	1,569 + 178
(n moles/gm)	CP-45,634	–	–	130 + 12 [a]
Lens	Control Group 1	21,203 + 1,530	–	–
Sorbitol	Control Group 2	–	–	25,600 + 2,373
(n moles/gm)	CP-45,634	–	–	2,683 + 278 [a]

[a] $p < 0.001$ compared to either Control Group 1 or Control Group 2.

Table 4

EFFECT OF CP-45,634 ON GALACTITOL LEVELS IN THE LENSES OF GALACTOSE FED RATS

Normal fed male rats were fed a 30% galactose diet for 7 days.Drug treated animals received CP-45,634 mixed with their good.On day 8, lenses were removed for galactitol determination.Values are means ± SEM; n = 5 for all groups.

Compound and Average Daily Dose	Rat Weight (grams)	Average Daily Food Consumption (grams/rat)	Average Daily Galactose Consumption (grams/rat)	Lens Galactitol (μ moles/gram)	% Inhibition
Control	208 ± 2	22.21	6.66	35.24 ± 6.66	---
CP-45,634 11.5 mg/kg	208 ± 3	21.70	6.51	1.52 ± 0.20 [a]	96
CP-45,634 23.5 mg/kg	211 ± 4	22.40	6.72	0.49 ± 0.13 [a]	99

[a] $p<0.001$ compared to control.

To study the effect of CP-45,634 on cataract formation in galactosemia, rats were fed a 30% galactose diet for 29 days and eyes were examined for lenticular opacities approximately twice each week. Control animals received only the galactose diet. Experimental animals received CP-45,634 mixed in the food to approximate daily doses of 5 and 10 mg/kg. Between the fourth and ninth day of the study, lenticular opacities developed in approximately 50% of the eys of the control animals (Figure 2). By day 15 almost 100% of the eyes of the controls showed some degree of opacity. By contrast no opacities were observed until day 14 in rats receiving CP-45,634. Between day 14 and 25 lenticular opacities were observed in only 10% or less of the eyes of rats receiving either dose of CP-45,634. On day 29, opacities were present in about 50% of the eyes of rats receiving CP-45,634 at 5 mg/kg. At that time, however, opacities were still limited to about 10% of the eyes of rats receiving CP-45,634 at 10 mg/kg.

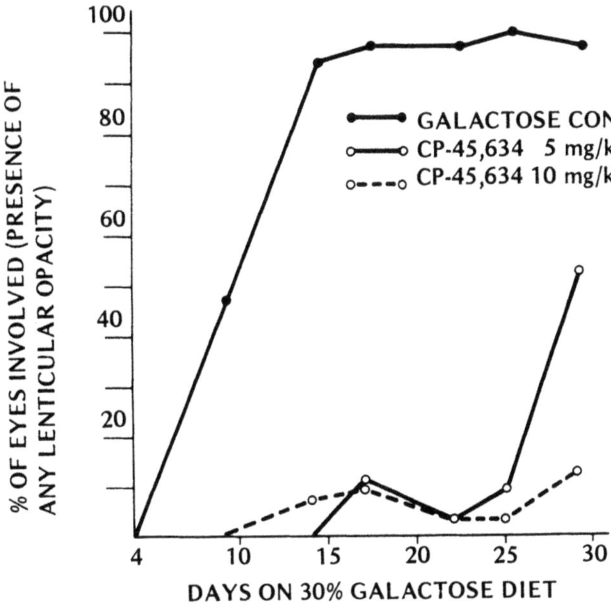

Fig. 2. Effect of CP-45,634 on cataract formation in galactosemic rats. Rats were fed a 30% galactose diet for 29 days and eye examinations were conducted approximately twice each week. Control animals received only the galactose diet. Experimental animals received CP-45,634 mixed in the food to approximate doses of 5 and 10 mg/kg.

DISCUSSION

In addition to the lens and peripheral nerves, the polyol pathway has been demonstrated in several other tissues in which diabetic complications occur. These include the retina, arterial endothelial cells and the renal papilla (7). Like the lens and peripheral nerves, these tissues do not require insulin for glucose transport and therefore are exposed to prevailing blood glucose levels. Since, however, aldose reductase has low substrate affinities, maximal rates of sorbitol or galactitol formation occur only under conditions of high intracellular glucose or galactose such as occurs in diabetes or galactosemia. Under such conditions products of the polyol pathway have been shown to accumulate in both the aorta (7) and renal papilla (1). The polyols formed accumulate because they are not efficiently metabolized and because they cannot readily diffuse across cell membranes (1). It is well established that sugar alcohol formation in the lens leads to hypertonicity and consequent accumulation of tissue water with lenticular swelling (1,3). Lenticular swelling and electrolyte imbalance eventually leads to a loss of osmotic integrity with large increases in intracellular sodium and water and the appearance of lenticular opacities (1). Tissue water accumulation secondary to elevations of sugar alcohol accumulation has also been implicated in the derangements associated with galactosemic and diabetic neuropathy (6) and atherosclerosis in diabetes (7). However, whether this "osmotic" hypothesis totally explains the mechanism by which increased flux through the polyol pathway may lead to certain complications remains to be established (6-7).

While known inhibitors of aldose reductase have been used to establish a role for the polyol pathway in the development of diabetic cataracts and peripheral neuropathy in animal models, their value in the clinical setting may be limited since they are only effective at relatively high oral doses (approximately 1 gm/kg/day (4-5). The data presented in this report show that the high potency of CP-45,634 in inhibiting partially purified aldose reductase, translates to a whole cell system and several whole animal models. In the isolated sciatic nerve preparation, CP-45,634 produced a 50% decrease in sorbitol accumulation at in vitro concentrations as low as 1×10^{-6} M. In diabetic rats, CP-45,634 both prevented sorbitol accumulation and reduced already elevated sorbitol levels at low oral doses. In acutely streptozotocinized rats, CP-45,634 at an oral dose of 0.75 mg/kg, t.i.d., almost completely prevented the accumulation of sorbitol in sciatic nerves. Also, at 0.25 mg/kg, t.i.d., a greater than 50% inhibition of accumulation was obtained when values are corrected for basal sorbitol levels. In rats which had been diabetic for two weeks, treatment with CP-45,634 at 2.5 mg/kg, b.i.d., for seven days dramatically reduced elevated sorbitol levels in both sciatic nerves and lenses. In sciatic nerves, sorbitol levels were essentially returned to normal. In no case could the effects of CP-45,634 on sorbitol levels in these models be accounted for by drug-induced depressions in blood glucose.

In galactosemic rats, lens galactitol accumulation over a seven day period was essentially abolished at oral doses of CP-45,634 approximating 10 and 20 mg/kg daily. The ability of CP-45,634 to markedly inhibit lens galactitol was reflected in its ability to delay cataract formation in this model. In rats receiving 10 mg/kg, the appearance of lenticular opacities were limited to only 10% of the eyes examined throughout the entire course of the study. In animals receiving 5 mg/kg lenticular opacities were also limited to about 10% of the eyes for 25 days. In galactose controls, some degree of lenticular opacity had developed in approximately 50% of the eyes by the ninth day of the study and almost 100% of the eyes

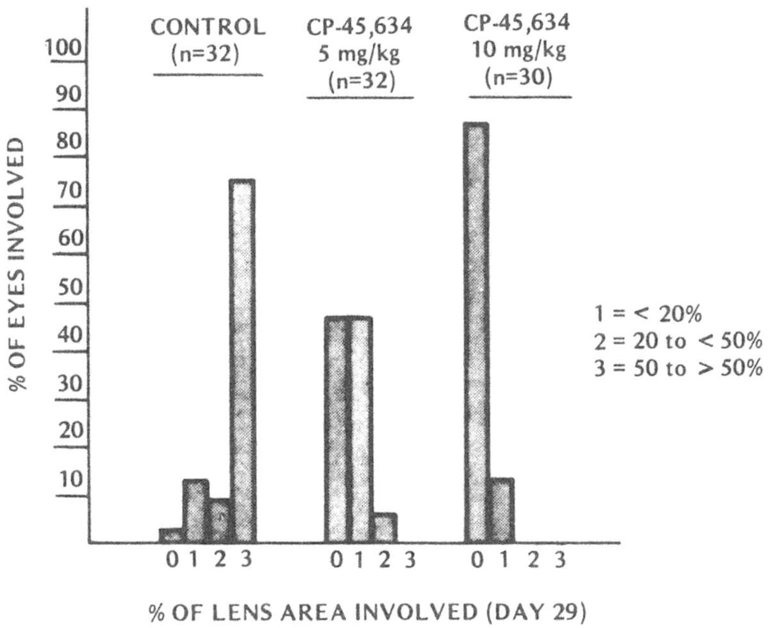

Fig. 3. Effect of CP-45,634 treatment on the severity of lenticular opacities in galactosemic rats.

were involved by the fourteenth day. The effectiveness of these low oral doses of CP-45,634 in delaying cataract development is even more apparent when the severity of lenticular opacities is considered (Figure 3). As an index of severity, the percentage of lens area involved was monitored. By day 29, 84% of the control lenses showed an area of involvement which was greater than 20%. This compares to 6% and 0% in the CP-45,634 treated animals receiving 5 and 10 mg/kg, respectively. In addition, 75% of the control lenses showed a greater than 50% area of involvement on day 29. This is in contrast to 0% in rats treated with either dose of CP-45,634.

Based on the above, the rationale appears strong for investigation of aldose reductase inhibitors with regard to their ability to prevent and/or ameliorate at least some of the complications of diabetes. CP-45,634 has been shown to be an orally active and highly potent inhibitor of aldose reductase in animal models and therefore has good potential for testing the role of the polyol pathway in the development of diabetic complications.

REFERENCES

1. *Gabbay, K.H. (1973). New Engl. J. Med., 288, 831.*
2. *Pirie, A. and Van Heyningen, R. (1964). Exp. Eye Res. 3, 124.*
3. *Ward, J.D. (1973) in Adv. Metab. Disorders Suppl. 2, Camerini-Davalos, R.A. and Cole, H.S. eds., Academic Press, New York and London, p. 425.*
4. *Varma, S.D. et al. (1977). Science, 195, 205.*
5. *Dvornik, D. et al. (1973). Science 182, 1146.*
6. *Gabbay, K.H. (1973) in Adv. Metab.Disorders Suppl. 2, Camerini-Davalos, R.A. and Cole, H.S. eds., Academic Press, New York and London, p. 417.*
7. *Winegrad, A.I. et al. (1973) in Adv. Metab. Disorders Suppl. 2, Camerini-Davalos, R.A. and Cole, H.S. eds., Academic Press, New York and London, p. 117.*
8. *Hayman, S. and Kinoshita, J.H. (1965) JBC 240, 877.*
9. *Clements, R.S. et al. (1969). Science 166, 1007.*
10. *Hayman, S. et al. (1969). Biochem and Biophys. Acta 128, 474.*
11. *Sweely, C.C. (1963). Am. Chem. Soc. 85, 2497.*
12. *Sippel, T.O. (1966). Invest. Ophthl. 5, 568.*

DISCUSSION

J. BARBOSA: *Dr. Krause, did you say that your genetically obese rats have less appetite? Was the food consumption lower than when they were on the enzyme?*

H. P. KRAUSE: *That's right.*

J. BARBOSA: *How do you interpret that?*

H. P. KRAUSE: *Well, that's very difficult to interpret, and, at this time, I think we can only speculate about this.*

J. BARBOSA: *Do you know if that happens on humans too, in human studies?*

H. P. KRAUSE: *We don't know.*

J. BARBOSA: *Dr. Peterson, although I think the data on preventing cataracts in these animals with sorbitol inhibitors is very conclusive, I'm not so impressed about the nerves. I would like to mention Dr. Winegrad's studies. I think he has shown, in his diabetic rats, that decrease of motor conduction velocity could be improved with relatively high myoinositol values. He further showed that, in spite of the high sorbitol content of the nerve, sorbitol was not related to the decrease in motor conduction velocity in rats.*

M. J. PETERSON: *Yes, I think there are some problems with the myoinsitol story. First, giving slightly more myoinositol than is required to improve neuroconduction velocity actually decreases it. Secondly, the different changes produced by myoinositol feeding on sensory and motor nerve conduction velocities, as shown by Dr. Clements are small in a situation where standard errors are fairly high. This bothers me. However, assuming that the myoinositol story is valid. I think one has to reconcile this with the fact that aldosereductase inhibitors, at least aldostatin (we are doing work with our own compound) has been shown to inhibit motor neuroconduction velocity in the galactosemic model. Therefore, if there is a connection, it may be that the loss in myoinositol may be a consequence of elevated increased flux through the polyol pathway.*

N. FREINKEL: *May I pursue this further? I think one of the postulates was that there is a finite capacity for retention of these higher sugars, so that you end up with one displacing the other, and the implication was that the elevation of intracellular fructose and sorbitol then affected a reduction of inositol. Afterwards, it was found that, with inositol supplementation, there was a preservation of the fructose and the sorbitol content of the nerve. Now, with the restoration of intracellular inositol content, the nerve conduction was restored. In this context, I wonder whether you have included measurements of polyol and inositol with your aldosereductase?*

M. J. PETERSON: *We didn't measure tissue inositol. With regard to what you said, I still think you are saying essentially that it is the build-up of sorbitol fructose which may inhibit or decrease...*

N. FREINKEL: *No, I'm saying that the ideas will be strengthened or refuted - whether there are inverse relationships with inositol, or whether there are reciprocal relationships with polyols and inositol.*

M. J. PETERSON: *Well, I would be the first to admit that the polyol hypothesis is just that - a rather good hypothesis, but mainly, I think we may have a tool to test the hypothesis with this compound.*

M. W. STEFFES: *Dr. Peterson, with islet transplantation, you cannot reverse cataracts, once they are established in diabetic rats. Have you looked, with this compound, whether cataracts once established can be reversed at all?*

M. J. PETERSON: *Well, that's a good question. We haven't done that yet, but I showed you the data in which, once the polyol is elevated, we can reduce it. We plan those experiments , but as yet haven't performed.*

K. D. HEPP. *I have a question regarding the aldosereductase inhibitor. Do you have evidence for an inhibition of other enzymes? It seems strange to conceive that it is just inhibiting one reductase.*

M. J. PETERSON: *We haven't systematicclly gone through to determine if the compound inhibits a variety of enzymes involved in carbohydrate metabolism. We have done radio-labelled glucose experiments, showing that the compound has really no effect on CO_2 production from radio-labelled glucose in various places, indicating that it's a relatively specific effect and not secondary to either some decrease in glucose uptake or some adverse effect on overall cellular oxidation of glucose. However, I should mention that most of these inhibitors of aldosereductase are fairly species-specific. This implies that these inhibitors may be rather specific for this enzyme. To answer* *your question directly, we haven't studied other enzymes per se, only overall oxidative metabolism.*

E. TUTWILER: *Dr. Krause, have you looked at the gastrointestinal side effects in terms such as diarrhea, which you might expect, since disease states where there is deficiency of amylase or sucrase there is generally diarrhea and other gastrointestinal side effects? Have you looked at this both in animals and man?*

H. P. KRAUSE: *As you saw, from one of the slides, with the threefold AD50 of the inhibitor, you will not find more carbohydrate in the large intestine; more carbohydrate would be necessary to see diarrhea, flatulence and meteorism in animals. In humans, we know there is some kind of meteorism and flatulence, but there might be a question of dosage. Perhaps, by reduction of dose, we could avoid degradation by bacterial enzymes of carbohydrates coming into the large intestine.*

GENETIC CONTROL OF TOLBUTAMIDE METABOLISM IN HUMANS

J. Scott, A.D. Henderson and
P.L. Poffenbarger*

Tolbutamide (1-butyl, 3-*p*-tolylsulfonylurea) has been in general use in the treatment of diabetes since 1956. Surprisingly little information has been published regarding the pharmacology of this drug. This dilemma achieved international recognition in 1970 when the University Group Diabetes Program (UGDP) published data indicating that tolbutamide, taken on a fixed dosage schedule over a period of years, significantly increased the risk of cardiovascular death. The studies reported here were designed to elucidate more clearly the pharmacology of tolbutamide. The results demonstrate strong genetic control of tolbutamide metabolism and imply that slow inactivators of the drug might be more susceptible to extrapancreatic effects by virtue of higher accrued blood levels on fixed dosage schedules.

TOLBUTAMIDE METABOLISM

Bänder and Sholz (1) first demonstrated that tolbutamide was oxidized to hydroxytolbutamide (1-butyl, 3-*p*-hydroxyphenylsulfonylurea) and carboxytolbutamide (1-butyl, 3-*p*-carboxyphenylsulfonylurea) by homogenates of rat liver and kidney. In a study by Thomas and Ikeda (2), ^{3}H-tolbutamide was given orally to eight normal males; 85% was excreted in 48 h in the urine, 9% in the feces. Hydroxytolbutamide (HTB) comprised 33% of the excretory product in the urine. In 1967 Tagg and co-workers reported that tolbutamide was metabolized by hepatic microsomes; hydroxytolbutamide was the major metabolite.

Figure 1 summarizes the scheme of tolbutamide metabolism eventually elucidated by McDaniel and co-workers (3) in the rat, and corroborated in humans by Schulz and Schmidt (4). According to this scheme, tolbutamide is first metabolized to HTB by the monooxygenase system of hepatic microsomes; HTB is then oxidized to carboxytolbutamide (CTB) by cytoplasmic enzymes. The microsomal oxidation to HTB is the rate-limiting step (4). A genetic polymorphism in this enzyme system could lead to marked variation in the rate of tolbutamide metabolism.

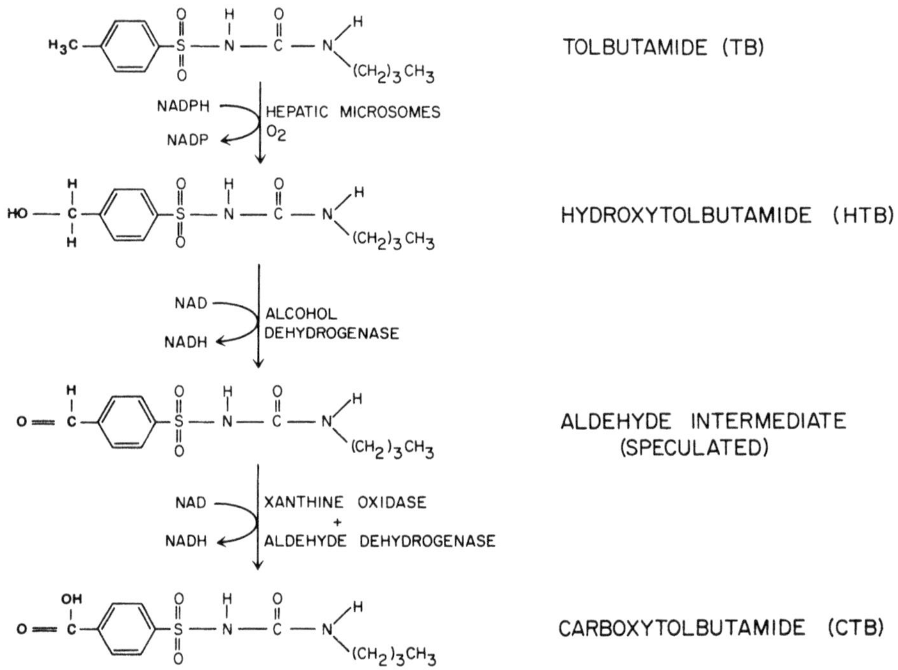

Fig. 1

TOLBUTAMIDE PHARMACOKINETICS

In 1973, studies by Shibasaki et al (5) on tolbutamide disposition resulted in the kinetic model appearing below. In this model, tolbutamide (TB) given intravenously is bound (93%) to plasma protein, namely, albumin, and only free TB is metabolized to HTB.

GENETICS OF THE HEPATIC MICROSOMAL MONOOXYGENASE ENZYME SYSTEM

The hepatic microsomal enzymes are a family of closely related hemoproteins known as cytochrome P-450. The term P-450 refers to the ability of the reduced enzyme to react with carbon monoxide yielding a complex with an absorption peak at 450 nm. Reduced

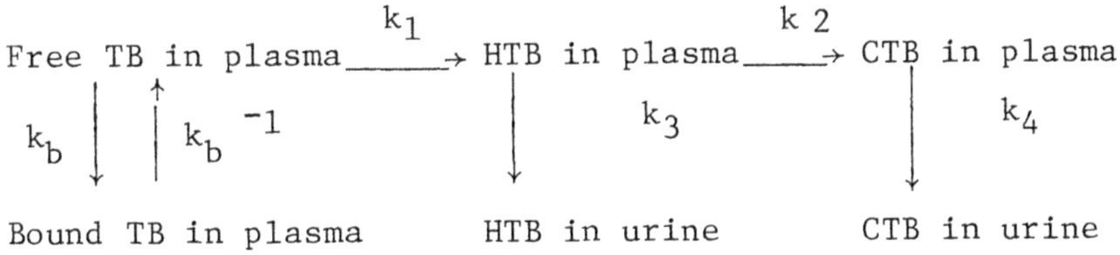

The value of principal interest to pharmacogeneticists is k_1 since this is the rate limiting step in the metabolism of tolbutamide.

NADPH and O_2 are required for enzyme function; one mole of O_2 is consumed for each mole of substrate oxidized.

A complete review of the molecular aspects of the cytochrome P-450 system is beyond the scope of this paper; suffice it to say, there are a number of microsomal monooxygenases. Table 1 summarizes some of the contemporary information regarding these enzymes. The major point is that there appears to be at least three microsomal monooxygenases, each differing in substrate and inducer specificity.

Table 1

THE MICROSOMAL MONOOXYGENASE SYSTEM

Enzyme	Alternate Term	Inducing Agent	M_r	Comments
P-450*a*	P-450; Form I*	ethanol	48,000	Consists of several peptides
P-450*b*	P-450; Form II	phenobarbital	60,000	Inhibited by SKF 525-A§ and by pentobarbitone
P-450*c*	P-448; P_1-450; P-446; Form III; aryl hydrocarbon hydroxylase	3,4-benzypyrene; 3-MC;Ψ TCDD;¶ β-naphthoflavone	54,000	Not inhibited by SKF 525-A§

*It is uncertain if the ethanol-inducible Form I of Comai and Gaylor (10) is identical to form P-450a of Johnson and Muller-Eberhard (11).

§SKF 525-A is the term for β-diethylaminoethyl diphenylpropylacetate.

Ψ3-methylcholanthrene.

¶2,3,7,8-tetrachlorodibenzo-*p*-dioxin.

Evidence for monogenic inheritance of control of monooxygenase activity in humans has been reported recently for the 3-methylcholanthrene-inducible P-448 system. Kellerman, et al (6) in a study of 57 subjects showed aryl hydrocarbon hydroxylase activity to separate into three distinct groups. A frequency histogram of half-lives of antipyrene, a drug which is metabolized by the P-448 enzyme, showed a trimodal pattern suggesting monogenic control. This type of study suggests a sufficient degree of substrate specificity within the monooxygenase system to permit a variant form of one enzyme to significantly alter the rate of metabolism of a particular drug.

TOLBUTAMIDE PHARMACOGENETICS

Definitive evidence for the specific monooxygenase involved in the first step in tolbutamide metabolism is not available; however, in 1975 we set about to define the influence, if any, of genetic control on tolbutamide metabolism in a study of 40 normal volunteers. Several aspects of this study will be reported elsewhere (7). The strategy employed was to define carefully the disappearance rate (K_d) of intravenously administered tolbutamide in this group of volunteers and construct a frequency histogram for K_d to test for possible monogenic control. If the frequency histogram were to demonstrate a statistically significant bimodal or trimodal pattern then family and twin studies would follow to either corroborate or disprove the genetic hypothesis.

The initial problem was to develop a sensitive method for measurement of plasma tolbutamide since the previously employed colorimetric procedures also detected plasma HTB and CTB. This was accomplished by a modification of the gas chromatographic method of Prescott and Redman in which we employed chlorpropamide as internal standard. Verification of the reliability of this procedure was obtained by mass spectrometry showing identical spectra between the extracted methylated derivative and methylated tolbutamide standard. The precision of the extraction and assay procedure was then tested over a plasma concentration range of 2.5 to 10 mg/100 ml. The coefficient of variation ranged from 1.76 to 6.02% as the tolbutamide concentration increased; mean coefficient of variation was 3.38%.

Next, in order to quantitate both HTB and CTB in urine the differential extraction and spectrophotometric procedure of Shibasaki, et al was adopted. CTB was donated by the Upjohn Company. It was necessary to synthesize HTB.

Plasma decay curves following tolbutamide administration were determined for up to 8 hours. Several pharmacokinetic parameters of drug behavior were analyzed; these included half-life ($t_{1/2}$), K_d, drug clearance rate, plasma tolbutamide concentration at 6 hours, plasma binding constant by equilibrium dialysis, and ratio of excreted HTB:CTB.

A nine-fold variation in K_d was found in 42 unrelated subjects (19 females, 23 males), with values ranging from 4.61×10^{-4} min^{-1} to 38.19×10^{-4} min^{-1}. This variation in rate of tolbutamide disappearance represents a range in drug half-life from 25 hours to less than 3 hours, with a mean $t_{1/2}$ of 6.89 hours. A comparison of K_d in a rapid and slow inactivator of tolbutamide is shown in Figure 2.

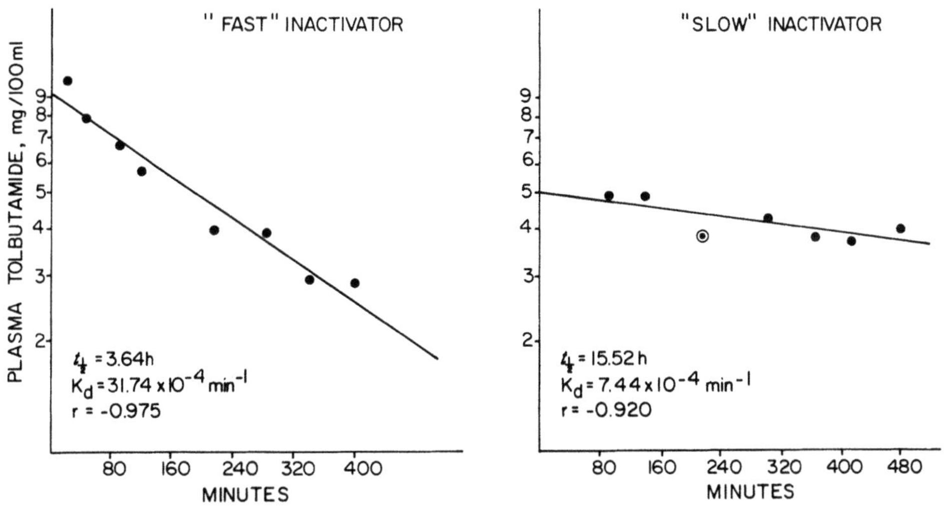

Fig. 2

No difference was found in K_d between males and females and no significant correlation between K_d and age was uncovered. Ages ranged from 16 to 66 years. Frequency histograms of the various pharmacokinetic parameters were constructed. Figure 3 shows the bimodal nature of the histogram for the 6 hour plasma tolbutamide. The practical value of this approach to analysis of the data is that the clinician might determine whether a maturity-onset diabetic is a fast or slow tolbutamide inactivator by drawing one plasma sample 6 hours following drug administration. Histograms of $t_{1/2}$ and drug clearance rate were skewed, particularly the clearance rate data. This is probably due to the fact that the apparent volume of distribution ($_aV_d$) is used in calculation

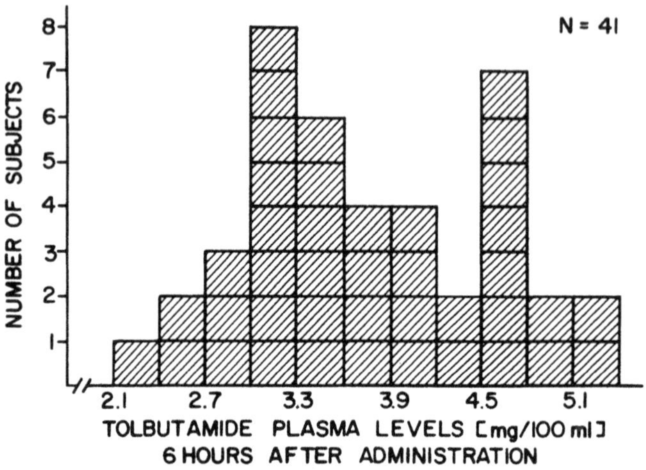

Fig. 3

of clearance rate and represents a non-genetic weighting of the data. It is interesting to note, in this regard, that data reported by Miller, et al indicated that plasma clearance and apparent volume of distribution of tolbutamide increased significantly with age; $t_{1/2}$ values did not. The most sensitive measure of genetic control was established by computer-fitted curves of the K_d frequency histogram; in this analysis, a trimodal model provided the best stastical fit of the data, indicating monogenic control of tolbutamide disappearance rate (7). This hypothesis was further corroborated by family and twin studies (7). These data provided evidence supporting autosomal transmission of fast and slow inactivation of tolbutamide, with approximately ¼ of the population "slow inactivators", ¼ "fast inactivators", and ½ heterozygotes manifesting intermediate K_d values.

In order to substantiate further the hydroxylation step as the rate-limiting site for genetic control the quantity of HTB and CTB in the urine was determined. The hypothesis entertained was that if the primary control in variations in rate of tolbutamide metabolism resided at the monooxygenase step, then subsequent carboxylation would show no effect: i.e., the excretion ratio of HTB:CTB should be similar in both slow and rapid inactivators. Figure 4 illustrates the plot of K_d versus the excretion ratio of HTB:CTB. No correlation was found, thus supporting the hypothesis. It should be noted that less than 2% of tolbutamide administered is excreted unchanged.

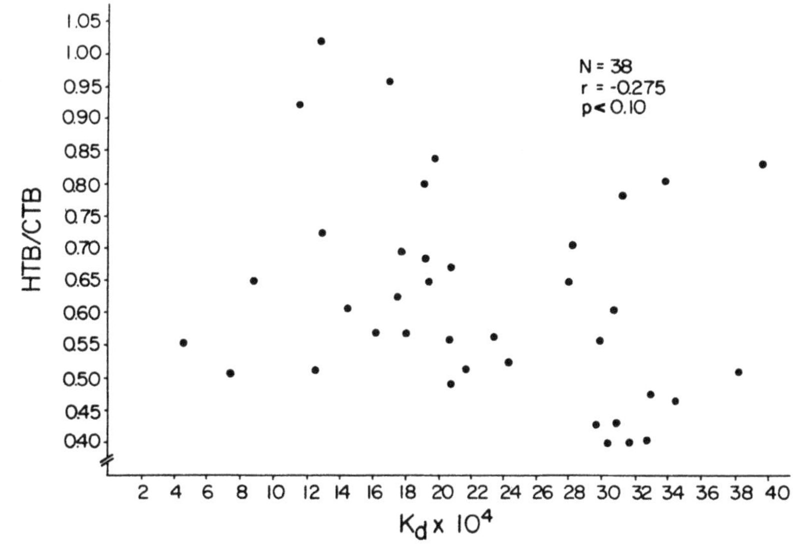

Fig. 4

Plasma protein binding of tolbutamide could also affect K_d by altering the amount of free drug presented to the liver and kidney, the organ sites for both hydroxylation and carboxylation. Binding variations might result from either genetic or drug-induced differences in the binding affinity constant. All subjects in this study had normal serum albumin concentrations and were not taking drugs; therefore, tolbutamide binding constants were determined by equilibrium dialysis. A summation of the binding data is shown in Figure 5. These data were compared to K_d; again, no relationship was found (7).

In practice, drug-induced variations in tolbutamide K_d might exert significant influences on tolbutamide blood levels either by influencing its binding to serum protein or by affecting hydroxylation rate, or both. In order to assess the former possibility, a number of commonly used drugs were obtained in pure powdered form from the appropriate pharmaceutical firm and tested for their effect on half-maximal binding of tolbutamide in an equilibrium dialysis system. Table 3 summarizes these results.

HTB was 10-fold less effective than CTB in displacing tolbutamide suggesting that the *p*-group on the benzene ring significantly affects binding affinity. It should be noted, however, that the plasma concentration of both HTB and CTB is 10-to 100-fold less than that of tolbutamide due to rapid renal clearance. Consequently, neither metabolite is likely to affect tolbutamide binding significantly in either slow or rapid inactivators. On the other hand,

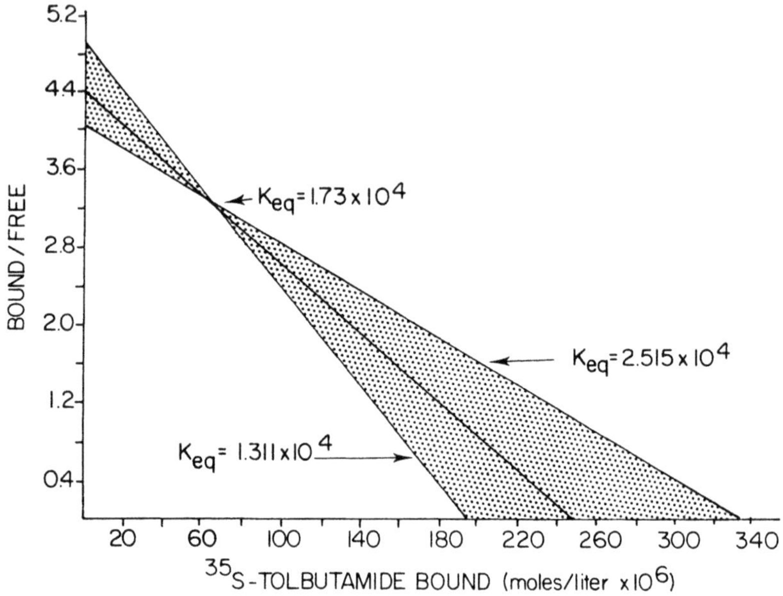

Fig. 5

Table 2

DRUGS INTERFERING WITH TOLBUTAMIDE BINDING TO SERUM PROTEIN

Drug	Concentration Range [M]	C_{50} [M]*
Tolbutamide	1.8×10^{-8} to 8.9×10^{-4}	1.2×10^{-4}
Hydroxytolbutamide	1.4×10^{-4} to 1.8×10^{-3}	10.7×10^{-4}
Carboxytolbutamide	1.8×10^{-8} to 1.3×10^{-3}	1.2×10^{-4}
Acetylsalicylic acid	1.1×10^{-9} to 1.1×10^{-3}	1.2×10^{-4}
Hydralazine	1.9×10^{-9} to 1.0×10^{-3}	2.1×10^{-4}
Probenecid	1.9×10^{-8} to 1.3×10^{-3}	2.3×10^{-4}
Trichloromethiazide	1.1×10^{-9} to 1.5×10^{-4}	3.2×10^{-4}
Sulfamethoxazole	1.3×10^{-9} to 6.9×10^{-4}	4.8×10^{-4}
α-Methyldopa	1.5×10^{-8} to 1.9×10^{-3}	No effect
Allopurinol	1.8×10^{-9} to 9.4×10^{-4}	No effect

*C_{50} is the concentration of the drug that produced half-maximal binding of ^{35}S-tolbutamide.

Table 3

PRELIMINARY DATA ON TOLBUTAMIDE HALF-LIFE IN MATURITY-ONSET DIABETICS BEFORE AND DURING TOLBUTAMIDE THERAPY

Patient	Sex	Age	Tolbutamide $t_{½}$ Before Tx (h)	Tolbutamide $t_{½}$ During Tx* (h)	Difference (h)
1	F	69	5.57	6.20	+0.64
2	F	41	3.30	3.73	+0.43
3	M	51	4.64	5.39	+0.75
4	F	64	5.38	3.34	-2.04

*Patients had received tolbutamide for at least 6 weeks prior to study and were not taking other medications except for Patient 4 who was taking α-methyldopa and thyroxine at the time of both *i.v.* tolbutamide tests. Patient 3 was a cigarette smoker; the others were not.

most drugs tested significantly affected tolbutamide binding. In practice, this would increase the concentration of free tolbutamide in plasma. Since the principal rate-limiting step in tolbutamide metabolism resides at the monooxygenase level, an increase in free plasma tolbutamide, due to competitive drug binding effects, might accentuate extrapancreatic tolbutamide effects. This consideration should be kept in mind, in addition to genetic control of tolbutamide metabolism, when considering dosage schedules.

Two questions remain with respect to genetic versus environmental influences over tolbutamide metabolism. These are: (1) the question of tolbutamide induction of the hepatic-renal tolbutamide monooxygenase, and (2) the verification that slow inactivators on oral tolbutamide actually have significantly higher plasma levels. Both questions are presently under study.

To date, the induction has not been confirmed, but one of the four subjects tested demonstrated a 2-hour reduction in tolbutamide half-life. The second question is being analyzed by comparison of tolbutamide K_d after intravenous administration to blood levels of tolbutamide after oral administration. If indeed the data demonstrate higher blood levels in slow inactivators, as similar studies of hydralazine and isoniazid would support, then the possibility that slow inactivators on the fixed-dosage regimen in the UGDP study were at greater risk for extrapancreatic toxic effects must be seriously considered.

REFERENCES

1. *Bänder, A., and Sholz, J. (1956). Deutsch. Med. Wschr. 81, 889.*
2. *Thomas, R.C. and Ikeda, G.J. (1966). J. Med. Chem. 9, 507.*
3. *McDaniel, H.G. et al. (1969). J. Pharmacol. Exp. Ther. 167, 91.*
4. *Schulz, E. and Schmidt, F.H. (1970). Klin. Wochenscr. 48, 759.*
5. *Shibasaki, J. et al. (1973). Chem. Pharm. Bull. 21, 1754.*
6. *Kellermann, G.K. et al. (1976). Clin. Pharm. Ther. 20, 72.*
7. *Scott, J. and Poffenbarger, P.L. (1979). Diabetes (in press).*

This work was supported by grants from the General Clinical Research Centers Program of the Division of Research Resources, National Institutes of Health (RR-73), NIH National Research Service Award GM 07204-02, and The Upjohn Company. Dr. D.J. McAdoo performed the mass spectrometric analysis. Mr. S.F. Micheletti performed the synthesis of HTB. Crystalline tolbutamide and carboxytolbutamide were provided by The Upjohn Company.

INSULIN RESISTANCE IN PATIENTS WITH INSULIN INDEPENDENT DIABETES MELLITUS: PARTIAL AMELIORATION BY THE SULFONYLUREA GLIPIZIDE

H. Lebovitz* and M.N. Feinglos

Insulin independent (adult-onset) diabetes mellitus is a distinct metabolic disorder. Evidence has accumulated which suggests that individuals with this disturbance have a marked resistance to insulin action (1) and an accompanying inability to overcome this resistance by exaggerated insulin secretion from their pancreatic beta cells (2). The exact nature of these abnormalities are unknown but some data are consistent with the insulin resistance being related to a decrease in insulin receptors on the plasma membrane of insulin sensitive tissues and the impaired insulin secretory response to an abnormality in a presumed glucose receptor on the plasma membrane of the beta cell. Therapeutic agents which ameliorate one or both of these abnormalities might be expected to be effective in controlling the hyperglycemia of insulin-independent diabetes.

Sulfonylurea drugs have been used in the management of insulin-independent diabetes since the early 1950s. Initial studies directed toward understanding the mechanism by which they lower blood glucose focused on hepatic and peripheral effects. The development of radioimmunoassays to measure plasma insulin allowed many investigators to show that acute administration of sulfonylurea drugs results in increased pancreatic insulin secretion. However, many clinical studies and several investigations in laboratory animals have shown that chronic sulfonylurea therapy is probably not associated with increased insulin secretion and that one or more extrapancreatic actions of the sulfonylurea drugs may be responsible for their antidiabetic action (3). The present report describes studies in patients with insulin-independent diabetes which indicate that a significant mode of action of one of the second generation sulfonylureas, glipizide, and presumably all sulfonylureas, is to potentiate the action of insulin and partially ameliorate the insulin resistance.

MATERIALS AND METHODS

Patients with untreated insulin independent diabetes mellitus were studied at the Clinical Research Unit of Duke University Medical Center. All patients had symptomatic hyperglycemia. Informed consent was obtained for all studies. On their first visit each patient was begun on a diet, containing 45% carbohydrate, calculated on the basis of his or her weight and activity level. This diet was continued throughout the study. Each patient underwent a 5 hour oral glucose tolerance test (100 g of glucose) and intravenous insulin tolerance tests (using 0.05, 0.1 and 0.2 units of regular pork insulin/kg of body weight) with blood samples drawn at 0, 5, 10, 15, 20, 25, 30, 45, 60, 90 and 120 min. Plasma glucose and insulin were measured on each sample.

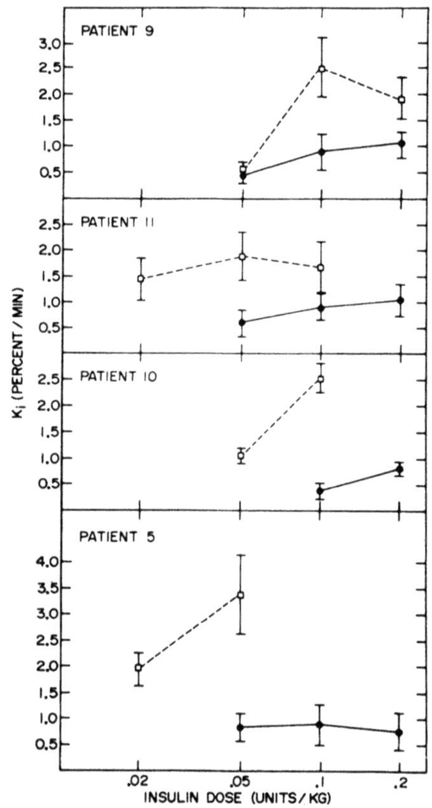

Fig. 1. Insulin-mediated glucose disposal in 4 patients treated with glipizide. The data are K ± 95% confidence limits for each insulin dose. The solid line is the untreated state. The dashed line is following 6 weeks of glipizide treatment which had restored the fasting plasma glucose to normal.

After a 1 to 2 week diet treatment period, the patients were assigned to either diet or diet plus glipizide (Pfizer Pharmaceutical, Inc.). The dose of glipizide (2.5 to 35 mg/day) was adjusted as needed to obtain normal fasting plasma glucose. After normal fasting plasma glucoses were achieved (usually 4 to 6 weeks of treatment), the initial studies were repeated. Studies were repeated at 6 months and where possible 1 year.

Insulin action on glucose metabolism was assessed by calculating the glucose disposal in response to exogenous insulin (K_I). (4). This number, expressed in percent/min., is a measure of the rate of fall in plasma glucose over time in response to specific doses of intravenous insulin and is derived from the slope of the initial, linear (20-30 min) portion of the regression line of ln plasma glucose vs time. 95% confidence limits were calculated by analysis of variance. The K_I (0.1U insulin/kg body weight) in a series of normal volunteers of comparable age to our patients ranged from 2.62 to 7.30 (mean ± SD 5.29 ± 1.62). (5) Statistical analyses were done by paired and unpaired Student's t tests.

RESULTS

Insulin Resistance in Insulin-Independent Diabetes Mellitus

Figure 1 illustrates the severe degree of insulin resistance which is present in patients with insulin-independent diabetes mellitus. The glucose disposal resulting from insulin administration in the untreated state (solid line) is markedly impaired. The lowest K_I observed in response to 0.1 U insulin/kg body weight in our normal control population is 2.62. As can be noted in Figure 1, all 4 patients have a K_I in response to 0.1 U insulin/kg of 1.0 or less. The dose response relationship between insulin administered and glucose disposal is very flat indicating that larger quantities of insulin are only slightly more effective. The insulin resistance of the insulin-independent diabetic is not the result of obesity, though obesity may contribute further to the insulin resistance. Patients 5 and 10 had body weights which were within ideal range while patients 9 and 11 were 37 and 87 percent above ideal body weight.

Tables 1 and 2 summarize the glucose disposal data in 5 patients undergoing diet treatment alone and 6 patients undergoing glipizide therapy. These data further illustrate the magnitude of the insulin resistance in the untreated state.

Effect of diet therapy on insulin resistance

All of our patients who were able to normalize their fasting plasma glucose on diet treatment were obese (48 to 80% above ideal body weight). Diet treatment consisted of a reduction in the

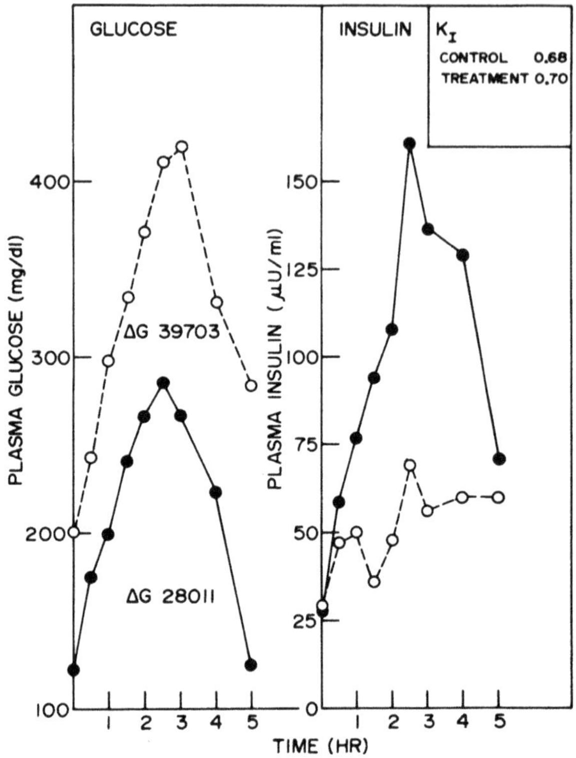

Fig. 2. The effect of diet treatment on the glucose and insulin response to 100g orally administered glucose. The dashed line is the untreated state. The solid line is after 6 weeks of diet treatment. The K_I for 0.1 U insulin/kg is given in the box.

Table 1

EFFECT OF DIET TREATMENT ON GLUCOSE DISPOSAL (K_I)

Five patients were studied prior to and after 6 weeks of treatment. K_I is percent per min. FPG is fasting plasma glucose and is given as mg/dl. Data are mean ± SE.

Treatment	FPG	K_I (0.05)	K_I (0.10)	K_I (0.20)
None	222 ± 33	0.55 ± 0.14	1.23 ± 0.21	1.42 ± 0.26
6 weeks	125 ± 12*	0.86 ± 0.23	1.49 ± 0.25	1.73 ± 0.27

*p <0.01

carbohydrate content of the diet to 45% and an attempt to restrict total calories.While the carbohydrate reduction was effective and probably accounted for the restoration of normal or near normal fasting plasma glucose, the caloric restriction was not successful as significant weight loss was not achieved. Table 1 shows that reduction of fasting plasma glucose to near normal by diet treatment had no significant effect on the insulin resistance.

Table 2

EFFECT OF GLIPIZIDE TREATMENT ON GLUCOSE DISPOSAL (K_I)

Six patients were studied prior to and after 6 weeks and 6 months of treatment with glipizide, K_I is percent per min. FPG is fasting plasma glucose and is given as mg/dl. Data are mean SE.

Treatment	FPG	K_I(0.15)	K_I(0.10)	K_I(0.20)
None	273 ± 23	0.43 ± 0.13	0.80 ± 0.10	1.04 ±0.11
6 weeks	110 ± 7*	1.64 ± 0.42+	2.40 ± 0.17*	
6 months	108 ± 8*	1.62 ± 0.29*	2.92 ± 0.41*	

+p <0.05
*p <0.01

Effect of glipizide treatment on insulin resistance

Table 2 shows that glipizide treatment restores the fasting plasma glucose to normal. The effect of the glipizide treatment on the insulin resistance is remarkable. The K_I in response to 0.1 U of insulin attains a mean of 2.40% at 6 weeks and 2.92% at 6 months. In 3 of the 6 patients, the K_I for 0.1 U insulin was in the normal range at 6 months. Figure 1 depicts the change in insulin action which results from 6 weeks of glipizide therapy. In all 4 patients, the magnitude of the glucose disposal is increased at each insulin dose and in 3 of the 4 patients the dose response curve is shifted to the left indicating that small doses of insulin are now effective.

The increase in insulin action observed in the glipizide-treated patients must be attributed to the drug. Only one of the 6 patients had a significant weight loss (36% above ideal body weight to 17%) while the others did not. The fasting plasma glucose attained in the glipizide treated group was similar to that in the diet treated group.

Comparison of effect of dietary therapy and glipizide therapy on endogenous insulin action.

Endogenous insulin action in patients with insulin independent diabetes can be assessed by determining glucose utilization and insulin secretion following a specific glucose challenge. We administered 100 g of glucose orally to our patients and calculated the plasma glucose area above the fasting plasma glucose and the plasma insulin area for 5 hours. The incremental glucose area ΔG is inversely proportional to glucose utilization. Insulin secretion is proportional to the insulin area since neither diet treatment nor glipizide altered the t ½ for insulin disappearance from the plasma compartment. Figure 2 illustrates such studies in an insulin independent diabetic patient treated by diet alone. In this patient, effective treatment restored the plasma glucose to normal, did not effect insulin mediated glucose disposal (K_I), increased glucose-stimulated insulin secretion dramatically and had a small beneficial effect on glucose utilization (29% decrease in ΔG). Figure 3 shows a similar study in a patient treated with glipizide. The sulfonylurea restored fasting plasma glucose to normal, markedly increased insulin-mediated glucose disposal (K_I), had no effect on glucose-stimulated insulin secretion and caused a striking increase in glucose utilization (63% decrease in ΔG). An even more convincing demonstration of the difference between the effects of diet and glipizide treatments are shown in Figure 4. This particular patient was originally seen with untreated diabetes and was managed by diet treatment. The patient subsequently went off the diet and returned to the untreated state. She was then treated with glipizide. Diet therapy did not effect the K_I, had no effect on glucose-mediated insulin secretion and had no effect on glucose utilization while it did lower the fasting plasma glucose to normal . Glipizide treatment increased the K_I, decreased glucose-mediated insulin secretion and significantly increased glucose utlization (decrease in ΔG 36%)/

These and similar data in other patients indicate that diet treatment without significant weight loss may lower the fasting plasma glucose to normal but does not significantly increase glucose utilization. Glipizide treatment, however, lowers the fasting plasma glucose to normal and significantly increases glucose utilization even when it does not increase glucose-mediated insulin release.

DISCUSSION

Glipizide treatment of insulin independent diabetes appears to ameliorate partially the insulin resistance associated with the illness. Studies in mice show that glipizide treatment causes an increase in insulin sensitivity that is due to an increase in insulin binding to the plasma membrane of insulin sensitive tissues. (6). This increase is insulin binding results from an increase in the number of plasma membrane insulin receptors rather than an increase

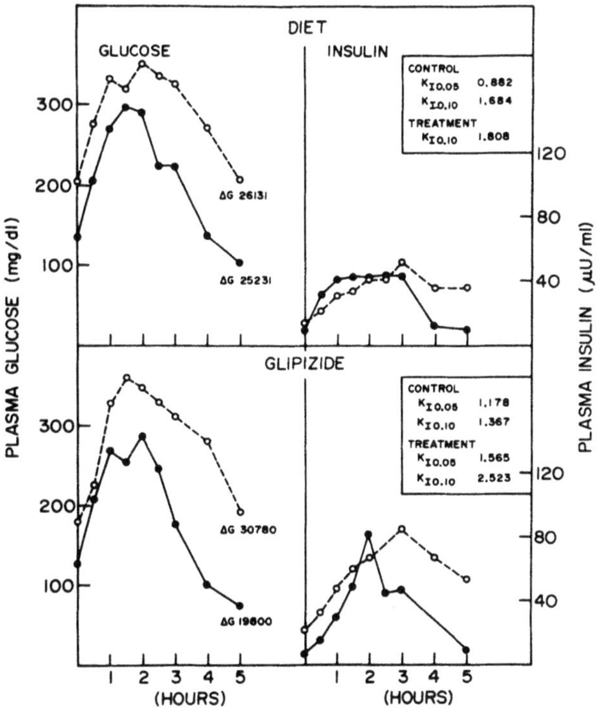

Fig. 3. The effect of glipizide treatment on the glucose and insulin response to 100g orally administered glucose. The dashed line is the untreated state. The solid line is after 6 weeks of treatment. The K_I for 0.1 U insulin/kg is given in the box.

in the binding affinity. It seems reasonable to assume that glipizide has similar effects on insulin receptors in patients with insulin independent diabetes and that this accounts, at least in part, for the increased sensitivity to insulin.

Since sulfonylurea drugs increase glucose-mediated insulin secretion during the early phases of treatment it is reasonable to hypothesize that the anti-diabetic action of sulfonylureas results initially from both increased insulin secretion and action. During prolonged therapy the insulin secretory action diminishes and perhaps the predominant anti-diabetic action is that resulting from the potentiation of insulin action. This hypothesis needs testing by more extensive and chronic studies. Perhaps a clearer understanding of primary and secondary sulfonylurea failures may be obtained from serial studies of the sulfonylurea-induced changes in insulin secretion and action.

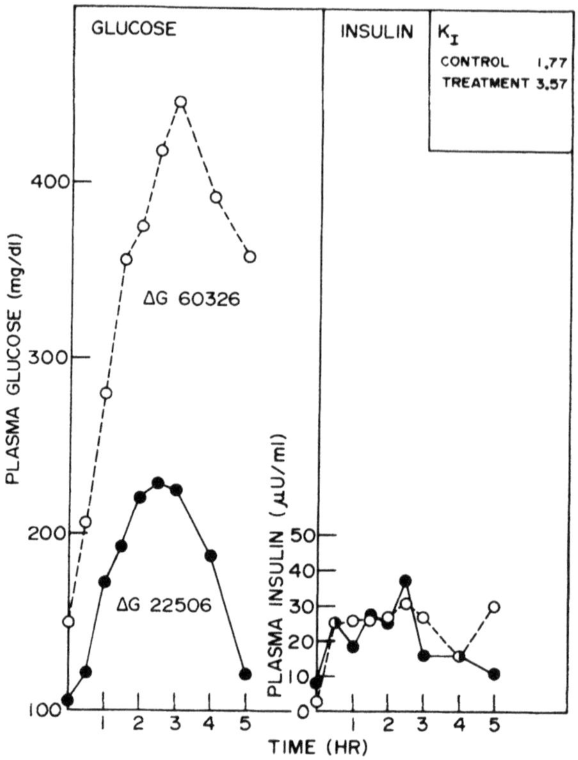

Fig. 4 A comparison of the effects of diet treatment and glipizide therapy in the same patient. The legend is the same as Figures 2 and 3.

SUMMARY

Studies in patients with insulin independent diabetes indicate that treatment with the second generation sulfonylurea glipizide results in partial amelioration of their insulin resistance and that this effect is significant in glipizide's antidiabetic action.

REFERENCES

1. *Reaven, G.M., et al. (1976). Am. J. Med. 60, 80.*
2. *Perly, M. and Kipnis, D.M. (1967). J. Clin. Invest. 46, 1954*
3. *Reaven, G. and Dray, J. (1967). Diabetes 16, 487*
4. *Lebovitz, H.E. and Feinglos, M.N. (1977). J. Clin. Endocrinol. Metab. 45, 601.*
5. *Lebovitz, H.E. and Feinglos, M.N. (1978). Diabetes Care 1, 189.*
6. *Feinglos, M.N. and Lebovitz, H.E. (1978). Nature 276, 184.*

These studies were supported by grants from Pfizer Pharmaceuticals, the National Institute of Arthritis Metabolic and Digestive Diseases (AM 01324) and by grant M01 FR 30 from the Clinical Research Center Branch Division of Research Facilities and Resources, U.S. Public Health Service.

DISCUSSION

Invited Discussant: S. PODOLSKY - *The purpose of our study in collaboration with Ann M. Lawrence, was to investigate the effects of fairly long term administration of a sulfonylurea agent on insulin and glucagon secretion in patients with maturity onset diabetes mellitus in whom there was tight control of hyperglycemia.*

Thirteen male patients with maturity onset diabetes were studied (mean age 56.1 years, age range 45-67 years). The mean estimated duration of diabetes was 4.3 years, with a range of 2 to 10 years. All patients weighed less than 120% of ideal body weight. Oral hypoglycemic agents were withdrawn and treatment maintained by diet alone for at least one month prior to the study. All patients were on an individualized American Diabetes Association diet calculated to attain or maintain optimal body weight; in addition each received a minimum of two individualized teaching sessions with a dietician at the beginning of the study.

A standard baseline oral glucose tolerance test with 100 g glucose was performed during the diet alone treatment period. Because of fasting hyperglycemia on diet alone therapy, the sulfonylurea chlorpropamide was begun in a daily morning dose of 250 mg. In patients whose fasting serum glucose levels continued to exceed 140 mg/dl after several months of chlorpropamide administration plus additional dietary instruction, the dosage of this sulfonylurea was gradually increased to a maximum quantity of 500 mg once daily. After eight months of individualized therapy designed to produce tight control of hyperglycemia, the GTT was repeated, with each patient taking his usual dose of chlorpropamide 90 minutes prior to the administration of the glucose load. Serum glucose levels were measured on a Technicon Autoanalyzer, and plasma insulin and glucagon were measured by radioimmunoassay. Bloods were drawn without discomfort from an indwelling 19 guage thin walled needle which remained in place during the studies (Podolsky, S. and Sivaprasad, R. (1972) J. Clin. Endocrinol. Metab. 35, 580).

Patient compliance to the dietary regimen was good. Adherence to the sulfonylurea regimen was excellent in all subjects. Mean body weight was unchanged over the study period.

There was gradual lowering of the elevated fasting serum glucose levels during the 32 weeks of sulfonylurea therapy. Normal fasting glucose levels were achieved for the group as a whole and for nine of the 13 patients.

Figure 1 shows the serum glucose response during the two glucose tolerance tests. In the baseline test glucose levels rose from a *level of 140.3 ± 10 mg/dl (mean ± SEM) to a peak level of 260.5 ± 18.2 mg/dl at 120 minutes. After control of hyperglycemia by the addition of chlorpropamide, the repeat GTT showed a mean fasting glucose level of 107.0 ± 8.4 mg/dl rising to a maximum of 225.7 ± 17.9 mg/dl at 120 minutes. There were significant differences in serum glucose values before and after chlorpropamide treatment at -10 min (p = <.05), 0 time (p = <.04), 30 min (p = <.01) and 60 min (p = <.01).*

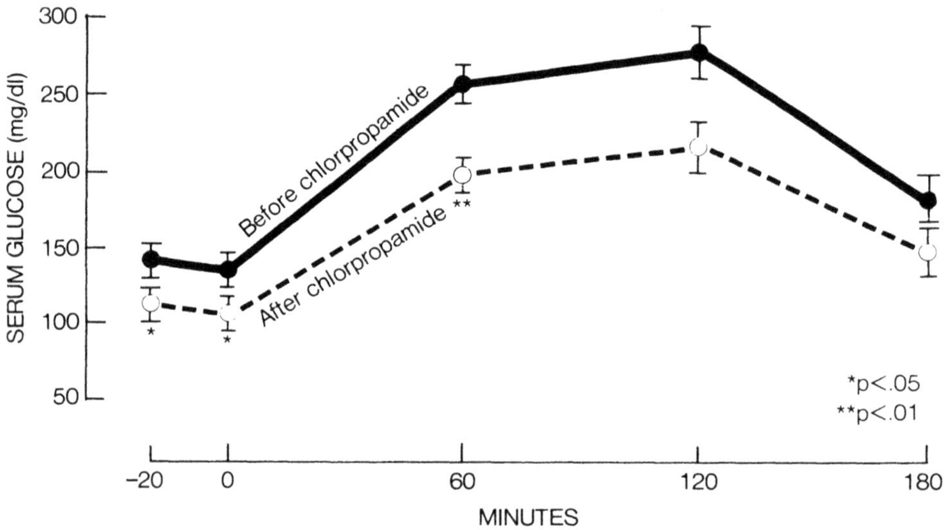

Fig. 1

Plasma insulin response before and after chlorpropamide therapy are shown in Figure 2. In the baseline test plasma insulin rose from 20.1 ± 2.5 uU/ml to a peak level of 75.2 ± 12.0 uU/ml at 120 minutes. There was no significant change in the repeat GTT, with plasma insulin rising from 18.9 ± 2.1 uU/ml to a maximum level of 70.0 ± 10.9 uU/ml at 120 minutes.

Plasma glucagon response before and after chlorpropamide therapy are shown in Figure 3. Fasting hyperglucagonemia occurred, before and after reduction of fasting hyperglycemia to normal with chlorpropamide therapy. There was a paradoxical glucagon rise associated with the hyperglycemic phase of both GTT's, with no significant difference between the two tests. Peak plasma glucagon level occurred at 60 minutes in each test, and fell insignificantly with therapy from 182.3 ± 29.4 pg/ml to 163.5 ± 26.4 pg/ml.

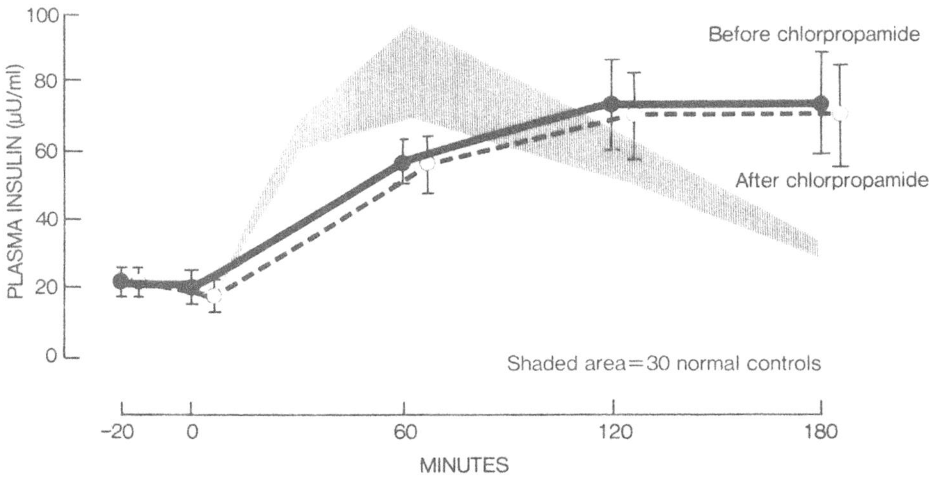
100
80
60
40
20
0
PLASMA INSULIN (μU/ml)
Before chlorpropamide
After chlorpropamide
Shaded area=30 normal controls
-20
0
60
120
180
MINUTES

Fig. 2

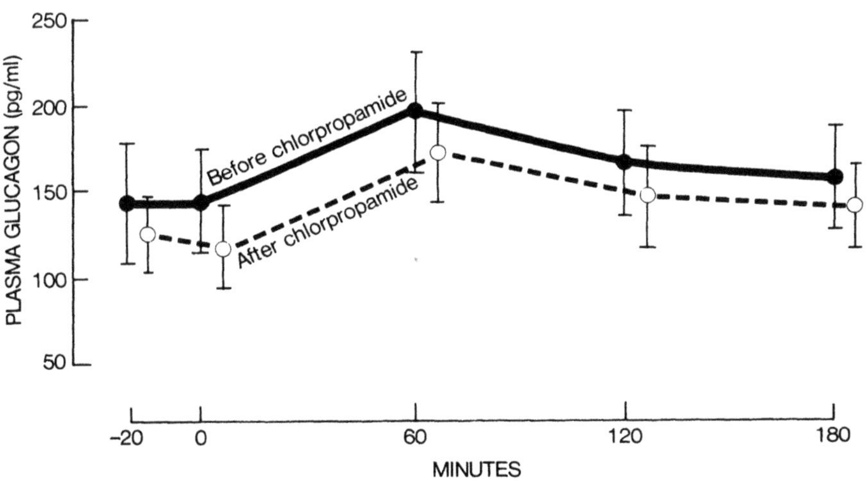
250
200
150
100
50
PLASMA GLUCAGON (pg/ml)
Before chlorpropamide
After chlorpropamide
-20
0
60
120
180
MINUTES

Fig. 3

Very good to excellent control of hypgerglycemia was achieved in this series of maturity onset diabetics by using chlorpropamide plus diet therapy. Lowering of fasting serum glucose levels beyond levels achieved by diet alone was evident after the first month of therapy with this sulfonylurea.

Although chlorpropamide therapy significantly lowered fasting serum glucose and serum glucose levels during the early phase of the glucose tolerance test, there was no change in fasting plasma insulin levels or insulin response to an oral glucose load, after such treatment. This data is in keeping with earlier studies which were performed after a shorter interval of drug therapy.

Glucagon levels did not change significantly for the group, but there were wide variations in individual responses. Neither the age, the duration of diabetes nor the state of control of hyperglycemia appeared to influence the pattern of the glucagon curve after chronic sulfonylurea administration. Whether elevated glucagon levels, such as those seen in our patients, causally contribute to the development of diabetes mellitus or strongly influence metabolic abnormalities in this disease remains controversial (Lawrence, A.M. and Abraira, C. (1979) in Clinical Diabetes: Modern Management, Podolsky, S., ed., Appleton-Century-Crofts, New York, in press.)

Recent studies indicate that sulfonylureas may act by affecting insulin receptor binding sites on circulating monocytes (Olefsky, J.M. and Reaven, G.M. (1976) Amer. J. Med. 60, 89) and there is considerable evidence that sulfonylureas may cause a decrease in insulin resistance and have other extrapancreatic actions. These mechanisms could account for persistent sulfonylurea induced lowering of elevated glucose levels without apparent alteration of circulating insulin or glucagon levels.

G. M. REAVEN: *I think the way Dr. Lebovitz made the dose respond is really elegant. Often, people have performed the insulin responsiveness by giving only one dose. I think this is a real advance and an important issue. My second comment is that findings, similar to those described by Dr. Lebovitz, have been shown by our group with chlorpropamide, in which the return towards normal of their glucose metabolism was associated with a definite return toward normal. I think there is a very nice correlation between the mice and people data, and we were using diabetic people. Lastly, the fact that Dr. Lebovitz could reduce the fasting glucose in his patients to normal levels and still have an impaired removal rate is a very important and dramatic issue, which suggest, at least, that this defect is really a basic defect and not secondary to the insulin resistance or to insulin deficiency.*

S. FAJANS: I'm sure that Dr. Reaven and Dr. Lebovitz are correct that there are a large number of patients with mature onset type of diabetes, who are insulin resistant. I don't think we should lose cognizance of the fact that everything is not 100% and that there are also individuals who are not insulin resistant. We've done insulin tolerance tests, such as Dr. Lebovitz, in a group of 12 young MODY non-obese patients, and their mean insulin responses to either .1 or .05 insulin per kilogram body weight were identical to a group of matched controlled subjects. As far as the mechanism of action is concerned: when we look at all of our young patients, who have been treated with chlorpropamide over many years and compare pre-and post-insulin responses to glucose during the glucose tolerance test, we can find no statistical difference for increased insulin secretion.

H. LEBOVITZ: Hemsworth first showed, and then Gerry (Reaven) reproduced with his method, that the insulin dependent patient really is not insulin resistant. We have a few young people, who have perfectly normal insulin responses in whom insulin secretion is so low that, although they haven't gone into ketoacidosis, in many other ways, they behave like a juvenile onset. Now, I think the problem is going to be the segregation of the groups of patients. I think Steve (Fajans) is right. There will be some heterogeneity.

DIABETIC GLOMERULOSCLEROSIS IN KK MICE AND ITS PREVENTION BY GLYBURIDE AND PYRIDINOLCARBAMATE

R. A. Camerini-Davalos, A. S. Reddi,
T. H. Ehrenreich, L. H. Strugatz and
W. Oppermann*

In earlier publications, we reported that the Japanese KK mouse develops human diabetic-like microangiopathy, namely glomerulosclerosis, retinopathy and peripheral gangrene due to small blood vessel disease. These studies were confirmed by other investigators. Diabetic glomerulosclerosis, which involves an excessive deposition of mesangial matrix, is a consistently demonstrable pathologic disorder in KK mice as early as 2 months of age. In older KK mice, the marked increase in the mesangial matrix results in the formation of glomerular nodules. Exudative-like glomerular lesions were also observed in these mice.

Electron microscopy of the kidney revealed an increase in mesangial matrix and thickening of the basement membrane. Usually, the mesangial accumulation was accompanied by cells, although in a few instances there were noted small, dense accumulations of mesangial matrix without mesangial cells. As the mesangium proliferates, it grows into the capillary wall and tends to become inserted between the basement membrane and the endothelium. In advances cases, the capillary lumen was partly occluded by the mass of mesangium. Electron-dense deposits were also seen in the mesangial matrix beneath the capillary endothelium, in the basement membrane, and occasionally partly occluding the capillary lumen. These appear to correspond to the exudative lesions seen in light microscopy.

In a recent report, Soret et al,(1) from Kalamazoo, described amyloidosis in the kidneys of his KK mice and suggested that this pathologic feature is misinterpreted as diabetic glomerulosclerosis. The authors believe that the KK mouse represents an animal model for the study of amyloidosis rather than diabetic glomerulosclerosis.

By contrast, our inbred colony of KK mice consistently demonstrates diabetic glomerulosclerosis, although the incidence varies from one generation to the other. In an analysis of 395 KK mice from several generations, 247 mice (63%) showed glomerulosclerosis, 33 (8%) amyloidosis and 4 (1%) pyelonephritis (2). The cause for these discrepancies is not apparent at the present time. However, certain differences do exist in regard to the maintenance of the colonies in Kalamazoo and New York. We feed them with the Old Guilford mouse laboratory chow, which contains 11% fat, compared to 4% in Purina mouse chow. The development of skin lesions, as described by Soret et al. in their KK mice, are rarely found in our KK. We observed such lesions when we placed 6 or more male KK mice in one cage. We attributed this to cannibalistic behavior of these mice. When we separated these mice and placed them in individual cages, the skin lesions disappeared. Furthermore, the possibility of these two colonies of KK mice representing entirely two different groups of mice, evolved as a result of selective breeding over several generations, cannot be excluded.

In this report, we summarize our results on the effects of two oral compounds, namely, glyburide (2), a sulfonylurea with blood sugar lowering effect and pyridinolcarbamate (3), an antiatherosclerotic agent without marked effect on blood sugar levels, in ameliorating and/or delaying the progression of glomerulosclerosis in KK mice.

MATERIAL AND METHODS

The KK mice, used in these studies, have been inbred in our laboratory since 1968. They were fed the Old Guilford mouse laboratory chow ad libitum. Both glyburide (Hoechst-Roussel Pharmaceuticals, Inc., Somerville, N.J.), and Pyridinolcarbamate (Banyu Pharmaceutical Co., Tokyo, Japan) were suspended in 0.154M saline containing 5% acacia. Glyburide was given in the amount of 0.5 mg/kg or 2.5 mg/kg from 2-12 months of age. Pyridinolcarbamate (PDC) was given in the amount of 250 mg/kg from 20 to 100 days of age. All mice were treated by oral intubation (0.1 ml/10 g) once a day for 7 days a week. A representative number of KK mice received 0.154M saline (0.1 ml/10 g) and served as controls for the treated groups.

Fasting blood sugars and oral glucose tolerance tests were performed in mice fasted for 18 h. with free access to water. These tests were carried out at intervals and at the time of sacrifice. For oral glucose tolerance tests, mice were given 3 g/kg of glucose and blood samples were collected from the orbital plexus at 30, 60 and 120 minutes. Blood sugar was determined by the ferricyanide method of Hoffman on the Technicon Autoanalyzer.

For light microscopy studies, the mice were sacrificed by decapitation, kidneys excised and a portion of the kidney was fixed in 10% neutral formalin. The tissues were embedded in paraffin and sections 2-3 u thick were cut. They were stained in periodic acid-Schiff (PAS), hemotoxylin and eosin, chromotrope silver methanamine or congo red. Histologic evaluation of glomeruli was done in a blind fashion, based on the following working classification (100±20 glomeruli counted).

Not significant (o)	No changes
	Few obsolescent glomeruli
	Diffuse glomerulosclerosis grade I
Mild (m)	Diffuse glomerulosclerosis grade II
Severe (s)	Diffuse and nodular
	Diffuse and nodular and/or deposits (exudative)

RESULTS

Figure 1 shows the prevalence of mild and severe glomerulosclerosis in untreated KK mice aged 2 to 18 months. As can be seen, about 60% KK mice demonstrate either moderate or severe glomerulosclerosis by 2 months of age. The severeity in glomerulosclerosis progressed with aging.

GLOMERULAR CHANGES IN RELATION

TO AGE (KK MICE)

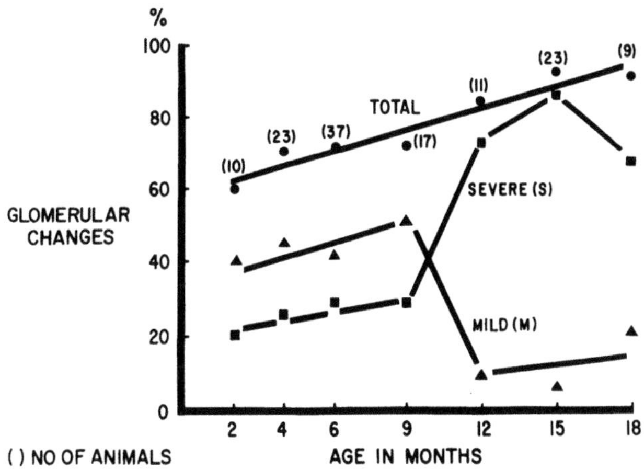

Fig. 1. Mild and severe glomerulosclerosis in KK mice aged 2 to 18 months. Numbers in parentheses indicate number of mice.

Figs. 2 and 3 demonstrate the degree of severity of glomerulosclerosis in KK mice. Electron microscopy revealed an increase in mesangial matrix, which in the early phases and in young animals did not result in widening of the mesangial space (Fig. 4). In older animals, the mesangium was further increased with marked widening of the mesangial space.

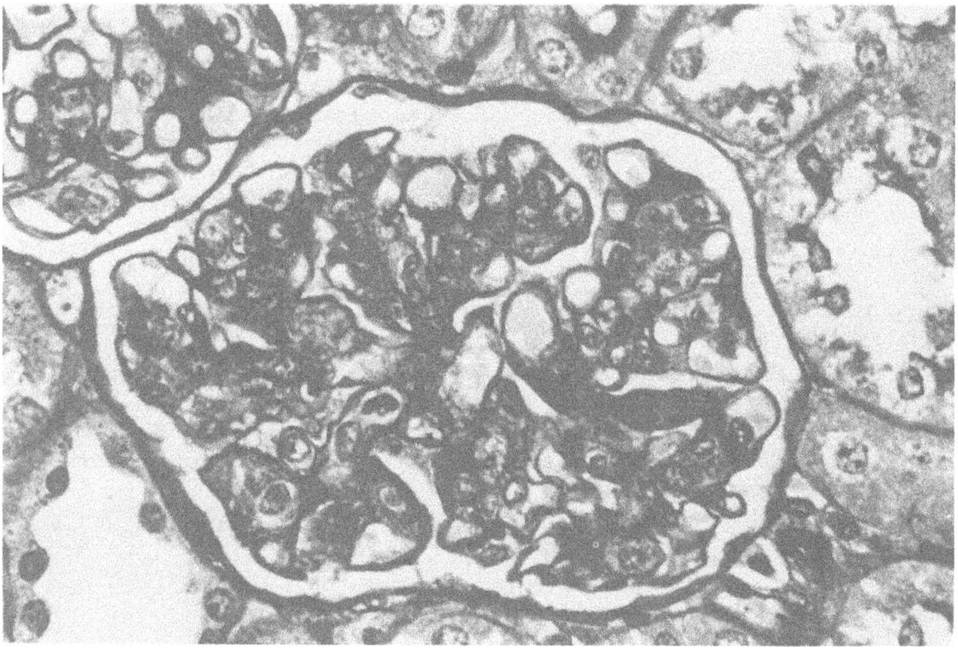

Fig. 2. Moderately severe, diffuse glomerulosclerosis, increase in mesangial matrix and cells with widening of the mesangial space. 15 months old animal PAS Stain x 800.

Table 1 gives general information on various species of mice in relation to the characteristics of diabetes. As may be seen in our laboratory only the KK mouse has glomerulosclerosis, which distinguishes it from other species of mice with mild hyperglycemia and hyperinsulinemia.

The effect of glyburide (0.5 mg/kg) on the prevalence of mild and severe forms of glomerulosclerosis is shown in Figure 5. After 2 and 4 months of treatment, the mice showed only 17% of mild glomerulosclerosis when compared to 42% in saline-treated mice. In mice treated for 7 and 10 months, 47% and 33% of mild glomerulosclerosis was found in comparison with 45% and 9% in saline-treated mice. The severe form of glomerulosclerosis

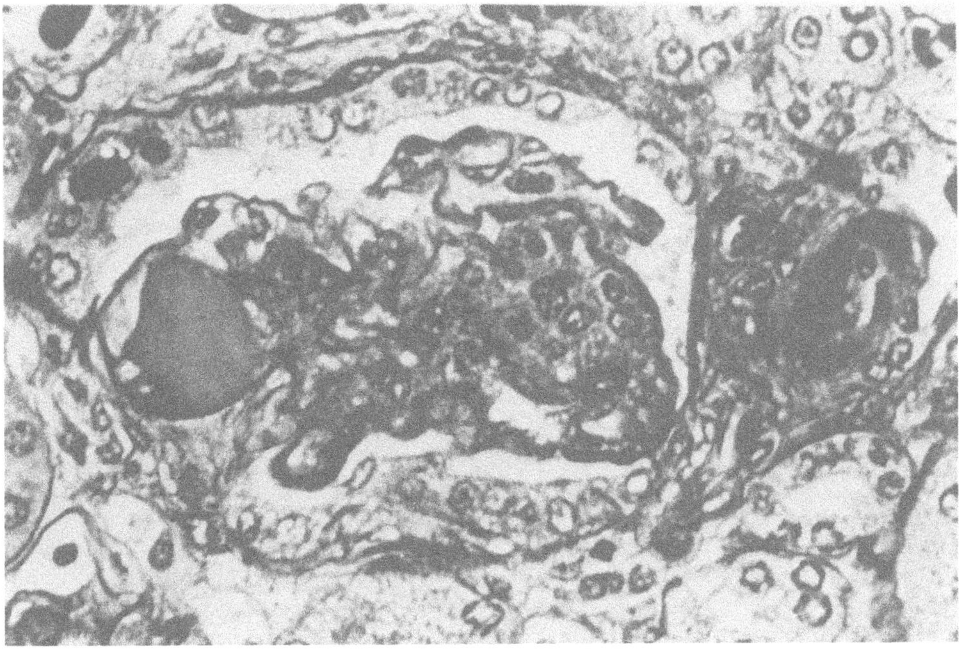

Fig. 3. Large exudative lesion apparently distending a capillary lumen. There is moderate increase in mesangial matrix and cells and striking segmental thickening of capillary walls. An arteriole near the glomerulus, probably the afferent arteriole, shows marked thickening of the wall with hyalinization, as well as narrowing of the lumen. KK mouse 15 months of age PAS Stain x 800.

was found only in one out of 6 (17%), none out of 12 (0%) and none out of 17 (0%) mice after 2, 4 and 7 months of glyburide treatment. After 10 months of glyburide treatment, only one mouse (33%) showed the severe form of glomerulosclerosis.

Fig. 6 shows the effect of 2.5 mg/kg of glyburide on the prevalence of mild and severe forms of glomerulosclerosis in KK mice. After 2, 4, 7 and 10 months of treatment, the mice had 50%, 0%, 55% and 43% of mild glomerulosclerosis, respectively. No severe glomerulosclerosis was found in mice treated for 2 and 4 months. However, after 7 and 10 months of drug treatment, the mice showed 5% and 28% of severe glomerulosclerosis, respectively, when compared to 35% and 73% in untreated mice.

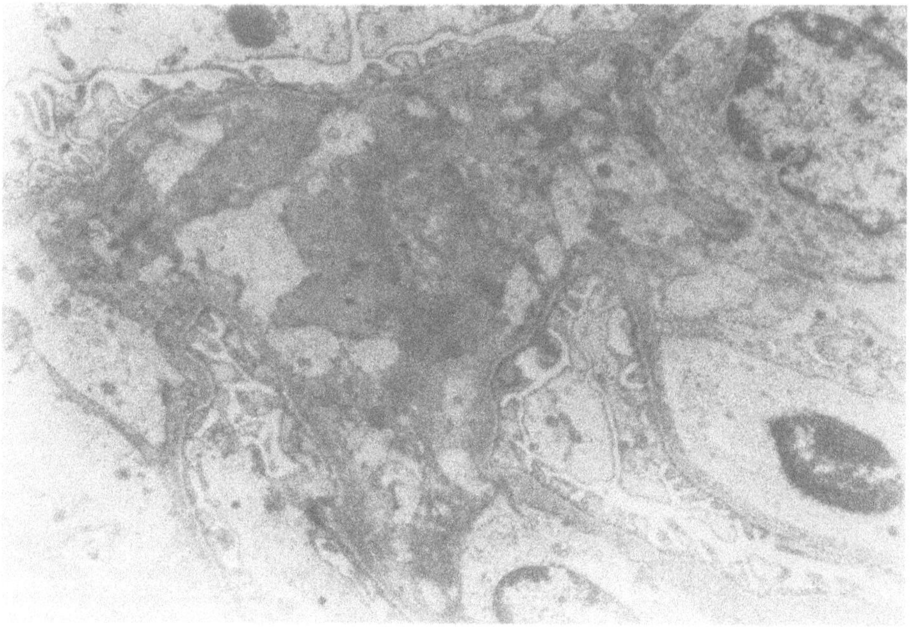

Fig. 4. Electron micrograph illustrating slight increase in mesangial matrix without widening of the mesangial space. KK mouse 3 months of age x 7800.

TABLE 1. Characteristics Of Various Strains Of Mice

MICE	GLUCOSE INTOLERANCE	HYPER INSULINISM	OBESITY	GLOMERULAR CHANGES
C57BL/6J	-	-	-	-
SWISS ALb.I	+	-	-	-
SWISS ALb.II	-	+	+	-
YELLOW (A^Y)	-	++	++	-
KK	++	+	-	+++

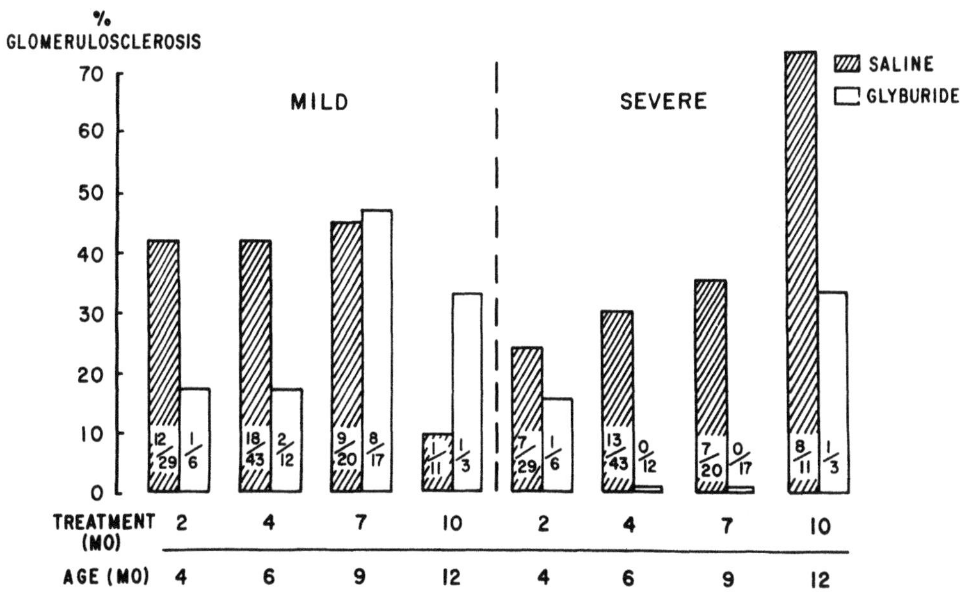

Fig. 5. Effect of prolonged treatment of saline and glyburide (0.5 mg/kg) on the prevalence of mild and severe forms of glomerulosclerosis in KK mice. Numbers in parentheses represent number of animals.

The oral glucose tolerance curves and glucose area levels in a representative number of saline and glyburide-treated (both doses) mice are shown in Figures 7 and 8. In some drug-treated mice, the tolerance to glucose was significantly improved, when compared to age-matched saline-treated mice (Figure 7). In other mice, no effect of glyburide treatment on blood sugar levels was found (Figure 8). In those mice with improved tolerance to glucose, no glomerulosclerosis was found. In other mice with no improvement in glucose tolerance, significant glomerulosclerosis was observed.

The prevalance of glomerlosclerosis in saline and PDC-treated KK mice, aged 70 and 100 days, is shown in Figure 9. As is evident, the severe type of glomerulosclerosis was predominant in saline-treated mice of both age groups. After 50 days of PDC-treatment (age of mice 70 days), the severe type was completely ameliorated to the mild type of glomerulosclerosis, but the other mice had no significant glomerular lesions.

Figure 10 shows the oral glucose tolerance of KK mice after 80 days of PDC-treatment. No difference in fasting blood sugar

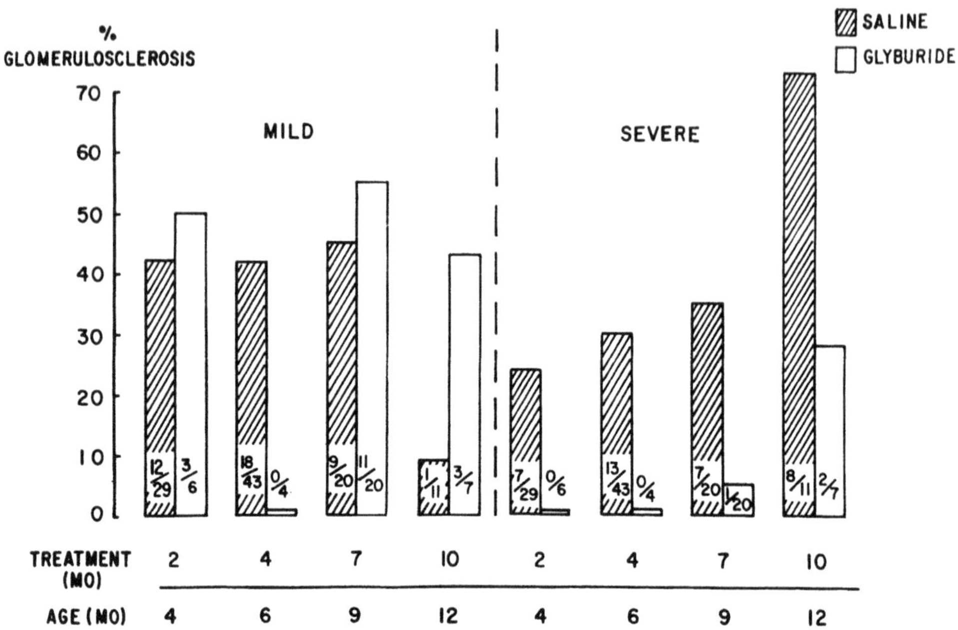

Fig. 6. Prevalence of mild and severe forms of glomerulosclerosis in saline and glyburide-treated (2.5 mg/kg) KK mice. Numbers in bars indicate number of animals.

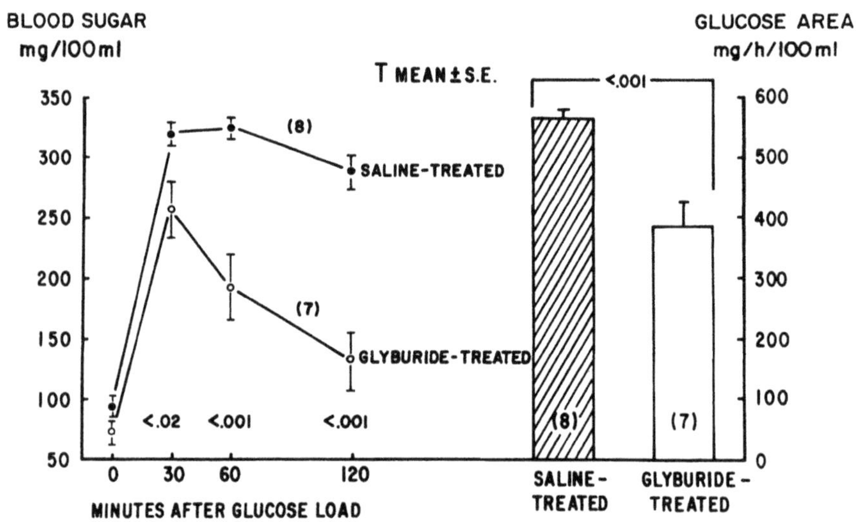

Fig. 7. Oral glucose tolerance tests and glucose area levels in saline and glyburide-treated (0.5 mg and 2.5 mg/kg) KK mice aged 4-12 months. Numbers in bars represent number of mice.

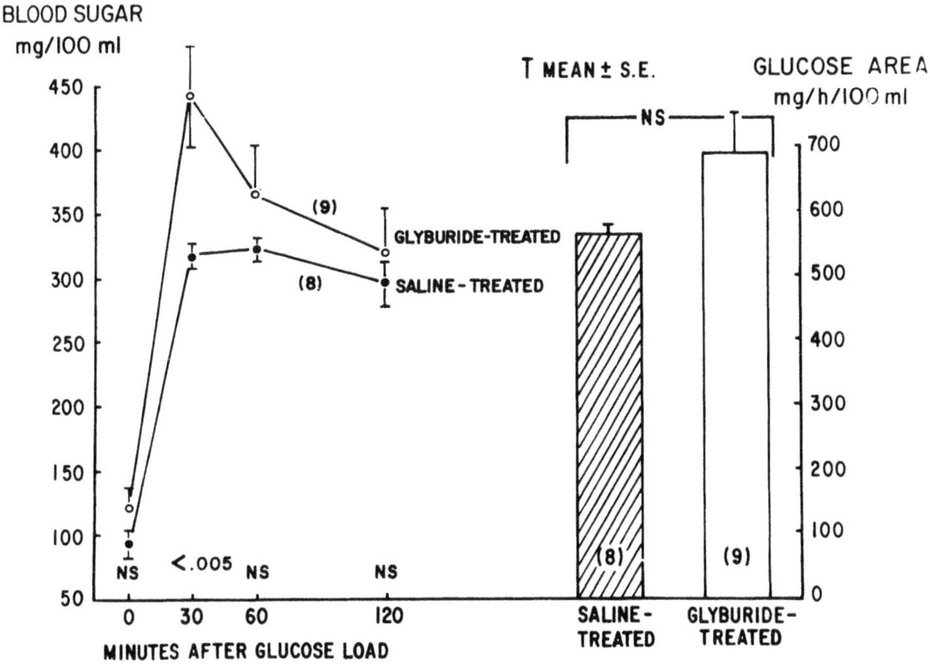

Fig. 8. Oral glucose tolerance tests and glucose area levels in saline and glyburide-treated (0.5 mg and 2.5 mg/kg) KK mice of 4-12 months of age. Numbers in parentheses indicate number of animals.

levels between saline and PDC-treated mice was observed. However, the blood sugar levels 30 and 60 minutes after glucose load were significantly decreased in PDC-treated mice.

DISCUSSION

The results shown in the present report clearly demonstrate that our colony of KK mice has increased accumulation of mesangial matrix, which in some cases presents in the form of nodules. Although the tissues were stained in PAS and chromotrope silver methanamine, the glomerular lesions can be clearly distinguished as diabetic glomerulosclerosis from amyloidosis, not only by experience, but also by visualization. Lesions that were suspicious of amyloidosis were stained with congo red. In view of these findings, our KK mice appear to be an ideal animal model for studies of genetic diabetic glomerulosclerosis.

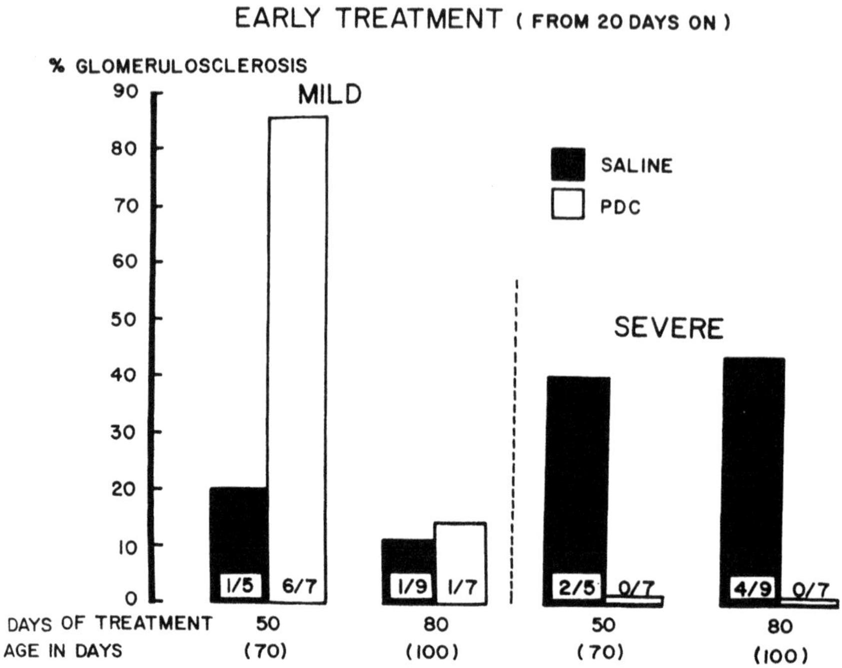

Fig. 9. Prevalence of mild and severe forms of glomerulosclerosis in saline and pyridinolcarbamate-treated KK mice. Numbers in bars represent number of animals.

The treatment of KK mice with two different types of oral medication shows that both agents are effective in preventing the progression of mild to severe forms of glomerulosclerosis. This is particularly important to human diabetics, where severe glomerulosclerosis may result in abnormal function of the glomerulus.

The delay in the progression of glomerulosclerosis in glyburide-treated mice appears to be related to the improvement in their tolerance to glucose. This is evident by data shown in Figure 7. By contrast, the mice that did not show improvement of their glucose tolerance had significant (89%) glomerulosclerosis. Although PDC-treatment significantly decreased blood sugar levels after 30 and 60 minutes of glucose load, it is unclear whether or not this slight improvement in carbohydrate tolerance is beneficial in the prevention of glomerulosclerosis in KK mice. However, results of Cotton et al. (4) show that PDC-treatment decreased blood glucose levels in streptozotocin-diabetic rats. Although the mechanisms of action of glyburide and PDC in preventing the progression of glomerulosclerosis in KK mice are not clearly understood at the present time, it is

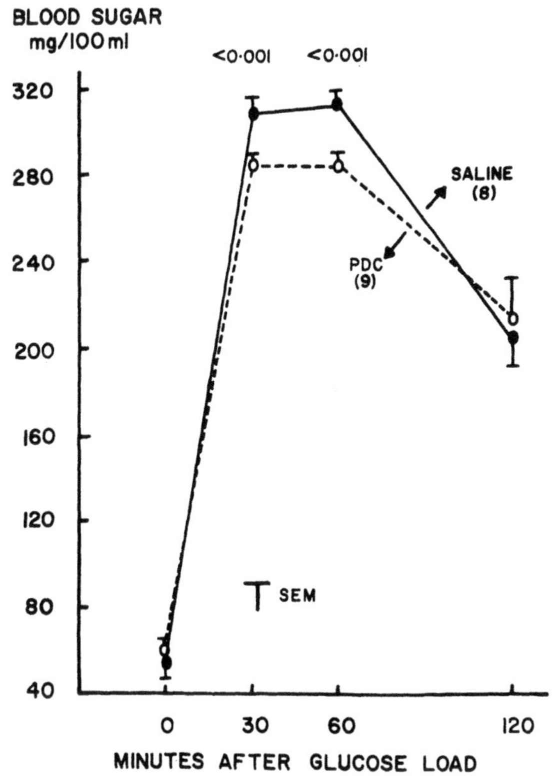

Fig. 10. Oral glucose tolerance tests in KK mice after 80 days (age of mice 100 days) of either saline or pyridinolcarbamate-treatment. Number of mice in each group is given in parentheses.

possible that part of the effect of glyburide (and PDC?) is related to the control of blood sugars and some of the enzymes involved in the snythesis or removal of the basement membrane or basement membrane-like glycoprotein in the mesangium.

REFERENCES

1. Soret, M.G., et al. (1977) Arch. Pathol. Lab. Med., 101:464.
2. Reddi, A.S., et al. (1978). Exp. Mol. Pathol., 29: 92.
3. Reddi, A.S., et al. (1977). Exp. Mol. Pathol., 26: 325.
4. Cotton, R.C., et al. (1973). In: Atherogenesis. Eds., T. Shimamoto, F. Numano and G.M. Addison, Vol. 2, pp. 384, Excerpta Medica, Amsterdam.

This study was supported in part by the General Research Support Grant RR-05398 from the General Research Support Branch, Division of Research Resources, National Institutes of Health, Hoechst-Roussel Pharmaceutical, Inc., Somerville, New Jersey, Japan Arteriosclerosis Research Foundation, Tokyo, Japan, and Hope for Diabetics Foundation, Inc., New York.

DISCUSSION

H. LEBOVITZ: *I'm a little confused. I thought that on Day 1 Dr. Camerini spoke about the KK mouse as a model for showing that the vascular lesions were independent of the glucose abnormalities. Am I wrong on that?*

R. CAMERINI-DAVALOS: *In the KK mice structural changes are present at 40 days and hyperglycemia is present on the 100th day.*

H. LEBOVITZ: *Well,then I'm confused by the presentation you made yesterday and the one today. Both, really, would seem to couple treatment of the diabetes with improvement of the lesions, which are reportedly independent of the glucose abnormality.*

W. OPPERMANN: *In our studies with glyburide, a sulfonylurea compound, we observed certain relationships between improvement in glucose tolerance and the prevalence of glomerulosclerosis. In those mice with improved tolerance to glucose, the glomerular lesions were not demonstrable. By contrast, the mice without any improvement in their tolerance had glomerulosclerosis, despite similar treatment. These findings suggest that control of hyperglycemia ameliorates or prevents the progression of diabetic glomerular lesions. This does not necessarily mean that hyperglycemia initiates the development of glomerulosclerosis in our KK mice.*

H. LEBOVITZ: *But you treat them and prevent....*

R. CAMERINI-DAVALOS: *May I answer that point? We do not believe that hyperglycemia is the causative factor for the vasculopathy. Since we do have vasculopathy in humans and in animals before hyperglycemia, it is hard to believe that hyperglycemia is necessary in the development of vasculopathy. That's why we accept that genetic and environmental factors are involved.*

E. TUTWILER: *This may be a very naive question, but in the genetically diabetic db/db mice, the sulfonylureas do not lower blood glucose. Do you have evidence in these KK mice that sulfonlylurea really lowered glucose?*

W. OPPERMANN: *We have definite evidence, in short and long-term experiments, that sulfonylureas decrease blood sugar.*

S. FAJANS: *I think most of us believe that the microangiopathy of diabetes is a combination of both genetic, as well as environmental, factors - the environmental factors being secondary to insulin insufficiency in hyperglycemia. I would like to ask Dr. Oppermann or Dr. Camerini if they have compared at 40 days the glucose tolerance tests of those who have glomerulopathy and those who have not?*

W. OPPERMANN: *Dr. Fajans, studies comparing glomerulosclerosis and hyperglycemia within KK mice are underway.*

M. COHEN: *Dr. Oppermann, you described a number of interesting enzymatic changes, which appear to be unrelated to the blood sugar and to the development of whatever the lesion is. My question is, do you have any evidence that these enzymatic changes, or changes in protein synthesis, have anything to do with the lesion which you describe? Secondly, is there some biochemical characterization of the lesion, which you observed in the kidney, which would provide convincing evidence that it's the same thing as that which occurs in human diabetic nephropathy?*

W. OPPERMANN: *To the first question: Yes, we believe so. At the present time, we do not have a definite answer for your second question.*

M.W. STEFFES: *Do you have electron microscopic data that these are mesangial changes? They do not look like glomerulosclerosis.*

W. OPPERMANN: *In the second Early Diabetes symposium 6 years ago, we published a data on EM studies. (Vascular and Neurological Changes in Early Diabetes - Academic Press, New York, 1973, p. 271).*

LONG TERM TREATMENT OF ASYMPTOMATIC DIABETES

J. A. Rull*, H. Dies, J. Schulte,
F. J. Gomez-Perez, J. Sanchez-Gochicoa,
J. Figueroa, O. Lozano-Castañeda

The treatment of asymptomatic diabetes with oral compounds is still under discussion (1-3). Clinical trials have produced conflicting results and, lately, the question of potential "toxic" effects has been raised (4). The prospective study reported here was initiated in 1965.

MATERIALS AND METHODS

The criteria for patient selection included: 1) more than 27 years of age; 2) normal fasting blood sugar; 3) absence of symptoms, and 4) no diabetic retinopathy. The diagnosis of asymptomatic diabetes was established either by a record of prior symptomatic periods with fasting hyperglycemia or by at least two consecutive diagnostic oral glucose tolerance tests (OGTT). Subjects in remission with a normal OGTT were also included. Recruiting was closed in 1970.

Randomization was accomplished through the clinical file number: even numbers were given treatment and uneven were kept as controls. All subjects received a diet, a sulfonylurea or a biguanide in variable dose, or placebo. The trial was conducted under usual clinical conditions: all patients were seen at least every three months and a fasting and 2 hour post-prandial blood sugar were obtained; an OGTT was performed annually without discontinuation of treatment; fundoscopic examination was done periodically.

Comparison of individual initial and latest OGTT was the basis of analysis. Each case was classified as follows: 1) normalization or improvement when a positive diagnostic test according to the criteria of Fajans and Conn (5) changed to normal or borderline; 2) stabilization, when no changes took place; and 3) progression, when a deterioration of OGTT or fasting hyperglycemia was observed. If gross hyperglycemia and glucosuria was found, the patient was considered a failure, and the necessary treatment was given. The diagnosis of retinopathy was made in the presence of microaneurysms, hemorrhages and/or exudates; vessels changes only were recorded as angiopathy.

RESULTS

331 patients were included up to 1970. 41% of the total group was lost during the follow-up period, but the percentage was the same in the treated and control groups. All further data refer to the 122 and 72 control subjects who remained. (Tables 1 and 2). The groups were similar with only a slight difference in the frequency of obesity.

TABLE 1 - CHARACTERIZATION OF THE GROUPS (I)

Group	1970-1978 (% lost)	Sex (F %)	Age Mean and range years	Obesity (%)
Treated	41.	64.	54. (27-78)	76.
Control	41.	71.	54. (28-76)	83.

TABLE 2 - CHARACTERIZATION OF THE GROUPS (II)

	Previous phase (%)		Duration	Previous treatment (%)			
	Asymp.	Sympt.	Mean and range years	None	Diet*	O.C.	I**
Total	19.6	80.4	4.5 (0-24	5.2	18.0	73.7	3.1
Treated	21.3	78.7	4.3 (0-20)	3.3	10.6	82.8	3.3
Control	16.7	83.3	4.9 (0-24)	8.3	30.6	58.3	2.8

*O.C.: oral compounds **I: Insulin

Patients taking biguanides weighed more than those taking sulfonylureas. Of the treated patients, 52% received tolbutamide, 31% some other sulfonylurea and 17% a biguanide (Table 3). No significant changes in weight were found, but there was a tendency to weight loss in those who failed and weight gain in well controlled subjects.

Although the tendency to progression (deterioration of OGTT) was less evident in the biguanide treated patients, Table 4 shows almost identical results in the control and treated groups.

TABLE 3 - TREATMENT DURING THE OBSERVATION PERIOD

Group	Duration (yrs) 5 to 10	10	Compliance to medication Good	Bad	Compliance to diet Fair	Bad
Treated	23.*	77.	70.	30.	55.	45.
Control	29.	71.	65.	35.	64.	36.
Sulfonylureas (83%)	22.	78.	73.	27.	55.	45.
Biguanides (17%)	29.	71.	59.	41.	55.	44.

*All figures represent percent values.

TABLE 4 - INDIVIDUAL RESULTS 1978

Group	Normalization	Improvement	Stabilization	Progression	Failure
Treated	9.*	5.	23.	33.	29.
Control	4.	7.	14.	39.	35.
Sulfonylureas	7.	6.	19.	36.	32.
Biguanides	22.	0.0	44.	17.	17.

*All figures represent percentages of each group.

Table 5 shows a sharp increase in the number of cases with retinal vessel changes and the appearance of background retinopathy in both groups, although the frequency of retinopathy is higher in the sulfonylurea treated group.

TABLE 5 - FREQUENCY OF RETINAL CHANGES

	Initial		Final	
	Angiopathy	Retinopathy	Angiopathy	Retinopathy
Treated	49*	0	75	14
Control	34	0	55	3
Sulfonylureas	38	0	60	14
Biguanides	11	0	15	0

*Number of cases

The study was not designed to investigate mortality, but Table 6 presents available data. As expected, vascular accidents and cancer were the leading causes of death. It is of interest that mortality has been the same in the control and treated groups.

TABLE 6 - DEATHS

		Deaths		
Group	Number	Vascular	Other	(Cancer)
Treated	6 (4.9%)	3	3	(2)
Control	5 (6.9%)	2	3	(2)
Sulfonylureas	4 (3.9%)	3	1	(0)
Biguanides	2 (10.5%)	0	2	(2)

DISCUSSION

In spite of slight baseline variations between the treated and controls, the two final groups were fairly similar. Patient drop-outs were very high, but this probably reflects the general tendency of patients to abandon long term programs under clinical conditions. There was compliance to treatment only in two thirds of the subjects, in agreement with known figures for long term programs. Only an occasional patient followed the prescribed diet, and dieting was considered "fair" when weight fluctuations were small.

Carbohydrate intolerance, as judged by the mean OGTT and by comparison of individual OGTT change during the whole observation period, revealed a tendency to progression in both groups (treated and controls). With the exception of the earlier years, the differences seen in some of the figures were small and, probably, represent only circumstantial fluctuations.

The high frequency of retinal changes, especially in the sulfonylurea treated group, is striking, even more so since some cases occurred in patients with both a normal fasting and OGTT throughout the study. Duration of the disease was the best single correlating factor and it is likely that the difference in frequency is due to chance and to the inclusion of some patients with a longer duration of diabetes in the sulfonylurea treated group.

Mortality figures are not totally reliable because they only included hospital deaths and no systematic investigation of mortality was conducted. It can only be stated that most patients from both groups died from vascular accidents and cancer.

REFERENCES

1. *Stowers, J.M. and Helgason, T. (1965). Diabetologia, 1:128.*
2. *Engelhardt, H.T. and Vecchio, T.J. (1965). Metabolism, 14:885.*
3. *Feldman, R. et al. (1973). Excerpta Medica Amsterdam, p:574.*
4. *The University Group Diabetes Program (1970). Diabetes, 19:747.*
5. *Fajans, S.S. and Conn, J.W. (1960). Diabetes, 9:83.*

METABOLIC FATE, VASCULAR OUTCOME AND THE EFFECT OF TREATMENT IN BORDERLINE DIABETICS

J. C. Pickup*, H. Keen, and R. J. Jarrett

Borderline diabetes is a state of impaired glucose tolerance which is sometimes equated with 'early diabetes'. The simplest definition of borderline diabetes, used in the Bedford (1) and the Whitehall Surveys (2,3) was a capillary blood glucose > 120 mg/100 ml and < 200 mg/100 ml 2 hours after a 50 g oral glucose load. This paper reviews the evidence that this state is really 'early' in the sense of its metabolic fate (i.e. that it evolves to unequivocal diabetes), how 'diabetic' is the condition (i.e. is borderline diabetes associated with macro- and micro-angiopathy, diseases which typify the diabetic syndrome) and finally the effect of treatment on metabolic worsening and vascular outcome.

CLINICAL FEATURES OF SURVEY PATIENTS AND TREATMENT PROTOCOL

The Bedford Survey was begun in 1962 and the Whitehall Study in 1968. About 20,000 individuals were screened in each group, in Bedford using a urine glucose 'prescreen' with an abbreviated test of glucose tolerance (2 hr post glucose load) on the urine positives; and, in the Whitehall Study, screening the whole population by standardized 2 hr post load (50 g glucose) blood sugar measurement. Final characterization was based on the two-hour blood sugar - if under 120 mg/dl it was non-diabetic, between 120 and 200 mg/dl borderline diabetes and above 200 mg/dl unequivocal diabetes mellitus. The subjects in the Bedford Survey were both male and female, age 20-79 years but Whitehall patients were exclusively male Civil Servants, working in London and aged 40-65 years. The prevalence of borderline diabetes, estimated from a random sample of Bedford citizens, was approximately 12%. In the Whitehall Study, a well-doctored population of limited age and sex composition, prevalence was considerably less at about 2.5%.

In both Surveys borderline diabetic subjects were randomly assigned to treatment (tolbutamide 0.5 g twice daily in the Bedford Study and phenformin S.A. 50 mg once daily for Whitehall subjects) or to their respective indistinguishable placebos. Both treatment and placebo groups were also randomly sub-divided into those who were recommended carbohydrate restriction (120 g/day) and those advised only "to cut down added sugar" (which they did anyway).

WORSENING TO DIABETES

Over the course of the long-term follow up (10 years in Bedford, 5 years in Whitehall) about 2% per year of each group of borderline subjects became diabetic by the study criteria. Approximately the same number per year reverted to normal carbohydrate tolerance. No form of treatment (tolbutamide, phenformin or carbohydrate restriction) statistically significantly influenced the rate of worsening of borderline diabetes (Table 1) though there were hints of reduction ($p > 0.05 < 0.1$) in the group treated with phenformin and CHO restriction.

Table 1. Worsening to Diabetes at the 5 Year Follow-up of the Whitehall Survey.

	PLACEBO	PHENFORMIN
Carbohydrate Restriction	13.3%	18.4%
	n = 45	n = 49
Recommended diet	18.2%	9.3%
	n = 44	n = 43

No significant differences between groups.

We have recently examined in the 5 year follow-up of the Whitehall Survey a number of baseline variables as possible predictors of worsening to overt diabetes (4). Neither treatment, family history of diabetes, evidence of arterial disease, smoking history, age, body mass index, systolic blood pressure, $\log_{10}$ triglyceride concentration nor cholesterol concentration were significant predictors of 'worsening to diabetes.' The only significant predictors were the initial blood glucose values (fasting, 1 hour and 2 hour post-load), although there was the suggestion that the least obese patients only deteriorated if they had a greater degree of glucose intolerance at baseline. In particular, weight loss was identical in those who did and who did not worsen to diabetes.

MACROVASCULAR OUTCOME

Cardiovascular morbidity was defined as new events over the follow-up period including clinical onset of angina, intermittent claudication or myocardial infarct (as defined by the standard WHO questionnaire) or ECG changes meeting requirements of the Minnesota Code.

After both 5 years and 8.5 years of follow-up of the Bedford subjects, the frequency of individuals developing items of cardiovascular morbidity showed a gradation from non-diabetics, through borderline diabetics to the unequivocal diabetics as newly detected at Survey (who had about 2.5 times the morbidity of non-diabetics). The gradient was also true of mortality (both total and cardiovascular). The gradient was particularly pronounced in women (Table 2). Tolbutamide significantly reduced the risk of cardiovascular morbidity in borderline diabetics who were under the age of 50 years and without pre-existing cardiovascular morbidity at entry to the study when placebo and treated groups were compared at 5 and 8½ years.

Table 2. Total and Cardiovascular Mortality at 10 Years (Bedford Survey)

	DIABETICS	BORDERLINE DIABETICS	CONTROLS	P VALUE
Total Mortality (Observed/Expected and No. of Subjects)				
Men	1.66 (51)	0.93 (130)	0.79 (104)	0.036
Women	1.66 (63)	1.15 (119)	0.38 (85)	0.0001
Cardiovascular Mortality				
Men	1.92 (51)	0.90 (130)	0.71 (104)	0.015
Women	1.77 (63)	1.21 (119)	0.25 (85)	0.0001

All deaths in the whole Whitehall cohort (approximately 24,000) were automatically reported and collated centrally. At 5 years of follow up, the mortality rate in those with glucose intolerance was 2-3 times higher than for the normoglycemic population - largely attributable to enhanced risk of cardiovascular death, though, in this group, there is the same enhancement of risk for the newly found borderline as for the unequivocal diabetics, a function perhaps of numbers and the restricted sex and age composition of the group.

MICROVASCULAR OUTCOME

Microangiopathy was assessed by direct ophthalmoscopy after pupillary dilatation in the two groups of borderline diabetics. Retinopathy was defined as the presence of one or more small red dots interpreted by the observer as microaneurysms in either eye. After 10 years in the Bedford and 9 years in the Whitehall Study no clinically significant diabetic retinopathy had developed in the borderline diabetics though a small number had at most 2 microaneurysms in one or other eye. In contrast, in Bedford about 6% of the newly found diabetics already had microaneurysms at entry and 32% had definite retinopathy at 6 years of follow-up.

CONCLUSIONS

Borderline diabetes should not be regarded as synonymous with 'early' diabetes. Few such subjects progress to unequivocal diabetes mellitus and this occurs particularly in those with the most severe initial degrees of glucose intolerence. Many revert to normal glucose tolerance. None of the forms of treatment studied significantly altered the metabolic fate of the borderline subjects. The group has clinical significance, however, in that cardiovascular mortality and morbidity were increased compared with controls. Tolbutamide treatment may have a role in the reduction of cardiovascular morbidity in borlerline diabetics but this could be shown only on the subgroup age under 50 years without cardiovasvular morbidity or hypertension at entry. The absence of microangiopathy (or, at least, retinopathy) in borderliners may be an indication and a hope that if blood glucose can be maintained below 200 mg/100 ml in diabetics this complication of the syndrome can be arrested, retarded or reversed.

REFERENCES

1. *Sharp, C.L., et al., (1964). Proc.Roy. Roc. Med. 57, 193.*
2. *Reid, D.D., et al., (1974). Lancet 1, 469.*
3. *Jarrett, R. J. et al., (1977). Brit. Med. J. 2, 861.*
4. *Jarrett, R.J. et al., (1979). Diabetologia, in press.*

LONG-TERM TREATMENT OF SUBJECTS WITH BORDERLINE GLUCOSE TOLERANCE

S. Carlstrom*, G. Persson, G. Sartor
and B. Schersten

A study of subjects with borderline glucose tolerance was started between the years 1962-1965. The diagnosis was based on the results of an oral glucose tolerance test (OGTT) in accordance with the criteria previously established (1).

MATERIAL AND METHODS

Subjects fulfilling our criteria of borderline glucose tolerance were divided at random into four groups: 51 subjects in the first group were given dietary instructions, 48 subjects in the second group were given dietary instructions and placebo tablets, 49 subjects in the third group were given dietary instructions and tolbutamide 1.5 gm daily and 59 subjects in the fourth group were left without treatment. The subjects were followed regularly, and at each visit they were given physical examination and an OGTT. Along with the group with borderline glucose tolerance (control) was followed. The mean ages of the groups at the beginning of the study are given in Table 1. At the 8-10 year visit, the subjects were given a thorough interview regarding smoking habits (Table 2), cardiovascular state, using the WHO-standardized questionnaire, with pulseplethysmography and with exercise tests (2).

At the 10-13 year visit, plasma insulin and plasma glycerol were followed during the OGTT. At this time, about half of the subjects in the tolbutamide group had discontinued their medication and, accordingly, this group was divided into two subgroups, one consisting of those who had continued tolbutamide treatment, and a second one consisting of those who had stopped the medication.

TABLE 1

	Mean age at start (years)	Death rate (all causes)	Cardio-vascular death rate	Progression to Overt diabetes	#
Borderline groups:					
Diet	56.0	16%	6%	10%	51
Diet plus placebo	57.9	29%	17%	11%	48
Diet plus tolbu-tamide	54.4	18%	10%	2%	49
Untreated	54.0	10%	8%	25%	59
Controls	43.5	13%	4%	0%	30

TABLE 2

The Lund-study (8-10 years follow up)

	Smokers %	#
Borderline groups:		
Diet	63	41
Diet plus placebo	52	38
Diet plus tolbu-tamide	54	37
Untreated	57	41
Controls	56	44

RESULTS

The results of the OGTT's of the separate groups at start of the study are summarized in figure 1, which shows the baseline OGTT's of the various groups. Regarding the fasting blood glucose concentrations there were no differences among the various borderline groups and no difference between the borderline and the normal control group. After the glucose load, however, the curves of the borderline groups separated significantly from the control group. Between the various borderline groups there were no differences during the OGTT's. This indicates that it is impossible to diagnose subjects with this type of borderline glucose tolerance using the fasting blood glucose concentration alone.

The results of the OGTT's at the 10-13 year visit are summarized in Figure 2. The mean blood glucose curves during the test are somewhat lower in all the borderline groups in comparison with those at the start of the study. Subjects who passed into a state of overt diabetes during the follow up period and those who were deceased, of course, were excluded. In the calculations, the subjects in the diet group and the diet-placebo group were considered together.

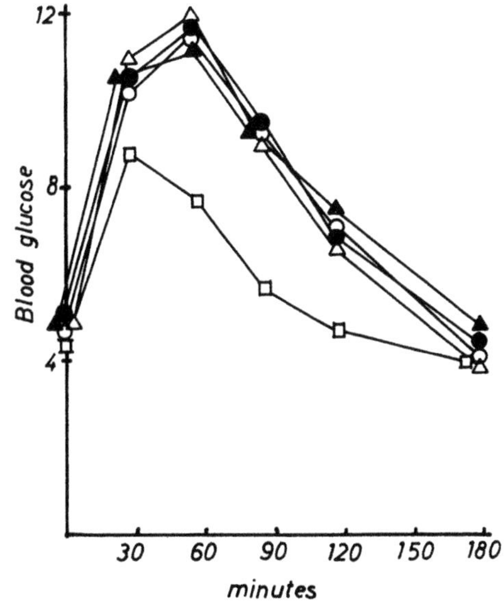

Fig. 1. The mean blood glucose concentrations during OGTT of the groups at start of the study.

△———△ *Diet,*
●———● *Placebo,*
○———○ *Tolbutamide,*
▲———▲ *Untreated,*
□———□ *Controls.*

The mean plasma insulin of the groups during the 10-13 year OGTT is shown in Figure 3. There is a tendency to higher levels in the borderline groups in comparison to the normal group. If, however, the plasma insulin concentrations are related to the blood glucose concentrations, i.e., the insulinogenic index - shown in Figure 4 - it is quite clear that the curve of the normal group reaches higher levels than those of the borderline groups.

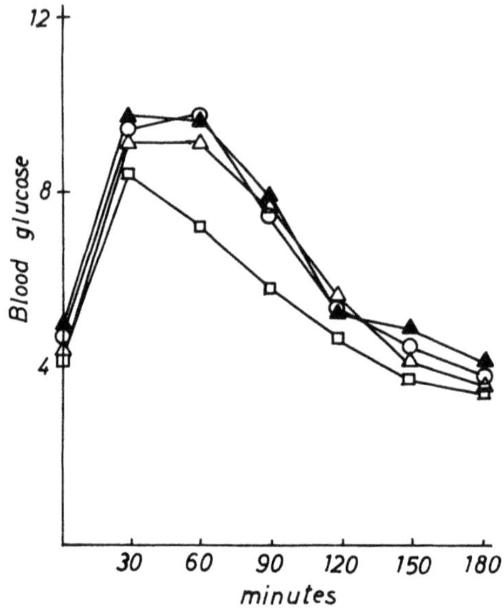

Fig. 2. The mean blood glucose concentrations during OGTT of the groups at the 10-13 year check up.

Δ———Δ	*Diet*
o———o	*Tolbutamide*
▲———▲	*Untreated*
□———□	*Controls*

Progression to overt diabetes in the separate groups is listed in Table 1. The highest figure was found in the untreated group, whereas the lowest figure was noticed in the tolbutamide treated group. Regarding death rate from all causes, there was no significant difference between the groups. However, the death rate from cardiovascular disease of the normal group was significantly lower than that of the borderline groups, separately or together. This confirms that cardiovascular mortality risk is higher in subjects with borderline glucose tolerance.

The mean diastolic blood pressure and the mean pulse rate of the different groups at the 10-13 year visit are presented in Table 3. There were no significant differences between the groups, but there may be a tendency to a lower mean figure in the tolbutamide treated grup in comparison with the other groups. Regarding the mean pulse rate figures, a significantly lower mean pulse rate was noticed in the tolbutamide treated group in comparison with all the other groups, including the normal control group.

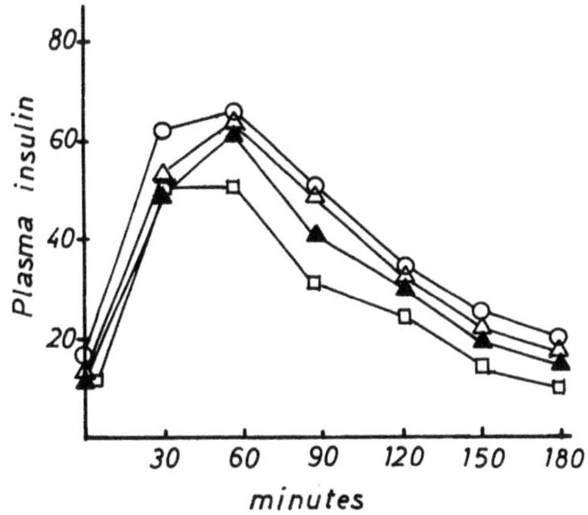

Fig. 3. The mean plasma insulin concentrations of the groups during OGTT at the 10-13 year check up.

△———△	*Diet*
o———o	*Tolbutamide*
▲———▲	*Untreated*
□———□	*Controls*

Concerning the percentages of cardiovascular complications, ascertained from interviews according to the WHO-standardized questionnaire (Table 4), there were significantly higher figures in the borderline groups than in the control group. That means that subjects with borderline glucose tolerance are at a higher risk to develop cardiovascular disease than subjects with normal glucose tolerance. This fact is further confirmed by the results of the pulse-plethysmography and the exercise tests (Table 4). The mean first flow after anoxia, determined with pulse-plethysmography, was higher in the tolbutamide group than in the other borderline groups, and this value was not separated from that of the normal control group. The percentage of ischemic ECG-changes was significantly higher in the borderline groups than in the normal control group. In addition, there was a tendency to lower percentages in the diet-placebo group and the tolbutamide group than in the other borderline groups.

The fasting venous plasma glycerol concentration and the fasting concentrations of plasma cholesterol and plasma triglyceride were determined at the 10-13 year visit. The results are summarized in Table 5. The mean plasma cholesterol concentrations were similar in the separate groups, but there was a significantly lower mean plasma triglyceride concentration in the group of subjects who had continued taking tolbutamide. The mean plasma glycerol concentration was also significantly lower in this group,

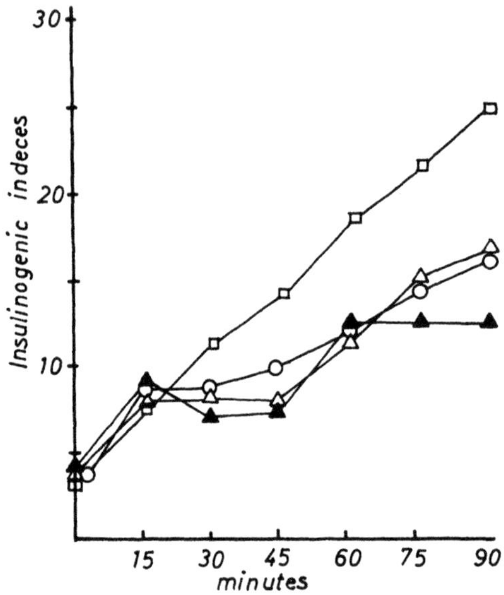

Fig. 4. *The insulinogenic index (Ii) of the groups during OGTT at the 10-13 years follow-up. (Ii) was estimated according to the following formulas:*

In the fasting state: $\frac{\text{Micro U insulin/ml}}{\text{Mmoles glucose/l}}$

During the test: $\frac{\text{Increment of insulin in micro U/ml}}{\text{Increment of glucose in Mmoles/l}}$

TABLE 3

	Diastolic blood pressure	Pulse rate at rest	#
Borderline groups:			
Diet	90 ± 1	77 ± 2	27
Diet plus placebo	88 ± 2	76 ± 2	24
Diet plus tolbutamide (cont.)	85 ± 2	63 ± 2	19
Diet plus tolbutamide (ceased)	90 ± 2	76 ± 2	19
Untreated	92 ± 2	70 ± 2	27
Controls	88 ± 1	71 ± 2	30

TABLE 4

	Cardio-vascular compli-cations (from inter-views)	Plethysm examina-tion (first flow ml min^{1} 100 ml^{-1})	Ischemic ECG-changes during exer-cise	#
Borderline groups:				
Diet	21%	22.9 ± 1.00	25%	41
Diet plus placebo	22%	23.8 ± 1.51	10%	38
Diet plus tolbuta-mide	14%	24.9 ± 1.27	11%	37
Untreated	30%	22.2 ± 0.94	19%	41
Controls	4%	25.9 ± 1.07	9%	44

and it thus seems that long-term treatment with tolbutamide has a lowering effect on both the plasma triglyceride and glycerol level. This effect apparently is not mediated by insulin, as the insulin concentrations were not different in the separate groups, and the finding may be interpreted as the result of an extra-pancreatic effect of tolbutamide treatment.

TABLE 5

The Lund-study (10-13 years follow up

	Fasting venous P-glycerol (mmoles/l)	P-cholesterol (mg/100 ml)	P-triglyceride (mmoles/l)	#
Borderline groups:				
Diet	0.41	258	1.18	27
Diet plus placebo	0.36	264	0.82	24
Diet plus tolbuta-mide (cont.)	0.22	254	0.73	19
Diet plus tolbuta-mide(ceased)	0.61	261	0.99	19
Untreated	0.44	262	1.18	27
Controls	0.21	246	1.04	30

SUMMARY

Subjects with borderline glucose tolerance are at a higher risk of suffering and dying from cardiovascular disease than subjects with normal glucose tolerance. Our data on the progression to overt diabetes and our data on cardiovascular morbidity and mortality suggests that tolbutamide treatment reduces these risks. In any case, we have no data supporting the theory that tolbutamide promotes cardiovascular damage.

REFERENCES

1. *Carlstrom, S., et al (1971). Acta med. scand. 189, 415*
2. *Persson, G. (1977) Acta. med. scand. suppl. 605*

DISCUSSION

Invited Discussant: J. R. WILLIAMSON: *If we examine the UGDP data on tolbutamide patients in the same way that I described yesterday for insulin treated subjects, we find that the outcome is the same; the frequency of cardiovascular deaths in the tolbutamide group is still much greater than in the placebo group. But, if we compare the frequency of cardiovascular deaths in the first 5 years of the UGDP with the frequency of cardiovascular deaths in the second 5 years, an interesting finding does become apparent (Table 1). The first five years corresponds to that portion of the study in which tolbutamide was administered, and the second five years runs from the discontinuation of tolbutamide to the termination of the study. What we find is that the cardiovascular death rate was essentially 5% in the placebo group in the first 5 years, compared to almost 14% in the second phase of the study. Thus in the second 5 years, the frequency of cardiovascular deaths almost tripled in the placebo group whereas there were no significant differences in the frequency of cardiovascular deaths in either of the two insulin treated groups for the two time periods. The increased frequency of cardiovascular deaths in the placebo group in the second five years is statistically significant at the P<.05 level. This difference could be due either to chance variation in the frequency of cardiovascular disease in the second phase. The finding that cardiovascular mortality for the entire duration of the study was the same in all three groups, i.e. the placebo group and both insulin treated groups, is consistent with both interpretations. If the difference in cardiovascular death rate in the two phases of the study in the placebo group is due to random fluctuation, then had the death rates in the 2 phases been reversed, there would have been no evidence of tolbutamide toxicity and the insulin variable treatment regimen would have shown some evidence of benefit.*

A number of other questions have been raised regarding whether excess cardiovascular deaths in tolbutamide treated subjects might have been due to increased cardiovascular risk factors, which were present in that group at baseline, and also to the fact that the drug was given in a fixed dose regardless of the patient's response. In view of Dr. Poffenbarger's elegant findings presented this morning, this latter criticism may be especially important. All these factors, coupled with the possibility of random fluctuation in the frequency of cardiovascular deaths in the placebo group, may well account for the apparent excess cardiovascular mortality associated with tolbutamide treatment. Dr. Poffenbarger's observations that premature ventricular contractions occurred in several patients during the course of their acute tolbutamide testing certainly is a cause for concern and would be consistent with tolbutamide toxicity. I would like to ask him if these problems arose in patients who were rapid or slow degraders of tolbutamide and if he has any information relating to the actual blood levels of tolbutamide in those patients who developed premature ventricular contractions?

TABLE 1

Frequency of Cardiovascular Deaths During the Tolbutamide (TOLB) and Insulin Phases of the UGDP Study in Subjects Who Did Not Dropout or Change Medication.[1]

	TOLB		INSULIN	
	%	(No)[2]	%	(No)
PLBO	5.0	(7/139)	13.8	(11/80)
TOLB	14.4	(22/153)	---	---
ISTD	11.6	(17/146)	7.8	(7/90)
IVAR	7.6	(12/159)	9.6	(11/114)

[1]Subjects who missed 4 or more consecutive quarterly examinations or who changed medication for the same time period were considered to be dropouts or medication changes, respectively (17).

[2]The first number in parentheses is the number of deaths, the second is the number at risk. Subjects who died of non-cardiovascular causes as well as from cardiovascular causes during the tolbutamide phase are eliminated from the number of subjects at risk during the insulin phase.

P. L. POFFENBARGER: *The interpretation of the UDGP data on the comparison of tolbutamide and placebo group, with respect to myocardial infarction, is that the number of individuals in the two groups, who experienced myocardial infarction, is not different. The number of individuals, who experienced fatal MI, is greater in the tolbutamide group. The fatality case rate is 50% in tolbutamide, compared to 18.2%, and the percent fatality is greatest in white females, a ninefold increase. With that brief background, we thought that sex or genetic factors might play a role in contributing to this apparent cardiovascular toxicity. What explains the increase in cardiovascular deaths in white females is the question. The white females are smaller in body size than males, and both are on a fixed 1.5 gm. per kilogram body weight tolbutamide. Therefore, their apparent volume for distribution of the drug will be smaller, so their blood concentration will be higher. The genetic study shows that 5% of that group will be slow inactivators and that they had high drug adherence rate. If you re-analyze the data, as Dr. Cornfeld has, with respect to individuals who have a very high medication adherence rate, the cardiovascular mortality difference increases by a factor of fourfold. The number of patients on whom we have done studies is limited. We found premature ventricular contractions during our studies in three subjects, which has been quite alarming. Two of them were slow and one was a rapid inactivator, who also smoked cigarettes during the study. Lastly, with respect to the Bedford study, they gave only 1 gm. tolbutamide per day, and I would predict that the level of tolbutamide would be lower on 1 gm. per day than on 1½ gms. per day. We might actually be dealing here with a very narrow therapeutic range for tolbutamide.*

T. PROUT: *The point I would like to make is about subdivision and the worries we all have about that. Dr. Poffenbarger has found difference in the females; this was also brought up by the biometric studies. We were aware of that and felt that it was a little unfair to subdivide and point up this difference. We did not have any additional internal consistency, but it does exist in the area. As far as the mortality question is concerned, and the problem of who was and who was not on tolbutamide, only one person in the mortality statistics was not on treatment at the time of our summation. The question of adherence is not a big one. Adherence was in fact greater in tolbutamide than in others. When one looks at this, something we did not put in our major paper because again subdivision is a bit of a problem, it changes analysis. Here, we see that the highest adherence was in fact associated with higher cardiovascular death rate, so it does seem to follow the use of the agent. The only thing that bothers me about Dr. Williamson's remarks is that his reanalysis failed to solve the problem.*

G. M. REAVEN: *There has been a tendency in the United States to make a fuss about what is and what is not diabetes, in terms of where you cut off the fasting glucose. What we've seen very elegantly, from both the Bedford study and the study in Lund, is that even people with mild glucose intolerance, call it what you will, are really at risk for cardiovascular disease and calling it diabetes or not is irrelevant. It doesn't mean that it goes away by not calling it diabetes. There are two other issues. First, the treatment of patients who have normal fasting glucose with sulfonylurea compounds. I'm not so sure that the way to mark these patients is by doing the oral glucose tolerance test. As I showed you yesterday, we take such patients and just give them food. The plasma glucose levels are indistinguishable from normal. Therefore, I'm not so sure that focusing on the damage of treatment by using GTT's doesn't serve a useful purpose. The last point is the very striking differences that Dr. Pickup showed between cardiovascular deaths in women with glucose intolerance, as compared to people who have normal tolerance. They have equally striking changes in triglyceride levels between males and females who are just out in the world. I'm wondering if you correlated your deaths with triglyceride levels?*

J. PICKUP: *Cholesterol levels were total. Triglyceride analysis is just being done in the Whitehall study.*

S. FAJANS: *I would like to continue in the vein that Dr. Reavens started on. The glucose tolerance is simply a more sensitive way, although it doesn't represent day to day blood sugar fluctuation. A young man on chlorpropamide, on the glucose test, went up to 400 mg, and I think everybody would accept that as diabetes, but after a mixed meal, his blood sugar level was absolutely normal. Dr. Pickup, you showed, as well as Dr. Carlstrom, that, in patients with tolerance or borderline diabetes, whatever you want to call it, there is increased risk of microangiopathy in contrast to normal control subjects. In other words, they are at risk; this is one of the diabetic features. The philosophical question is why should we eliminate thinking of diabetes in this group, when there is both abnormal glucose tolerance tests and the predisposition to earlier deaths from vascular complications which mark diabetes? Finally, you showed us that 3.3% "only" have retinopathy. The general population doesn't have a 3.3% retinopathy. So, you are actually showing that even that complication, which is not specific for all diabetics, is increased in the population. I would suggest that your borderline diabetics, or, if you like, impaired glucose tolerance, are then indeed a subclass of diabetic patients by very conventional criteria, namely, accelerated vascular disease and abnormal glucose levels.*

J. PICKUP: *All we are saying is that, over the followup period, nobody developed clinically severe diabetic retinopathy in that particular group, although they certainly did so in the overt diabetics. In other words, there is a qualitative, as well as quantitative, change here. The overt diabetics get severe retinopathy, and several were actually blind at the end of the 10 year study. The other part of the question pertains to the problem of defining really what is meant by diabetic control. There is no more evidence that it is blood sugar which is doing the damage than anything else, such as lactate. So, we only happen to choose this particular marker of diabetes because, at the beginning of the study in 1962, it was just the easiest measure. However, it's quite true that one should also be looking at all of the other intermediate metabolites and one knows, of course, that there are plenty of people who have normal mean blood sugar and fasting blood sugars with proliferative retinopathy. We all have plenty of patients like that.*

H. LEBOVITZ: *Plenty? Does everybody else have plenty? I've seen an occasional patient.*

J. PICKUP: *Well, in our series, we've got about 10 patients who have mean fasting blood sugars, which one would consider reasonable control, yet have proliferative retinopathy. There is obviously something very strange about these people, and one can speculate for hours about exactly what is going on regarding other metabolites, hormones and things which are abnormal.*

T. PROUT: *There was on death, I think that was unreported in the first study. It had not been reported because of delay in getting data on a patient who died. One of the missing patients, I believe, I'm not sure of the data, but there was nothing overt about that.*

B. METZGER: *Dr. Pickup, in analyzing the appearance of retinopathy, have you been able to determine whether smoking or hypertension are coexisting factors accelerating the appearance of retinopathy?*

J. PICKUP: *In our particular study, there is no correlation between smoking or hypertension and the development of retinopathy, but that analysis has only been made in the borderline and not in the overt diabetics.*

S. CARLSTROM: *I didn't mention that, but we have examined our borderliners for retinopathy, and we found 4% with small red dots in the retina. This examination was made after about 8 years, so I don't have recent data now.*

E. PFEIFFER: *Some of the speakers showed lowering of the triglycerides and no increase in the insulin levels in cases treated with tolbutamide. I think this very clearly does not point against mobilization of the surplus of insulin because it is only possible to discover the increased insulin levels when you measure it immediately after the administration of the drugs in the morning hours and not in the fasting state. In overt diabetes, as far as we have seen and heard in all the other surveys, there is greater mortality rate than in borderline cases. Is this correct or not? In the long run, this means that the sulfonylurea cases should develop a lower mortality if they do not progress to the overt diabetes condition.*

J. PICKUP: *Well, tolbutamide only had an effect in a particular subgroup of diabetics; those who were under 50 years of age, who didn't have cardiovascular morbidity when they started. Other than that, there was absolutely no significant differences.*

J. HOET: *I would like to ask if, in the borderline cases, there has been any attempt to evaluate the exercises which the people have been doing? It seems that everything but exercises has been taken into consideration.*

S. CARLSTROM: *We haven't done a study on that, but we have exercise tests in all our borderline cases, and we know there are physical fitness exercises.*

J. PICKUP: *We've made no analysis on the borderline group exercise.*

G. M. REAVEN: *Perhaps I missed something on what Pfeiffer was saying, that the data implied there was a decrease in progression with the treated group. My impression is that no one showed that these drugs inhibit a progression of the diabetes.*

S. CARLSTROM: *I think it is our study you are talking about. We had 2% onsets of overt diabetes in the tolbutamide treated group, in comparison to 15% in the other borderline groups.*

G. M. REAVEN: *I'm sorry, but Pickup did not show what Rull showed. That is still obviously a clotted question.*

J. PICKUP: *Yes, that is quite right. In our study, there was no effect of any form of treatment on worsening to overt diabetes.*

G. M. REAVEN: *There is no need to believe, although atherosclerotic lesion ends up the same in terms of the artery, that the metabolic events which led to it are identical. It may well be that in different subgroups of patients different metabolic lesions would lead to atherosclerosis. So, it would be nice if all of these people who do epidemiology, would make lots of measurements, including free fatty acids, which would be a very important thing to know in terms of atherosclerotic heart disease.*

S. CARLSTROM: *Our data on triglyceride and plasma glycerol showed lower mean levels in the tolbutamide treated group. We were a little astonished with that, and I would very much like to hear any comments on that. This effect of tolbutamide, to lower plasma glycerol and plasma triglyceride, seems not to be mediated through insulin, as the insulin curve is the same in the separate borderline groups.*

GLIPIZIDE: A NEW SECOND GENERATION SULFONYLUREA

E. Norris*

Glipizide (Fig. 1), indicated for the treatment of nonketotic maturity onset diabetes, is among the newest of the second generation sulfonylureas and is characterized by increased potency resulting in clinical effectiveness at relatively low milligram doses.

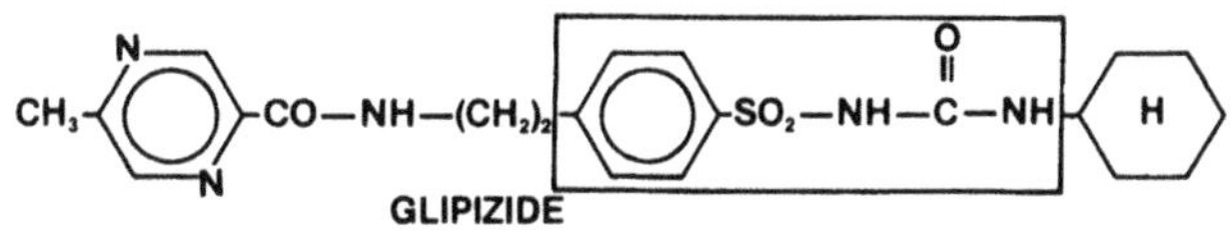

Fig. 1. Chemical structure of glipizide

PHARMACOLOGY

The pharmacologic properties of glipizide differ significantly from other members of this class. Although the plasma half-life of glipizide is short, less than 3 hours, it has a sufficiently long duration of action such that a single dose may often be adequate to control hyperglycemia over a 24-hour period (1). A review of selected clinical studies of glipizide will illustrate the features of the drug that makes it particularly useful in the treatment of maturity-onset nonketotic diabetes.

Both absorption and elimination of glipizide are rapid, uniform and complete following oral administration in man. After a single 5 mg dose, the plasma concentration of glipizide can be expected to peak at about 2 hours and then rapidly fall off. (Fig. 2). At 9 hours, plasma glipizide levels are only 20% of peak levels, and at 24 hours, plasma levels approach zero. (2, 3). Chronic administration does not appear to alter these parameters. Glipizide is metabolized mainly in the liver; the majority of the drug (88%) is excreted as inactive metabolites in the urine, with a small percentage (about 5% to 10%) excreted in the feces (4).

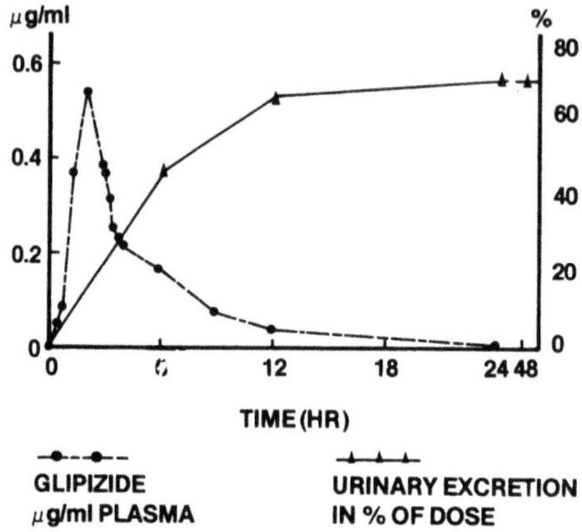

Fig. 2. Glipizide plasma levels and urinary excretion in one patient (from Cochet et al., 1975 (2)).

The onset of hypoglycemic activity of a 5 mg oral dose of glipizide is rapid with a measurable decrease in blood glucose evident after half an hour (5). Plasma immunoreactive insulin (IRI) levels peaked within half an hour (5) (Fig. 3).

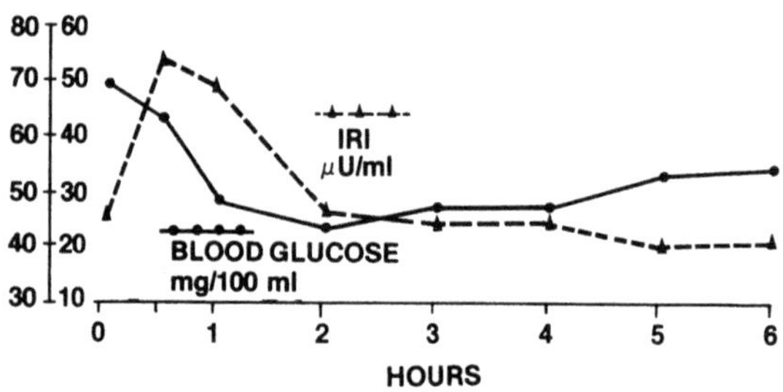

Fig. 3. Blood glucose and insulin levels following glipizide administration (5 mg orally) in 8 healthy patients. (From Pedrazzi et al., 1971 (5)).

In addition to its rapid onset of action, glipizide can maintain its clinical effectiveness throughout the day. Corrall et al. (1) found that a single 5 mg or 10 mg morning dose of glipizide given to diet-failed maturity-onset diabetics was sufficient to control the glucose challenge of 3 meals ingested over a period of 10 hours. Blood glucose levels were lowered significantly after each of the 3 meals in glipizide-treated patients; similarly IRI levels rose appropriately after each of the 3 meals (Fig. 4). Thus, glipizide remained effective in controlling glucose challenges long after peak plasma levels had been achieved. By comparison, in a control group of patients treated by diet alone, blood glucose and IRI levels failed to respond adequately.

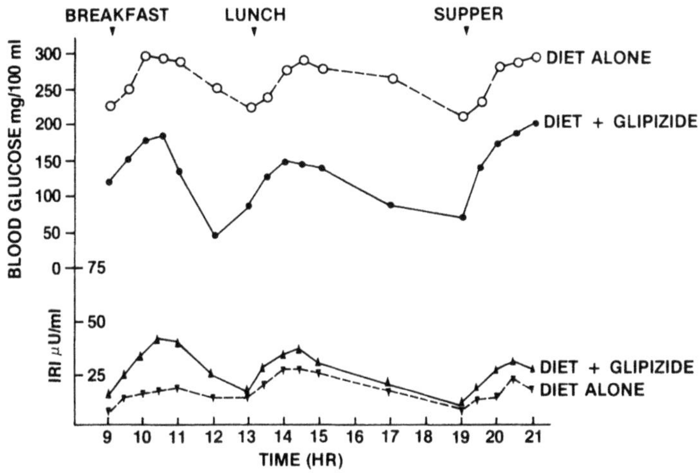

Fig. 4. Blood glucose and insulin levels in 6 patients given standard diet following a single morning dose of glipizide. The average dosage was 7 mg per patient with a range of from 5-10 mg/day. (From Corrall et al., 1976 (1)).

A further study by Corrall et al. demonstrated that, when maturity onset diabetics received glipizide but were deprived of meals, blood glucose levels stabilized at safe levels (Fig. 5). Insulin peaks, which were previously noted following meals, did not occur in fasting patients, and no instances of hypoglycemia were reported.

Thus glipizide has prompt, uniform and complete absorption, (1,4) rapid onset of action and a more physiologic response in its effect on patients' blood glucose and insulin levels. Essentially, glipizide appears to have the ability to induce a response to a specific demand. If there is a glucose challenge, glipizide will produce a rapid hypoglycemia effect. If there is no challenge, the drug will have only a minimal effect on blood glucose levels (1).

Additionally, the work of Lebovitz, presented at this symposium, illustrates another extremely interesting property of glipizide, an ability to potentiate insulin action and thus make the same quantity of insulin considerably more effective in the diabetic patient (6).

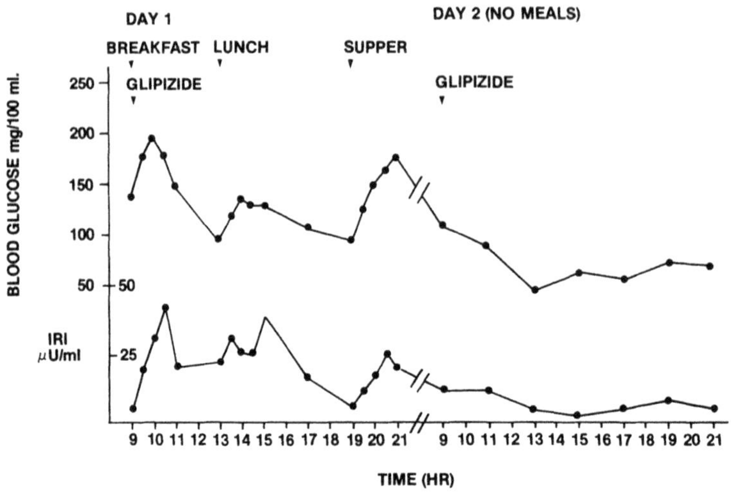

Fig. 5. Blood glucose and IRI levels in 6 diabetic patients treated with glipizide with standard diet on day 1 and no meals on day 2. The average daily dosage of glipizide was 8.3 mg, with a range of 5-10 mg per day. (From Corrall et al., 1976 (1)).

Further work in this area may more precisely characterize the mechanism of action of glipizide.

CLINICAL EXPERIENCE

Efficacy

The overall clinical efficacy of glipizide is demonstrated by a comprehensive series of 29 clinical studies conducted in the United States, Latin America and Europe. A significant reduction in fasting and 2-hour postprandial glucose levels (FPG and PPG) in relation to established baseline values, as well as an absolute reduction in plasma glucose, were demonstrated in a majority of the glipizide-treated patients who had sufficient data to permit evaluation (7).

Most of the studies were designed either as single or double-blind parallel comparisons of glipized with other sulfonylureas and with placebo. A total of 360 patients with confirmed nonketotic, maturity-onset diabetes mellitus who received glipizide were evaluated for drug efficacy. The mean age was 56.0 years, with a range from 28 to 78 years. Patients took glipizide for periods ranging from 1 to 39 months in daily doses of 1.25 mg to 40 mg. The majority of diabetics receiving glipizide had the disease for at least 5 years, with a mean duration of 6.1 years (7).

The mean baseline FPG, as determined during the initial diet-screening period, was 221 mg%. Efficacy of glipizide therapy was evaluated using clinical control criteria as measured by the mean of the patient's last 3 FPG values, and when available, PPG data. Glipizide therapy was shown to produce acceptable (FPG ≤ 180 mg%) control of FPG levels in 67% of patients. Of those controlled, 70% came under excellent or good control, with a FPG ≤ 150 mg%. (7)

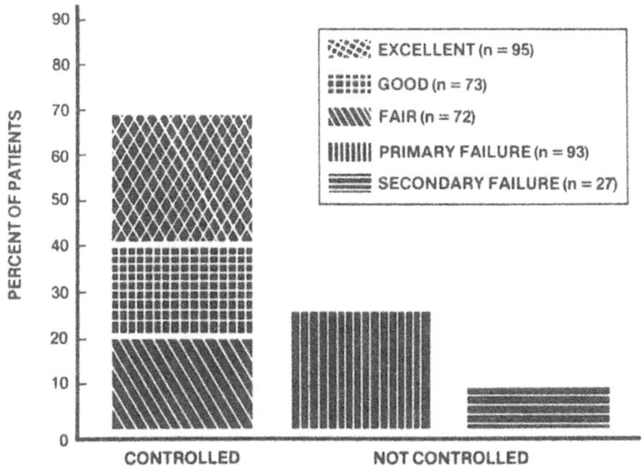

Fig. 6. Overall fasting plasma glucose responses to glipizide therapy. (From Sachs et al., 1977 (7)).

A similar response to glipizide therapy was found based on PPG levels, with 75% of patients coming under control (PPG < 220 mg%). In general, response of glipizide therapy based on FPG levels was well correlated with response based on PPG levels. (7)

The degree to which glipizide lowered plasma glucose was also evaluated. FPG was lowered in all patients from a mean of 221 mg% to 171 mg% (23%), and PPG was decreased from 256 mg% to 185 mg% (28%). For those patients considered under control using FPG criteria, the overall mean reduction in FPG values was 31% of baseline; for those patients considered under control using PPG criteria, the overall mean reduction in PPG values was 33% of baseline. (7)

Dose/response

A daily dose of 20 mg or less was sufficient to control about 60% of all successfully controlled patients with once or twice daily dosing. Furthermore, 71% of patients who came under excellent or good control were in this dosing regimen. Eighty-one percent of the patients were controlled with 30 mg or less per day. (7)

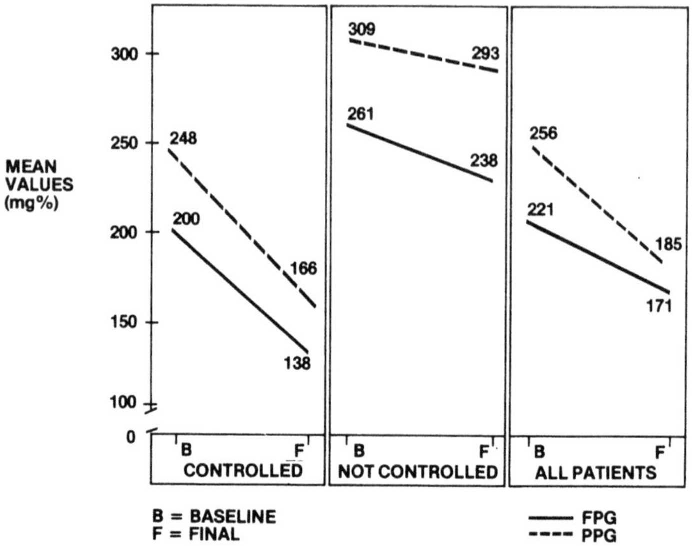

Fig. 7. Mean reduction in fasting and postprandial plasma glucose in glipizide-treated patients.

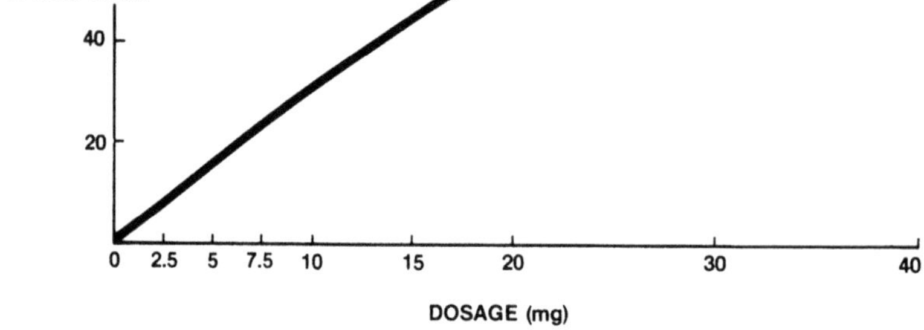

Fig. 8. Range of dosages (mg) used for those responding successfully to glipizide therapy. (From Sachs et al., 1977 (7)).

LONG-TERM SUCCESS RATE

The ability of glipizide to maintain effective control of blood glucose levels during long-term therapy was demonstrated by Parodi and Caputo in a study of 72 patients who received glipizide for a period of over four years. (8)

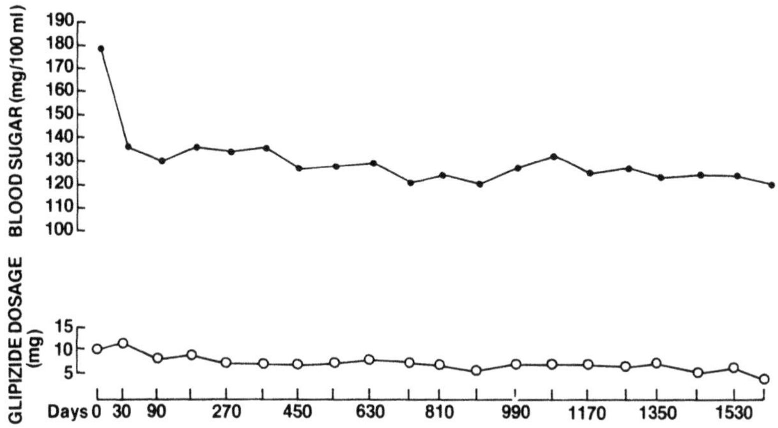

Fig. 9. Mean blood sugar levels and glipizide dosage in 72 patients. (From Parodi and Caputo, 1974 (8)).

Safety profile

Careful monitoring of 702 patients in 35 clinical studies has demonstrated that the incidence of side effects was low. Of the small percentage (11.8%) of patients reporting side effects that might be attributable to glipizide therapy, the most commonly reported ones were those generally seen in maturity onset diabetics taking sulfonylurea agents. Few adverse reactions were reported by greater than 1% of patients. (7) (Table 7)

Table 1. Adverse Reactions Reported by 1% of Patients (7)

Dizziness	2.25%
Lack of Energy	2.13%
Drowsiness	1.75%
Dermatologic Reactions	1.42%
Nausea	1.38%
Diarrhea	1.25%
Headache	1.25%
Sweating	1.25%

Thirty-nine patients (5.6%) reported symptoms that could have been attributed to hypoglycemia. Blood glucose determinations were made in 6 of these patients and in only one instance could hypoglycemia be documented. (7)

While numerous laboratory parameters were monitored in most of the 702 patients on glipizide therapy, the incidence of abnormal test results (either higher or lower than normal) was low. Those abnormalities that were recorded were felt by the investigators to be of no clinical significance as evidenced by the fact that no patient had to discontinue glipizide therapy due to abnormal laboratory tests. (7)

Dosage and administration

As with any sulfonylurea, dosage must be individualized based upon clinical response. Thus frequent blood glucose determinations, during dose titration and throughout maintenance, remain the key to successful management of the diabetic patient. The recommended starting dose is 5 mg given once daily before breakfast. Dosage adjustments should ordinarily be in increments of 2.5 mg to 5 mg daily, as determined by blood glucose response. At least several days should elapse between titration steps. The recommended total daily dosage range of glipizide is 5 to 40 mg given in a single or divided doses depending upon total daily dose required. Many patients may be able to be controlled on a once a day, before breakfast, dosage regimen. This tends to be most effective in patients requiring 20 mg or less daily.

REFERENCES

1. *Corrall, R.J.M., et al. (1976). Acta Therapeutica 2, 77.*
2. *Cochet, B., et al. (1975) Schweiz. Rundschau. Med. (PRAXIS) 64, 562.*
3. *Data on file 1978 Pfizer Laboratories, Pfizer, Inc.*
4. *Fabre, J., et al. (1973). XIIth International Congress of Therapeutics, Geneva, Sept. 24.*
5. *Pedrazzi, F., et al. (1971). Arzneim. Forsch. (Drug Res.) 21, No. 2, 220.*
6. *Lebovitz, H.E., et al. (1977) J. Clin. Endocrinol. Metab. 45, 601.*
7. *Sachs, R., et al. (1979) Marco Island Symposium on Glipizide, 1977. Excerpta Medica (In Press).*
8. *Parodi, F.A., and Caputo, G. (1974). Curr. Med. Res. Opin. 3 Suppl. 1, 31.*

EFFECT OF THE ORAL HYPOGLYCEMIC AGENT PIROGLIRIDE TARTRATE ON INSULIN AND GLUCAGON SECRETION IN VIVO AND IN VITRO

G. F. Tutwiler*, H. C. Fawthrop, R. T. Krill
and S. Pek

Pirogliride [N-(1-methyl-2-pyrrolidinylidene)-N'-phenyl-1-pyrrolidine carboximidamide] whose structure is shown below is a new oral hypoglycemic compound which differs structurally and mechanistically from the sulfonylureas and biguanides (1,2). However, the mechanism responsible for its blood glucose lowering action is

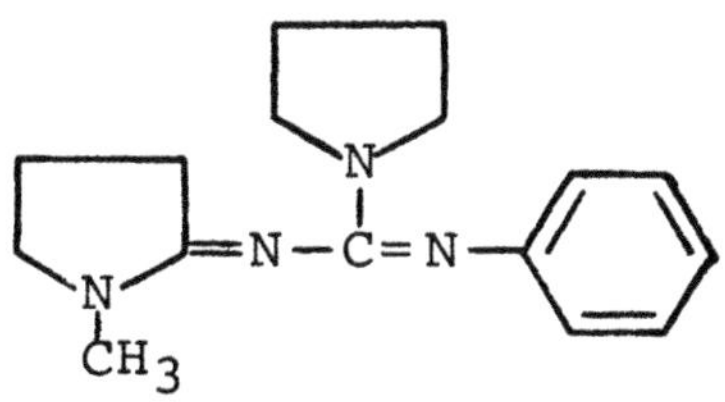

not understood. Unlike the sulfonylureas, oral administration of pirogliride to fasted dogs did not increase peripheral plasma insulin and it lowered the blood glucose in db/db mice and streptozotocin diabetic rats. However, a role for insulin secretion in the hypoglycemic effect was not ruled out, since, among other findings (1), pirogliride failed to lower the blood glucose in depancreatized dogs. This finding indicated perhaps that either the presence of some insulin is required for the compound's activity or that it may be suppressing glucagon secretion. Therefore, in order to explore these possibilities, the effects of pirogliride on plasma glucagon and insulin levels *in vivo* and their secretion *in vitro* were studied.

MATERIALS AND METHODS

In Vivo Studies

Drug effects on resting levels of insulin and glucagon, in fasting healthy beagle dogs (7-12 kg) of either sex were studied using procedures and dietary conditions described previously (1,2). For arginine infusion experiments, the left jugular vein and carotid artery were cannulated in healthy mongrel dogs anesthetized with pentobarbital sodium (39 mg/kg, i.v., Spencer-Mead, Inc.). Following surgery, each dog received an intramuscular injection of antibiotic (Combiotic[R], Chas. Pfizer and Co.) and each was fasted overnight prior to the start of the experiment. L-arginine hydrochloride (Sigma Chemical Co.) adjusted to pH 7.4 was infused via the venous cannula at a total dose per infusion of 0.33 g/kg: one-half given as a bolus and one-half given at a constant rate of approximately 0.2 gm/min for ten minutes. Ninety minutes following the termination of the first infusion, drugs dissolved in water or the vehicle were given by oral intubation and 60 minutes later, a second infusion of arginine was administered using the previous protocol. Arterial blood samples were collected in heparinized tubes and plasma separated by centrifugation. Plasma levels of glucose were analyzed by the hexokinase method. Plasma was then stored at -20°C until analyzed for glucagon by the method of Unger using the 30-K antiserum, and for insulin using kits purchased from Corning.

In Vitro Studies

A perfusion system was used to study the release of pancreatic islet hormones. The details of the surgical procedures, the perfusion apparatus, radioimmunoassays and the artificial perfusion media have been reported previously (3).

RESULTS AND DISCUSSION

In Vivo Studies

Pirogliride has been reported (1) to significantly lower the plasma glucose concentrations of fasting beagle dogs in a dose-dependent manner without significantly altering immunoreactive insulin. In order to evaluate the effect of this drug on the resting levels of immunoreactive glucagon, 10 additional fasted dogs were given various doses of pirogliride (10-40 mg/kg, p.o. and 5-10 mg/kg, i.v.). While pirogliride lowered the plasma glucose concentrations of all dogs by 20 to 50%, peripheral plasma levels of glucagon were lowered only marginally (15%) in three of the dogs. However, plasma glucagon levels were generally found to be increased following the nadir of plasma glucose. An example of a typical dog experiment is graphically illustrated in Figure 1. Presumably, the increases in plasma glucagon that were observed are a compensatory response to the blood glucose lowering action of pirogliride since hypoglycemia is known to be a powerful stimulant of glucagon secretion. Similar increases in glucagon have also been observed (unpublished results) following the peak hypoglycemic effect of piroglibride in non-diabetic man.

It is well recognized that intravenous infusion of arginine, alanine and mixtures of amino acids can stimulate the secretion of glucagon and insulin in dogs and man. Therefore, the effects of

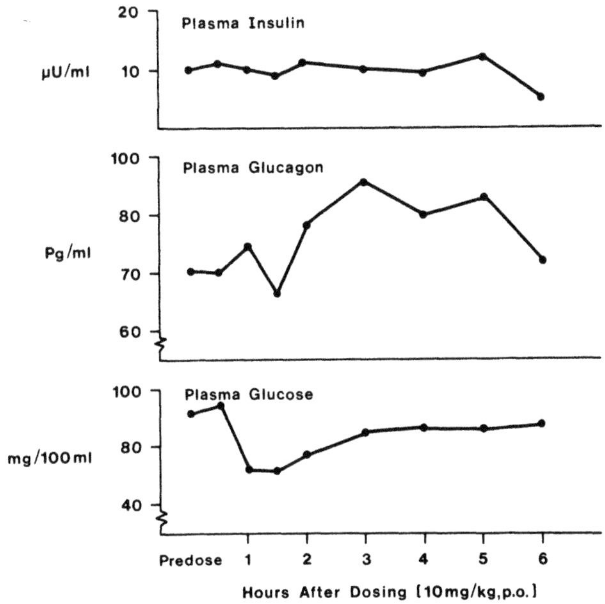

Fig. 1. The effect of pirogliride tartrate (10 mg/kg, p.o.) on glucagon, insulin and glucose concentrations of a fasted beagle dog.

pirogliride on glucagon secretion was also studied in dogs given intravenous doses (0.33 gm/kg) of arginine. As illustrated in Figure 2, administration of pirogliride failed to produce a statistically significant decrease of baseline or arginine stimulated glucagon levels compared to animals dosed similarly with the vehicle (H_2O). However, as shown in Figure 3, the resting insulin levels and insulin levels following the second arginine infusion were increased significantly. Thus, an insulin secretory effect of pirogliride which had not been seen previously (1) was observed in the above experiments. As expected, plasma glucose declined following pirogliride treatment. However, in spite of the higher plasma insulin observed in the present experiments the magnitude of the decrease in plasma glucose following pirogliride was similar to experiments (1) done in the absence of arginine infusion. Tolbutamide (20 mg/kg, p.o.) was also studied in this model. It failed to alter glucagon levels and its insulin stimulatory effect was the same as seen in experiments done in the absence of arginine infusions.

In Vitro Studies

The effect of piroglíride on insulin and glucagon secretion was also studied using the isolated perfused rat pancreas. In the presence of 5.6 mM glucose, exposure of the pancreas to pirogliride for periods of 1-20 minutes produced an inconsistent secretion of both insulin and glucagon which was not dose-dependent. Examples of typical experiments using 10^{-4}M pirogliride and tolbutamide are illustrated in Figure 4. At best, the magnitude of

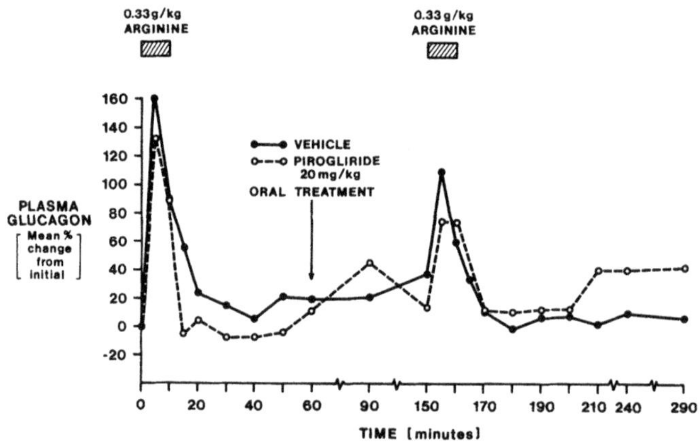

Fig. 2. Effect of pirogliride tartrate upon plasma glucagon levels of fasted dogs given arginine infusions. (Arginine was given intravenously over two ten minute periods separated by 140 minutes; pirogliride or vehicle was given 60 prior to the second infusion of arginine. Four dogs each were given vehicle and pirogliride).

the insulin release in response to pirogliride was found to be 10-20% of that seen with equimolar amounts of tolbutamide. Thus the quantitative effects of pirogliride and tolbutamide on insulin secretion fail to explain the 3-4 fold greater potency of pirogliride (1) as a hypoglycemic agent in rats. Also, the relevancy of these modest increases in non-stimulated insulin secretion to pirogliride's hypoglycemic effect can be questioned since an analogue of pirogliride, N-(1-methyl-2-pyrrolidinylidene)-N'-(4-methylsulfonylphenyl)-4-morpholinecarboximidamide, which does not produce hypoglycemia produced at 10^{-4}M a similar small increase in insulin and glucagon secretion.

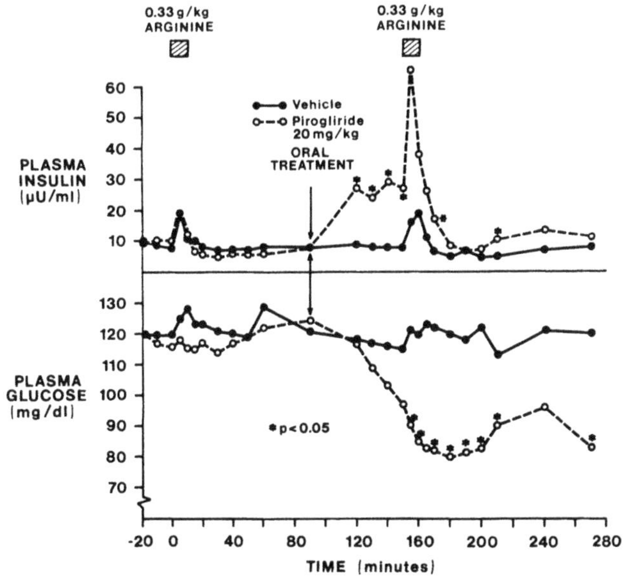

Fig. 3. Effect of piroglíride tartrate on plasma insulin and glucose levels of fasted dogs given arginine infusions. (See figure 2 for experimental details).

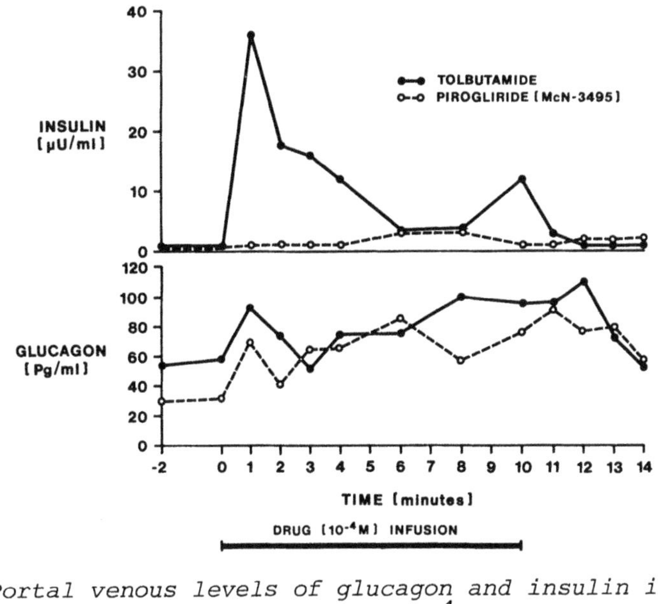

Fig. 4. Portal venous levels of glucagon and insulin in response to a 10-minute perfusion of 10^{-4}M piroglíride or tolbutamide in the presence of 5.6 mM glucose.

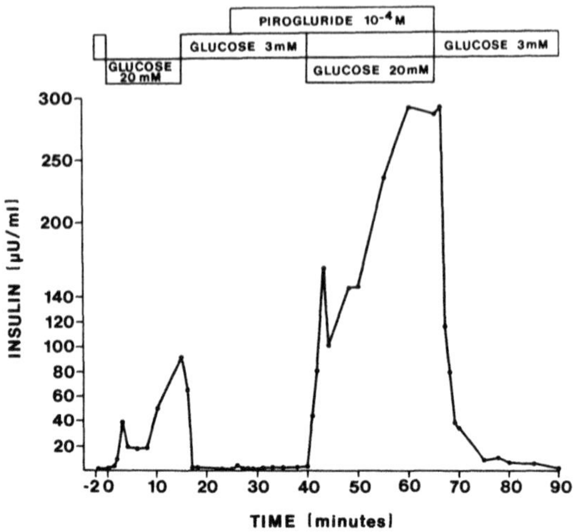

Fig. 5. Effect of piroglíride on glucose stimulated insulin secretion using the perfused rat pancreas.

However, an insulin secretagogue action of pirogliride was clearly apparent when insulin secretion was stimulated using glucose. As shown in Figure 5, when 10^{-4}M pirogliride was perfused prior to and during perfusion with 20 mM glucose, both phases of glucose induced insulin release were augmented greatly. Since perfusion of the pancreas with tolbutamide has generally been reported (4,5) to leave the pancreas refractory to glucose, the β-cytotrophic action of pirogliride may be qualitatively as well as quantitatively distinct from that of tolbutamide.

In Conclusion

Previous findings that pirogliride, unlike the sulfonylureas, lowers the blood glucose of db/db mice and streptozotocin diabetic rats (1) and produces a number of direct metabolic effects *in vitro* (6) suggested that the hypoglycemic action of pirogliride was the result of non-pancreatic mechanisms. However, the present results suggest that an insulin secretogogue effect may also be among the mechanisms of its hypoglycemic action. Diminished glucagon release is not, however, a mechanism. Also it appears that the effects of pirogliride on insulin secretion *in vivo* and *in vitro* were different from those of the sulfonylurea, tolbutamide.

REFERENCES

1. *Tutwiler, G.F., et al., (1978). Diabetes 27, 856 .*
2. *Tutwiler, G.F. and Bridi, G. (1978). Diabetes, 27, 868.*
3. *Pek, S., et al. (1975). Prostaglandins 10, 493.*

4. *Lenzen, S. (1978). Diabetes 27, 27.*
5. *Grodsky, G.M., et al., (1969). Excerpta Medical Int. Cong. Series 149, 11.*
6. *Tutwiler, G.F. (1978). Fed. Proc. 37, 745.*

GLICLAZIDE IN THE TREATMENT OF DIABETIC RETINOPATHY

F. Regnault*

According to present theories, capillary obliteration is the first clinical sign of diabetic retinopathy. It induces hypoxia in the neighboring zones and this, for some, is the common denominator of most manifestations of diabetic retinopathy. Should these theories be confirmed, disturbances in the platelet behaviour might be considered as one of the main pathogenetic mechanisms of diabetic retinopathy.

A recent synthesized oral anti-diabetic compound, gliclazide, structurally different from the sulphonylureas, has the novel action of changing platelet properties. It would appear that gliclazide, studied under various experimental conditions, controls abnormal functional hyperactivity in platelets and reduces the number of platelet-released factors (1,2). Having confirmed in previous studies the drug's efficacy in diabetes, we investigate the influence of this product on the course of diabetic retinopathy.

METHODS

Patients participating in the study were chosen on the basis of the following criteria:

Diabetes: type I (non insulin dependent) and type II (insulin dependent),

Retinal condition at initial examination:

either retinopathy at a non-proliferative stage,

or retina intact, but long-standing diabetes of at least 7 years .

Two randomly selected therapeutic groups were formed: a gliclazide-treated group and a control group. The same anti-diabetic treatment was prescribed throughout the trial. Treatment was changed in cases of poor diabetic stabilization and the patient eliminated from the trial. Fluorescence angiography and a retinography were carried out at the start of the treatment, then every six months after. The planned duration of treatment was 3 years.

According to retinal condition, each therapeutic group was subdivided into three groups:

intact retina;

angiographic retinopathy, i.e., lesions detectable only on angiographs;

clinical retinopathy with lesions visible on retinographs.

Ophthalmologic results were evaluated on fluorescent angiography pictures taking into account the overall changes, in all retinal vascular lesions (capillary occlusions, micro-aneurysms, capillary dilations, exudates) recorded at each examination (3):

aggravation

no change

improvement

Comparative statistics on the distribution of results in both therapeutic groups were carried out using the X^2 test.

RESULTS

Sixty-five patients whose features are shown in Table 1 were treated (mean duration of 32.5 ± 2.5 months).

The distribution of the oral anti-diabetic treatment in the 59 patients with retinopathy was the following:

GLICLAZIDE GROUP		CONTROL GROUP	
Gliclazide alone or combined with biguanide:	23	Sulphonylureas alone or combined with biguanide:	14
Gliclazide + Insulin :	8	Insulin :	14

TABLE 1

	GLICLAZIDE GROUP	NORMAL GROUP
Sex	19 males	20 males
	15 females	11 females
Age (years)	54 ± 4.3	50.1 ± 2.2
Known duration of diabetes	8.8 ± 2	10.1 ± 2.2
Retinal vascular state		
Normal	10	8
Retinopathy	54	53

In this report only the observations of patients with retinopathy at the beginning of the study have been considered. After random allocation, those two groups were comparable in regard to patient's features and metabolic state.

Diabetic Control

After treatment, the changes noted in body weight and fasting blood glucose levels are slight and without any statistical difference the two groups. In maturity-onset diabetes, the results were:

	GLICLAZIDE GROUP	CONTROL GROUP
Fasting blood glucose (g/l)	1.37 ± 0.12 ↓ 1.43 ± 0.15	1.36 ± 0.19 ↓ 1.57 ± 0.22
Body weight (kg)	68.65 ± 3.68 ↓ 68.35 ± 3.54	68.78 ± 6.23 ↓ 69.18 ± 6.43

Evolution of the Retinopathy

The results were based on the changes noted in the different retinal vascular abnormalities: capillary occlusions, microaneurysms, venous dilations, exudates. Coefficients were given according to the angiographical classification:

0	A	B	C	D
0	1	2	3	4

in order to realize a quantitative approach of the data (multifactorial discriminant analysis of Fisher*). A qualitative evaluation of the global evolution of the retinopathy was also performed.

Evolution of the Retinal Vascular Abnormalities

The changes noted in the grade of severity of each lesion are shown in the next table:

	Occlusions	Microaneurysms	Dilations	Exudates
GLICLAZIDE GROUP	- 6	- 10	- 1	+ 4
CONTROL GROUP	- 1	+ 6	+ 9	0

The discriminant analysis indicates a significant difference in the evolution of retinopathy in the two groups ($p < 0.01$).

The different retinal abnormalities are favourably influenced in the gliclazide group.

Global Evolution of Retinopathy

The results are distributed as follows:

in patients with diabetes (type I)

*We are indebted to Prof. Fondarai for this kind collaboration

	Worsening	No change	Improvement
GLICLAZIDE GROUP 39 ophthal. obs.	9 (23%)	14 (36%)	16 (41%)
CONTROL GROUP 27 ophthal. obs.	16 (59.3%)	6 (22.2%)	5 (18.5%)

In patients with diabetes type I + type II :

	Worsening	No change	Improvement
GLICLAZIDE GROUP 54 ophthal. obs.	13 (24.1%)	18 (33.3%)	23 (42.6%)
CONTROL GROUP 53 ophthal. obs.	29 (54.6%)	14 (26.4%)	10 (19%)

In the gliclazide treated group, the percentage of improvement is twice higher and the percentage of worsening twice lower than in the control group. The X^2 test confirms the statistical difference of evolution between the two groups ($p < 0.01$) and indicates that this difference concerns the percentage of improvement ($p < 0.01$) as well as the percentage of worsening ($p < 0.01$).

CONCLUSIONS

In the reported trial, after random allocation of treatments the two groups were comparable in regard to the relevant clinical details of the patients and to the history of diabetes. During the trial, only minor changes took place in the metabolic state. No statistical differences were found between the groups concerning the modification of body weight and glycemia. Therefore, the ophthalmological evaluation based on fluorescein angiography showed a marked and significant difference in the evolution of retinopathy characterized by a percentage of improvement twice higher and a percentage of worsening twice lower in the gliclazide group.

Since the two tested groups differed mainly as to which oral anti-diabetic was administered, the results obtained after a

32.5 months study support the view that gliclazide significantly influences the course of diabetic retinopathy by delaying and preventing the onset of retinal vascular lesions.

REFERENCES

1. *Vainer, H. and Verry M. (1974). Thrombosis Research, 4, 523.*
2. *Verry, M., et al. (1974). Entretiens de Bichat, Therapeutique.*
3. *Regnault, F., et al. (1973). Classification angiographique de la retinopathie diabetique. Bull. Soc. Ophtal. 1, 71.*

We wish to thank Professor Canivet and Doctors Deuil, Mundler, Puech and Barre and the ophthalmologists Doctors Rietzler, Bons and Lavat for their collaboration to this study.

DISCUSSION

J. ANDERSON: *Dr. Regnault, I wonder if any of your patients had proliferative retinopathy and whether you saw any retinal hemorrhage as a result? You indicated two patients had to be referred to an ophthalmologist. Is that a concern with this agent? Have you noticed anything in this regard?*

F. REGNAULT: *In our trial, we did not find any retinal hemorrhages which can be attributed to the treatment.*

S. PODOLSKY: *Dr. Regnault, I wonder whether this drug interferes with platelet adhesion in vitro, or platelet aggregation, or some other one of the many in vitro tests?*

F. REGNAULT: *The only thing I presented was the clinical effect of this drug and, as far as the mechanism is concerned, I cannot give you any conclusive data.*

P. L. POFFENBARGER: *Dr. Tutwiler, following the administration of your drug, have you measured insulin-like activity in any of the dog or human studies?*

E. TUTWILER: *No, we haven't looked at that at all, I'm sorry.*

E. PFEIFFER: *Dr. Norris, how many of your patients were on insulin before you switched them to oral agents?*

E. NORRIS: *In the U.S. studies, I think very few, if any, of the patients have previously been on insulin. They almost all, if not all, have been either previously treated with sulfonylureas, or were newly diagnosed diabetics. In some of the European studies, there were patients who had previously been on insulin. There were some studies done with the intravenous form of glipizide and, from a kinetic point of view, the oral and intravenous forms seem to act similarly, a rapid peak and a rapid fall-off. So, in that regard, it would more mimic tolbutamide, but the activity seemed to last longer than tolbutamide.*

M. de GASPARO: *I would like to ask Dr. Norris and Dr. Tutwiler if their compound bound to some plasma fraction and if this binding is accompanied with inactivation of the drug? Also, Dr. Tutwiler, have you measured the insulin release in the portal vein in vitro, and finally, is there any action of this compound on adrenaline?*

E. NORRIS: *As far as protein binding of glipizide is concerned, it is very highly bound, something over 90%.*

E. TUTWILER: *Obviously, piroglíride hasn't been studied as extensively as some of the other drugs. I know it is protein bound but not as extensively as the sulfonylureas by any stretch of the imagination. As far as your questions about portal vein insulins are concerned, we've not yet looked at those. I would just comment that we do not believe that the drug affects the adrenal, because the drug is still very hyperglycemic in adreanlectomized animals. We've shown a number of direct effects for the drug on certain isolated tissues. One of these that's quite exciting to us is that, at very low concentrations, the drug has a direct effect to enhance glucose metabolism. Very recently, we've gotten some more exciting data which also appears to do this on the islets. If we can confirm this, it might explain the effect on insulin secretion. At this point, we think that the drug is really working by bimodal or multimodal mechanism.*

N. FREINKEL: *Dr. Tutwiler, have any other nutrient secretogogues been tested with regard to potentiation? Dr. Norris, you showed us nice data around the clock sampling for insulin, but is there any data available with regard to acute phases in insulin release? In other words, the precise kinetics, not at the hourly intervals which were shown on the illustration, but with any kind of nutrient challenge, say 5-6-7 hours after a preceding oral dose of the agent?*

E. TUTWILER: *We were surprised at the effect we got in the arginine infused dog, because we had not seen increases in the insulin levels before, and suddenly, after an arginine infusion, we gave the drug and there were increases which now were clearly discernible. I know there have been various reports in the literature that arginine can potentiate insulin secretogogues. We are interested in looking at that.*

E. NORRIS: *Dr. Freinkel, to the best of my knowledge, those data are not available.*

C. HELLERSTROM: *We have maintained isolated mouse islet in tissue culture in the presence of two micromoles of glucose over a period of 1 week to 10 days and 2 micromoles of glucose corresponds to about 18 micrograms per mm. We could see an increased insulin release only during the first 3 days of exposure, and then there was no difference at all in the release of insulin to the culture medium. We were, however, alarmed by the fact that, at the end of the culture period, there was a statistical significant inhibition of insulin biosynthesis in islets which have been exposed to the drug. Also, there was profound degranulation and depletion of insulin, so the outcome of these experi-*

ments would indicate that only in the acute exposure can you see an increased insulin release. After that, there is a kind of adaptation to the drug.

H. LEBOVITZ: *There are other studies wherein it was found that patients, treated chronically for a year on glibenclimide, had decreased insulin levels in blood and a decreased percentage of proinsulin. The questions were raised as to whether there was inhibition of proinsulin biosynthesis in the chronically treated patients. That data can only be interpreted from the numbers which are available.*

M. de GASPARO: *I wonder if there is good data on possible cell neogenesis after oral compounds:*

C. HELLERSTROM: *We have studied this problem in culture islets, and I can only report that there was no increase whatsoever for one week after tolbutamide.*

R. CAMERINI-DAVALOS: *Dr. Norris, I was under the impression that there were some experimental studies with glipizide in isolated heart in rats, measuring many parameters without major changes. Am I correct?*

E. NORRIS: *Yes.*

H. LEBOVITZ: *Yes, there have been no cardiovascular effects reported. Likewise, there are some acute insulin secretory studies, which I think were acute bursts, but I can't remember the exact data.*

R. CAMERINI-DAVALOS: *Right, there were acute experiments done regarding the levels of insulin in the chronic treatment of early diabetes.*

B. METZGER: *I'd like to ask about the possibility of hypoglycemia. I was impressed that, in the slide which Dr. Norris showed, the level of glucose fell in the second 24 hours, when the glipizide was given without meals. Then, on one of his slides, he showed postprandial reactive hypoglycemia, with blood sugars falling into the range of 50.*

E. NORRIS: *You are correct in your reading of the graphs, and what is significant is that none of the patients reported any symptoms related to hypoglycemia.*

H. LEBOVITZ: *We have had one or two patients who got a very brisk early insulin response after they were just started on the drug for the first 2 months. Some of those patients, who had both a very brisk insulin response to glucose plus a marked potentiation of insulin action, actually got reactive hypoglycemia. We put them on a low carbohydrate diet for a short period of time, until the insulin secretion began to fall back down, and then it disappeared.*

M. J. PETERSON: *Dr. Tutwiler, Dr. Norris showed that there is little insulin release in fasted men with glipizide administration, but that after meals there is rather good release, and I'm just wondering if you've studied your drug under similar circumstances?*

E. TUTWILER: *It hasn't really been studied well enough. I really don't want to comment on that. There have been some increases in fasted men, but I don't know if we have enough data to make a comment.*

THE EFFECT OF REPETITIVE EXERCISE ON DAILY CONTROL OF GLYCEMIA IN INSULIN-DEPENDENT DIABETIC PATIENTS

R.Coce, R.Femenic, Z. Skrabalo and M.Vranic*

In the postabsorptive state, glucose needs of the muscle are met by a precisely matched release of glucose from the liver (1). The precise nature of this coordination is not yet known, but many regulatory components have been investigated systematically. Glucose production increases under the influence of decreased levels of insulin and increased levels of glucagon (2) and catecholamines (3). A number of endogenous factors can affect glucose utilization: muscular activity factors (4), nonsuppressible insulin-like activity (5), changed sensitivity of insulin receptors (6), hypoxia (7) and changes in cytoplasmatic calcium levels (8). The relative importance of these factors is not established, but they may act as amplifiers of insulin, which(on the basis of in vivo and in vitro data) is considered to be essential for stimulation of glucose uptake during exercise (1,9). It is also indicated that increased blood flow and augmented capillary area can provide an adequate amount of insulin to the muscle, even when its concentration in blood is low (1). Catecholamines can interfere with glucose uptake by the muscle directly by increasing muscle glycogenolysis and indirectly by increasing lipolysis and then enhancing oxidation of fatty acids in the working muscle (for review see reference 10)

The studies, in dogs and man, led to the conclusion that the effect of exercise on glucose homeostasis in diabetes can be related in part, to levels of insulin in plasma. (Fig. 1, reference 10)

a) When insulin is below basal levels during exercise, as documented in normal dogs (4) and humans (11), increments of glucose production and utilization are of the same magnitude and plasma glucose does not change. The same phenomenon also occurs in depancreatized dogs infused intraportally with insulin where measured IRI levels were below basal levels (1). Normoglycemia and increased glucose turnover were also seen in diabetics infused peripherally with insulin, IRI levels in such patients could not be measured because of the presence of insulin antibodies (11). The increased flux of

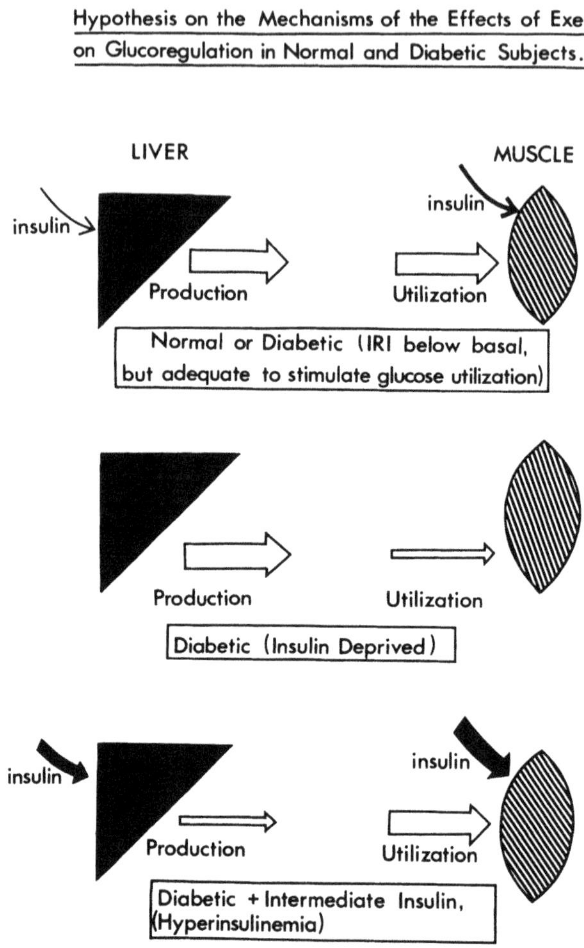

Fig. 1

glucose into the exercising muscles of diabetic patients (11, 12,13) presumably due to the presence of low but adequate circulating insulin levels, could indeed be metabolically advantageous to the diabetic.

b) In insulin-deficient states, exercise fails to stimulate glucose utlization (1,9,14), hence the exercise-induced increase in glucose production (1,14) leads to a rise in blood glucose levels. Under these conditions, exercise has a deleterious effect on glucose homeostasis. An essential role of insulin in regulating glucose uptake in the working muscle thus becomes apparent.

c) If exercise is performed following the subcutaneous injection of insulin, insulin levels frequently are above normal, and in addition, the delivery of exogenous insulin into the circulation can be accelerated inducing a further increase in plasma insulin levels. Glucose production rates are inhibited (or do not rise appropriately) due to hyperinsulinism during exercise and, hence, the increased peripheral glucose utilization leads to a fall in blood glucose levels (11,15). The hypoglycemic reactions are not likely to occur in the fasted state, when the liver is the only source of glucose, and an excess of insulin can block production of newly formed glucose. The exercise-induced increase in IRI was seen in depancreatized dogs (15), in diabetics treated with lente insulin, in whom IRI concentrations could be measured as these diabetics did not develop insulin antibodies (11), in patients injected subcutaneously with iodinated radioactive crystalline insulin, where the disappearance of radioactivity was monitored externally (16), and in rats and men injected with tritiated crystalline insulin, where the appearance of tritiated insulin was monitored in plasma (17,18).

The hypothesis regarding the significance of plasma IRI in the control of glycemia in diabetic patients (Fig.1), is related mainly to the postabsorptive state, in which the liver represents the only source of glucose necessary to match the energy needs of the exercising muscle. It was the aim of preliminary studies reported here, to find out whether exercise could affect the daily control of glycemia in diabetics injected with long acting insulin and given 6 meals per day.Generally,one can expect that insulin treated diabetics will have peripheral hyperinsulinemia in the resting state, as has been documented in depancreatized dogs (15). In contrast to normal subjects, exogenous insulin is not suppressed by exercise, but as reviewed above, its mobilation can be enhanced. It was of interest to find out the immediate and prolonged effects which exercise might have on postprandial plasma glucose in insulin-injected patients.

MATERIALS AND METHODS

Subjects studies

Six male insulin-dependent diabetics were studied in the Zagreb Diabetes Institute. The subjects were non-obese and had diabetes diagnosed 13-25 days before the commencement of the study. They were hospitalized during the period of the two studies. They were in good nutritional balance and were on weight-maintaining diets (40% carbohydrate, 40% fat and 20% protein). There was no clinical or laboratory evidence of diabetic complications, and hepatic, renal, cardiac and circulatory functions were normal. A normal exercise electrocardiogram was a pre-requisite to participation in the study. Anthropomorphic data on the subjects and details of their diabetic history are given in Table 1.

Table 1

ANTHROPOMORPHIC DATA OF THE PATIENTS

Patient	Age (yrs)	Sex	Height (cm)	Weight (kg)	Duration of diabetes (insulin treatment) before the rest & exercise studies	Insulin (type)	Dose (U/d)	Diet (calories)
1	25	M	198	91	18/21	Lente	12	2000
2	24	M	175	85.5	19/23	Regular	12	1300
						Lente	20	
3	26	M	178	65.5	25/29	Regular	16	2000
						Lente	20	
4	44	M	182	75.2	22/30	Reular	12	2500
						Lente	20	
5	55	M	177	82	15/18	Regular	24	2000
						lente	20	
6	37	M	176	66	13/18	Regular	16	2500
						Lente	20	

On the morning of the study, a double lumen catheter was inserted into a forearm vein for continuous blood glucose monitoring (in 3 patients for 14 hours and in the other 3 patients for 21 hours). Another catheter was introduced into a contralateral forearm vein for sampling of blood for measurements of concentrations of C-peptide, pyruvate, lactate, FFA and glycerol. At 7:00 a.m., the patients were given their usual dose of insulin, as indicated in Table 1. Their daily caloric intake was divided into 6 rations: breakfast (8:00 a.m.), snack (10:00 a.m.), lunch (1:00 p.m.), snack (4:00 p.m.), dinner (7:00 p.m.), and the last snack (9:00 p.m.). During the first protocol, the patients were lying comfortably in bed throughout the test period. Three to seven days later, the same protocol was followed except that 30 minutes after the first snack, and 1 hour after lunch and dinner respectively, the patients were exercising on an ergometer bicycle for 20-30 minutes at a work load of 70-100 watts (approximately 50% Vmax). Continuous blood glucose monitoring was maintained throughout the exercise periods.

Processing of blood samples

The continuous monitoring of plasma glucose was performed using a Technicon auto-analyzer with a glucose oxidase technique; glucose measurements were averaged for each 30 min period. The instrument was standardized internally with glucose solutions and externally by calibrating with at least two simultaneously obtained plasma samples also analyzed with a glucose oxidase technique. Lactate (19), pyruvate (20) and glycerol (21) were determined enzymatically and free fatty acids were determined by the method of Dole and Meinertz (22). Plasma C-peptide was determined by the radioimmunossay kit (RIA-mat, Byk-MallincKrodt).

RESULTS AND DISCUSSION

In the morning of the study, the mean plasma glucose levels from 7:30 to 1-:30 a.m. (time of first exercise period on the day of exercise) varied in the 6 patients between 170 and 320 mg%. The plasma glucose concentrations were randomly distributed between the 2 days of study. In 2 patients, the plasma glucose levels were higher on the day of experiment, in three patients on the day of rest and in one patient they were equal on both days.

Table 2

MEAN PLASMA GLUCOSE LEVELS (BETWEEN 7:30 A.M. - 1:00 P.M. AND 1:30 - 9:00 P.M.) IN 6 INSULIN DEPENDENT DIABETICS RESTING OR SUBJECTED TO THREE EXERCISE PERIODS

Patient	Glucose (mg%)			
	7:30 a.m.-1:00 p.m.		1:30 p.m.- 9:00 p.m.	
	Rest	Exercise	Rest	Exercise
1	135	161	143	98
2	165	196	181	105
3	189	168	138	100
4	276	209	228	172
5	219	141	119	86
6	315	248	264	181
Mean $\pm$ SEM	217 ± 28	187 ± 16	162 ± 16	124 ± 17
Paired t test	t=1.47 (not significant)		t=6.60 ($p<0.001$)	

Table 2 shows the mean plasma glucose concentrations in each patient during rest and exercise periods respectively. The first exercise period did not affect plasma glucose; there was no significant difference between the rest and exercise days between 8:30 a.m. - 1:00 p.m. Exercise periods, however, lowered plasma glucose consistently in each patient in the period between 1:30 - 9:00 p.m. This difference is highly significant statistically (paired t-test). It is remarkable that despite the intake of meals, in 4 exercising patients, the mean plasma glucose values were within normal limits. The other 2 patients were hyperglycemic, but glycemia was markedly reduced when compared to the resting days. The mean values of all exercising patients were 40 mg% lower than in resting conditions.

Figures 2-4 show individual data in three patients.

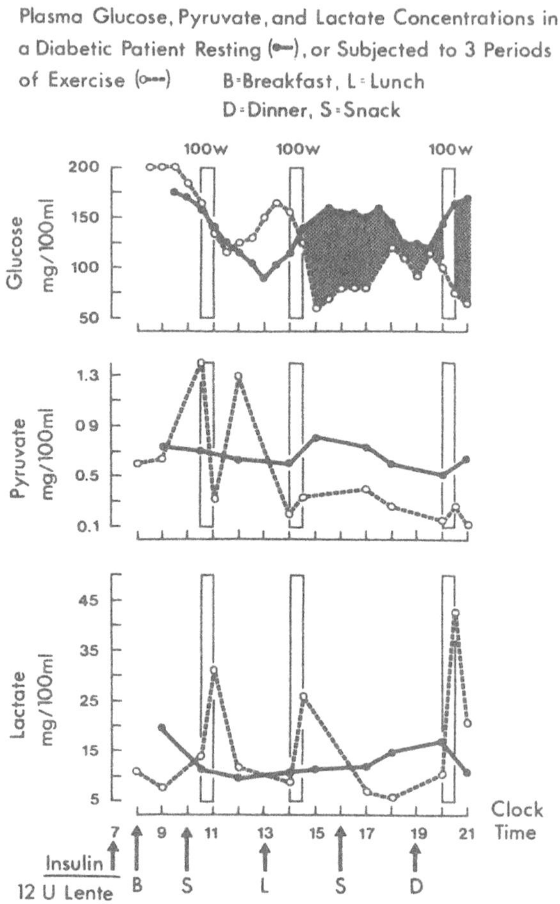

Fig. 2

Figure 2 (patient number 1) and Figure 3 (patient number 3) clearly illustrate that the first exercise period did not exert an effect on glycemia, but a markedly improved glycemic profile was observed from the second exercise period until the end of the study. Figure 4 (patient number 4) illustrates a study in which glucose monitoring was continued for 24 hours. The exercise regimen stabilized the glucose profile which on the resting day, had indicated a pattern of large glucose gluctuations. The effect of exercise was evident up to 1:00 a.m. The three figures also illustrate the responses of lactate and pyruvate . These gluconeogenic precursors were fairly stable during the day when the patients were resting and food intake did not affect this pattern. However, in all patients, each exercise period induced a marked, but transient, increase in lactate concentration and in 2 patients the concentration of pyruvate was

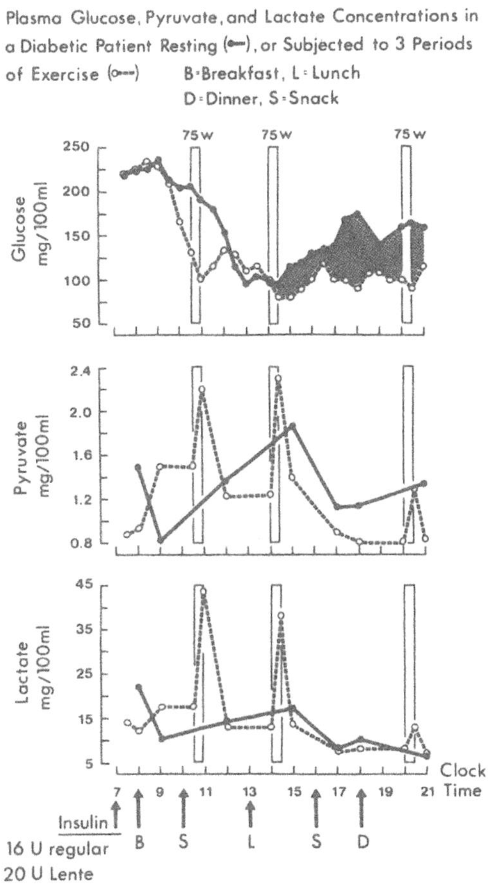

Fig. 3

also affected in a similar manner. In 7 out of 18 exercise periods, physical activity induced an increase in FFA concentration whereas exercise did not affect glycerol levels.

C-peptide concentrations could be detected in all patients. In three patients (1,3,5), C-peptide was present in normal concentrations (2-3 ng/ml), whereas in the remaining three patients (2,4, 6) C-peptide was below normal (1.0-1.7 ng/ml). Characteristically for the diabetic state, the concentration of C-peptide was not increased after food ingestion; a marginal response to meals was noted only in one patient. Exercise did not have any effects on C-peptide plasma values.

Thus repetitive exercise has indeed improved glucose control in all 6 patients studied, but only after the second and third exercise periods. This beneficial effect was not confined to the time of exercise but persisted for a period of at least 12 hours. These data

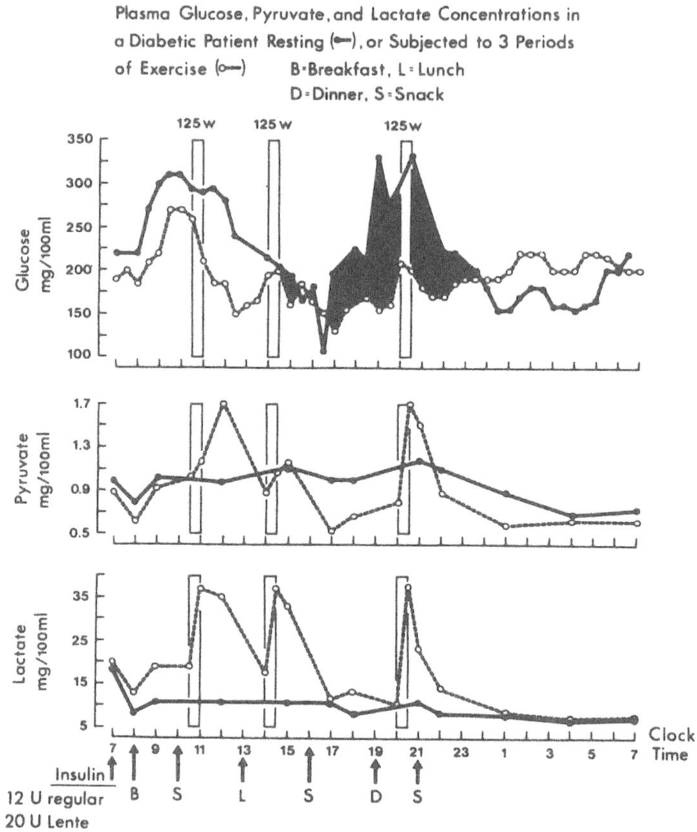

Fig. 4

are preliminary and are now being extended by including diabetic patients in which the sequence of studies will be reversed; that is exercise studies will precede those in resting patients. In addition, normal controls will be included to compare the control of glycemia in diabetics to normals subjected to the same exercise and diet regimen.

The diabetic patients were treated with insulin for 14-30 days prior to the studies in order to minimize formation of insulin antibodies. In order to study the role of insulin in glucoregulation of these patients, it will be necessary to complete IRI measurements in those patients, where absence of antibodies has been documented. The measurements of C-peptide indicate that in all diabetic patients studied, the deficiency of the endogenous source of insulin has been documented, because C-peptide was not affected either by food intake or by exercise. The increased levels of pyruvate and lactate during exercise indicate that glucose was only partially oxidized when fuel oxidation in the muscle was substantially increased.

The surprisingly prolonged effect of repetitive exercise on control of plasma glucose cannot be explained at present, but a number of possibilities can be mentioned. It may be that the increased sensitivity of insulin receptors observed during exercise (6) may persist for a period of much longer duration than the period of exercise itself. Likewise, the increased blood flow and enlarged capillary area may affect availability of insulin and substrates to the muscle (1) for a prolonged period of time perhaps through adaptive enzymatic changes. Furthermore, it is well known that exercise decreases motility of the gastrointestinal tract and therefore, can delay food absorption. A blunting of the food absorption peaks could also account for better control of glycemia in diabetics when insulin release is correlated with food absorption. Such a persistent effect is consistent with decreased insulin requirements in diabetics chronically subjected to periods of increased physical activity.

In summary then, our preliminary experiments indicate that repetitive exercise can exert a prolonged beneficial effect on control of glycemia in fed insulin-dependent diabetics. The mechanism of such an effect remains to be explored. It is noteworthy that hypoglycemic reactions did not occur during or after the 18 exercise periods in the 6 diabetic patients studies.

REFERENCES

1. *Vranic, M. et al (1976) J. Clin. Invest., 57,245*
2. *Issekutz,B. and Vranic, M. (1978) Diabetes, 27, suppl. 2, 454*
3. *Issekutz,B. (1979) Diabetes, 28 (in press)*
4. *Goldstein, M.S., et al (1953) Am. J. Physiol., 173, 212*
5. *Couturier,E. et al (1971) Horm. Met. Res., 3, 382*
6. *Soman,V. et al (1978) Diabetes, 27, suppl. 2, 449*
7. *Randle,P.J. and Smith,G.H. (1958) Biochem. J., 70, 501*
8. *Hollowsky,J.O. and Narahara,H.T. (1967) J. Gen. Physiol., 50,551*
9. *Berger, M. et al (1975) Biochem. J., 146, 231*
10. *Vranic,M and Berger, M. (1979) Diabetes, 28 (in press)*
11. *Zinman,B. et al (1977) J. Clin. Endocrin. Metabl.,45, 641*
12. *Felig,P. and Wahren,J. (1975) N. Engl. J. Med., 293, 1078*
13. *Sanders, C.A. et al (1964) N. Engl. J. Med., 271, 220*
14. *Vranic,M. and Wrenshall,G.A. (1969) Endocrinology, 85, 165*
15. *Kawamori,R. and Vranic,M. (1977) J. Clin. Invest., 59, 331*
16. *Koivisto,V.A. and Felig,P. (1978) N. Engl. J. Med., 298, 77*
17. *Berger,M. et al (1978) Diabetologia, 15, 133*
18. *Berger,M. et al (1979) Diabetes, 28 (in press)*
19. *Gutman,I. and Wahlefeld,A.W. (1974) In: Methoden der enzymatischen analyse 3. Auflage, Band II, Verlag Chemie, Weinheim,1510*
20. *Czok, R. and Lamprecht (1974). In: Methods of Enzymatic Analysis, 2nd English ed. Verlag Chemie Wienheim and Academic Press,Inc., New York and London 4, p. 1446.*

21. Eggstein, M. (1966). Klin. Wschr., 44, 267.
22. Dole, V.P. and Meinertz, H.J. (1960). J. Lipid Res., 1, 199.

DISCUSSION

G. M. REAVEN: *We have taken "chronic exercise rats" and looked at insulin sensitivity in perfused organs. Muscle uptake of glucose, under a low dose of insulin, was greatly accelerated as a result of chronic exercise. On the other hand, the liver became relatively insulin resistant to the same dose, and that might again fit into your scheme.*

N. FREINKEL: *I want to ask what your current thought is as to exercise per se, promoting glucose utilization via insulin and just providing a permissive action?*

M. VRANIC: Well, *I think the word "permissive" means really what one tries to attribute to it. The fact is that glucose utilization in the muscle can be greatly promoted if you have insulin around, and the circulating insulin can be quite low, but not below a certain level. In dogs, it is about 5 to 6 microunits, which is still enough. Most people agree now that it is most probably due to enhanced blood flow and the enhanced capillary area in the muscle that, despite that the circulating insulin is low, more insulin nevertheless can enter into muscle. It may be that it is not only a permissive effect, but that it is regulatory if more insulin comes into the muscle. The other very important observation comes from Felig. Namely, exercise for 2 or 3 hours can increase sensitivity of receptors for insulin.*

H. LEBOVITZ: *Do you have any experiments in which you've given insulin intravenously as you have given somatostatin, rather than in long acting form?*

M. VRANIC: *Yes, this worked. We did it in dogs and in humans. In dogs, we infused peripherally. Glucose production increased, and the increase of glucose utilization was practically normal, both in dogs and in juvenile humans.*

H. LEBOVITZ: *Do you really think that there is no effect of exercise itself directly on the muscle? This is all an insulin mediated effect?*

M. VRANIC: *I don't think we can say that. All we can say is that there is a low amount of circulating insulin and we can speculate that there is a very elaborate scheme. In this scheme, you can include muscular activity factors like the one of Goldstein and calcium shifts. So, there must be a number of factors, induced by exercise, which act in addition to insulin.*

H. LEBOVITZ: *In the perfused muscle of the chronically exercised animal, one can show no effect of increased glucose uptake without having insulin availble.*

T. DECKERT: *With regard to Lebovitz' remark, in every case of juvenile diabetes, who could not produce any C-Peptide under exercise in the artificial pancreas, the infusion rate of insulin went down. This means that physical exercise will increase the glucose uptake.*

M. VRANIC: *Yes, but that was not so in the artificial pancreas of the group in Toronto, where the juvenile diabetics were infused. It depends a lot on the type of exercise. It depends on many things.*

ISOLATION AND PRESERVATION IN VITRO OF HUMAN PANCREATIC ISLETS INTENDED FOR TRANSPLANTATION

C. Hellerström*, B. Nilsson, S. Sandler,
A. Andersson, A. Agren and B. Petersson

Transplantation of pancreatic B-cells to diabetic patients would be an ideal way of restoring glycemic control and probably protecting against the development of vascular complications. While this goal has been achieved by syngeneic transplantation of isolated islets to diabetic animals (1), a number of problems have arisen in the clinical situation (2). Whole-organ pancreatic transplantation is followed by both immunological reactions and surgical complications. Obviously, some of these problems can be avoided by the use of isolated islets, but the yield of islets, by present isolation techniques, from a single human pancreas is insufficient for transplantation purposes (3). However, if isolated islets from several donors could be preserved in a visable state, it should be possible to collect a sufficient number of islets for meaningful transplantation to diabetic patients. It is the purpose of the present survey to briefly describe methods for preservation of islets either in tissue culture or at subzero temperature.

I. ISOLATION AND PRESERVATION OF ADULT HUMAN ISLETS IN TISSUE CULTURE

In 1972, we described a method for tissue culture of isolated mammalian islets, which has now been applied to the maintenance of human islets in vitro (3-4). The principles of the technique are as follows: Islets are isolated by collagenase digestion and transferred to plastic tissue culture dishes containing 5 ml culture medium TCM 199 supplemented with 10% calf serum, antibiotics and 5.5 mM glucose. More recently, we have used as an alternative culture medium RPMI 1640, which seems to offer a better preservation of the insulin response to glucose. The cultures are incubated at +37°C in a gas phase consisting of 5% CO_2 in humidified air. The medium is changed after 3 days and subsequently every second day. At the end of the culture period, islets are harvested mechanically by means of a "rubber policeman" and further processed for morphological or biochemical studies.

The viability of human islets in the culture system described above has been evaluated in a series of experiments using a total of 55 pancreatic glands obtained from brain dead kidney donors in the age range 8-65 years. In agreement with findings in other laboratories, the isolation of human islets presented serious technical problems, and the yield of islets remained limited, varying from about 100 up to several thousands of islets per gland. Furthermore, with the conventional collagenase isolation technique, it was difficult to process an entire gland in a reasonable period of time, and we therefore developed a digestion/filtration chamber, which considerably streamlined and improved the isolation procedure. The principles and use of the device are described in Fig. 1. This procedure consistently increased the yield of human islets, and also allowed the simultaneous digestion of an entire human pancreatic gland.

The morphological and metabolic properties of the isolated human islets were evaluated after 1 or 3 weeks in culture (3). Electron microscopic studies indicated a well preserved ultrastructure with few necrotic or damaged cells. The in vitro oxygen consumption of the islets proceeded at a constant rate for more than two hours and was of the same order of magnitude as previously observed in fresh mouse islets. An increase in the glucose concentration of the medium caused an immediate enhancement of the respiratory rate, again in agreement with previous observations in mice (4).

It was worthy of note that islets maintained for one week in culture responded to glucose with a marked increase of the insulin release and a significant suppression of the glucagon secretion. Perifusion experiments with one-week cultured human islets indicated that the temporal pattern of glucose-stimulated insulin release resembled that which has been previously demonstrated with rat and mouse islets. Furthermore, gel filtration of extracts of cultured islets which had been incubated for 3 hours with ^{3}H-leucine or ^{3}H-phenylalanine showed a marked incorporation of radioactivity into proteins eluting with either the proinsulin or insulin markers. The elution pattern indicated that proinsulin was being converted to insulin at a rate very similar to that previously found in the rat. This pattern of incorporation was seen in extracts of islets cultured either for one or three weeks.

These combined studies indicate that viable islets can be isolated from the pancreas of adult donors and maintained in tissue culture. Indeed, by this means, human islets have been kept for more than 5 months without significant decrease in the insulin response to glucose or glucose plus theophylline (5).

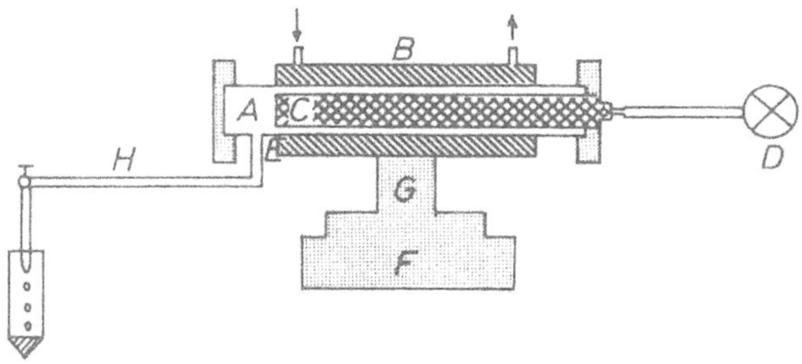

Fig. 1. Digestion/filtration chamber used for isolation of human pancreatic islets. The unit consists of a chromatography column (A) (Model K26, Pharmacia Fine Chemicals, Uppsala, Sweden; 2.6 x 23 cm) fitted with an outer water jacket (B) and an inner filter chamber (C), made from nylon net (250 μ mesh width). The transparent column is connected to a peristaltic pump (D) (Minipuls 2, Gilson, Aronville-les-Gonesse, France) and has an outlet (E) which is kept closed during the digestion. The filtration/digestion chamber is attached to a shaker (F), which can accommodate up to four similar chambers. The shaker moves in an opposite direction to the column and can be tilted (G) to allow filling and emptying. Before digestion, the pancreas is finely diced and suspended in about 100 ml Hanks' solution, supplemented with 5.5 mM glucose, 25 mM HEPES and antibiotics (penicillin 100 U/ml; streptomycin 0.1 mg/ml). After addition of 5 mg/ml collagenase, 25 ml of the tissue suspension is transferred to the filter chamber (C) and violently shaken (250 strokes/min). The temperature is maintained at +35°C by water circulating through the jacket. After 5-7 min of shaking, samples of fluid from the space outside the filter are taken for examination under the stereomicroscope. When isolated islets appear, usually within 10 min, the chamber is emptied and the collagenase solution replaced by pumping pre-warmed Hanks' solution through the tube (H). After separation, by centrifugation of the tissue suspended in the collagenase solution, the Hanks' solution is pumped out and the supernatant from the collagenase suspension reintroduced into the digestion chamber. This cycle is repeated for about 20 min or until no more islets or tissue fragments are recovered. The digested tissue specimens are quickly washed several times in Hanks' solution and put on ice before further separation of islets by hand picking and explantation into culture dishes.

II. PRESERVATION OF FETAL HUMAN PANCREAS IN TISSUE CULTURE

Although the techniques described above seem to be useful for both isolation and storage of pancreatic islets of adult man, the limited supply of donor pancreas and the still consistently insufficient yield of islets make meaningful attempts at transplantation very difficult. An alternative approach might be the use of fetal human pancreas with a high growth potential, which may sufficiently expand the B-cell volume to meet the insulin demands of a transplanted diabetic patient. Work in experimental animals indicates that pancreatic tissue obtained from rat fetuses is able to completely reverse severe diabetes in syngeneic recipients (6-7). Furthermore, pioneering work by Milner et al (8), Fujimoto & Williams (9) and Goldman & Colle (10) suggests that human fetal endocrine pancreas can survive in tissue culture. We have now extended these studies with a view to a more detailed characterization of the function in culture of the fetal pancreas.

Pancreas material was obtained from 18 human fetuses with estimated gestational ages of 15-24 weeks. The pancreas was dissected within an hour of legal abortion, induced by prostaglandin, and diced into minute pieces before being suspended in culture medium TCM 199 supplemented with 20% calf serum, antibiotics and, except otherwise stated, glucose to a final concentration of 5.5 mM. The culture dishes were subsequently maintained for 6-13 days at +37°C in a gas phase of 5% CO_2 in humidified air. The medium was changed after the first 36 hours and subsequently every day.

A histological examination of pancreatic specimens at the end of the culture period showed numerous well preserved islet cells scattered within a connective tissue stroma containing very few acinar cells. Hormone extractions of pancreatic specimens indicated the occurrence of insulin, glucagon and somatostatin already in the freshly excised pancreas. However, during the culture period the concentration of insulin and glucagon increased 14 times and that of somatostatin 36 times suggesting an excellent preservation of the endocrine pancreatic cells. This observation, also, suggests the degeneration of other cell types but should not be taken as evidence for a selective growth of endocrine tissue. The insulin release to the medium on the first and eleventh day of culture is shown in Table 1. Whereas an increase of the glucose concentration failed to stimulate the insulin release on the first day of culture ($p > 0.05$) there was a significant stimulation on the eleventh day of culture ($p < 0.01$). Addition of glucose in the presence of theophylline strongly stimulated insulin release at both these time points. However, under these conditions, the rate of insulin release was consistently higher on the eleventh than on the first day of culture

TABLE 1

Day of culture	No of observations	Additions to the culture medium		
		3.3mM glucose	16.7 mM glucose	16.7 mM glucose + 10 mM theophylline
1	8	1.6±0.2	2.7±0.7	10.1±1.3
11	8	1.7±0.1	3.9±0.6	16.2±1.8

Insulin release from cultured human fetal pancreas. The pancreatic specimens were incubated in the culture dishes at +37°C for three successive 4-hour periods in TCM 199 containing antibiotics and the concentrations of glucose, or glucose plus theophylline, given in the Table. Serum was omitted during these experiments. The insulin released to the incubation medium is expressed as ng/h/mg wet weight of tissue explanted on day 1.

($p < 0.001$), suggesting a net increase of the B-cell mass during culture. In further studies, cultured explants were incubated with radioactive amino acids in order to study the biosynthesis of insulin and glucagon. Absorption of immunoreactive material in pancreatic extracts to Sepharose-bound insulin and glucagon antibodies demonstrated a significant synthesis of both insulin and glucagon in the cultured specimens. These combined data confirm that human fetal pancreas can survive in culture over extended periods of time.

III. PRESERVATION OF ISLETS AT SUBZERO TEMPERATURE

Long-term storage of isolated islets intended for clinical transplantation would be considerably simplified if the tissue could be stored frozen without loss of viability. So far, however, knowledge seems to be limited as regards cryopreservation of isolated islets Ferguson et al (11) reported that subzero storage of rat islets, frozen in the presence of dimethylsulphoxide (DMSO), was compatible with a preserved insulin response to glucose after thawing. More recently, Rajotte et al (12) concluded from their observations on rat islets, that these specimens appeared to survive freeze-thawing, although their data on the islet response to glucose gives no firm support for this conclusion. However, Brown et al (6) using cryopreserved fetal rat pancreas observed a complete reversal of diabetes in isologous recipient rats after transplantation of only one fetal pancreas.

We have recently studied isolated mouse pancreatic islets in order to evaluate, in quantitative terms, the preservation of insulin biosynthesis and release after storage at subzero temperature (-196°C). For this purpose islets were isolated with collagenase and maintained for 2 days in tissue culture using RPMI 1640 supplemented with 11.1 mM glucose and 10% calf serum as culture medium. The islets were then frozen at 0.4-0.8°C/min, in the presence of 1 M DMSO, until they reached a temperature of -80°C and were subsequently stored at -196°C. Thawing was performed rapidly (<1 min) to ± 0°C, followed by dilution of the DMSO-containing cryoprotective medium. The islets were cultured for another 2 days in the identical conditions prior to freezing and subsequently studied with regard to insulin release and biosynthesis.

Initial experiments showed that the rates of freezing and thawing are critical to the recovery of morphologically intact islets. Thus, the slow freezing and quick thawing procedures indicated above are compatible with almost 100 per cent recovery

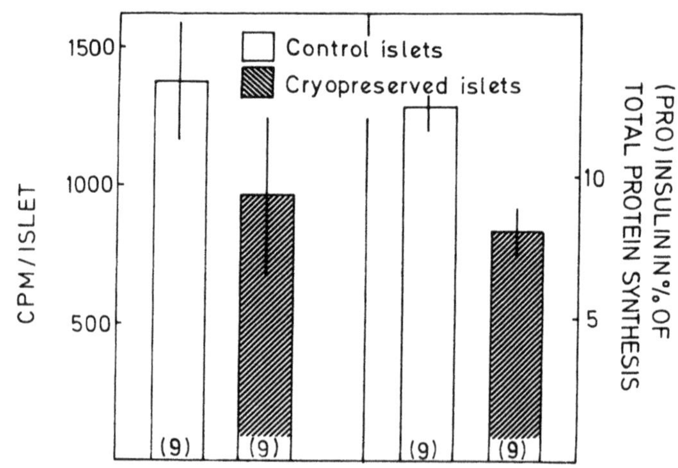

Fig. 2. Biosynthesis of (pro) insulin after cryopreservation of isolated mouse islets. Insulin and total islet protein biosynthesis were measured using an immune-binding technique. The glucose concentration of the incubation medium was 16.7 mM. Means ± S.E.M.

of the cryopreserved islets. When exposed to glucose (15 mM) and theophylline (5 mM) in a perifusion system, these islets released insulin biphasically, although at a lower rate than non-frozen control islets. Similarly, the cryopreserved islets synthesized insulin in response to glucose, the average rate being about 70 per cent of that observed in the control islets (Fig. 2).

These studies suggest that isolated islets can be kept at subzero temperatures without major loss of their specific functions. However, the techniques used for freezing and thawing still have to be refined in order to maintain complete viability of the stored specimens.

REFERENCES

1. *Lacy, P.E. (1978). Diabetes, 27, 427*
2. *Gliedman, M.L., et al (1978). Diabetes Care, 1, 1*
3. *Andersson, A., et al (1976). J. Clin. Invest. 57, 1295*
4. *Andersson, A., Hellerström, C. (1972). Diabetes, 21, 546*
5. *Høiriis-Nielsen, J., et al (1978). Diabetologia in press*
6. *Brown, J., et al (1977). In "Diabetes" (Bajaj, J.S. ed.) Excerpta Medica, Amsterdam, 535*
7. *McEvoy, R.C. Hegre, O.D. (1977). In "Diabetes" (Bajaj, J.S. ed.) Excerpta Medica, Amsterdam, 556*
8. *Milner, R.D.G., et al (1977). In "Pancreatic Beta Cell Culture" (Wasielewski, E. von, Chick, W.L. eds.) Excerpta Medica, Amsterdam, 143*
9. *Fujimoto, W.Y., Williams, R.H. (1972). Endocrinology, 91, 1133*
10. *Goldman, H., Colle, E. (1976). Science, 192, 1014*
11. *Ferguson, J., et al (1976). Diabetologia, 12, 115*
12. *Rajotte, R.V., et al (1977). Cryobiology, 14, 116*

Financial support was given by the Swedish Medical Research Council, the Nordic Insulin Fund, the Swedish Diabetes Association, Expressens Prenatalforskningsfond and the University of Uppsala.

THE DEVELOPMENT, ENHANCEMENT AND REVERSIBILITY OF DIABETIC GLOMERULOPATHY

M. W. Steffes*, D.M. Brown and S.M. Mauer

Evidence in man clearly demonstrates the dynamic nature of diabetic glomerulopathy, even very early in the disease. Osterby and Gundersen (1) documented increased glomerular volume and peripheral glomerular capillary surface area in human kidneys within the first few months after onset of diabetes. In an earlier study (2), Osterby found increased glomerular basement membrane (GBM) thickness within the first 1.5-2.5 years of diabetes. Mauer et al. (3), studying normal kidneys transplanted to diabetic recipients, observed within 2-4 years of transplantation, deposition of albumin and IgG in a linear fashion along the GBM, tubular basement membranes and Bowman's capsule, In addition, at this time afferent and efferent hyaline arteriolar changes and, often, diffuse mesangial thickening were noted. Studying renal function in patients with diabetes of recent onset (even prior to treatment with insulin in some patients), Mogensen (4) documented increased kidney size, elevated glomerular filtration rate (GFR) and enhanced glomerular permeability to albumin (with and without exercise). Following initiation of therapy with injected insular these early changes revert towards normal. Although establishment of good control may improve the functional changes of diabetes (4), no evidence exists in man as to the reversibility of morphologic lesions once established in the diabetic kidney.

The inbred Lewis rat, made diabetic with streptozotocin, provides an animal model of diabetes and accompanying glomerulopathy resembling that in man. Lesions in the diabetic rat paralleling those in man have been described with respect to increased glomerular volume and filtration surface (5), GBM thickening (6), diffuse thickening of the mesangium, enhanced mesangial staining for smooth muscle antigens and glomerular hyaline (exudative) lesions - containing immunoglobulins and complement and capable of fixing heterologous complement (7). Deposition of the IgG and albumin occurs in a linear pattern along the GBM in man (3) and contrastingly IgG, IgM and complement are localized in a mesangial distribution in the rat (7). Functionally, the diabetic rat presents with early albuminuria (8) (measured by immunoassay) as does man. The morphologic and functional changes outlined above occur within the first 6 months of diabetes in the rat. Islet transplantation in the rat, early in the diabetic process (6-8 months) permits evaluation of the relationship between normalized insulin and glucose levels following islet transplantation (Fig. 1) (9) and the progression of the renal alterations.

ISLET TRANSPLANTATION AND DIABETIC NEPHROPATHY

Parallel to the normalization of glucose in the transplanted rat, the IgG, IgM and complement staining in the mesangium decreases rapidly to normal intensity (Fig. 1) (7). By light microscopic examination, the PAS-positive mesangial matrix thickening also decreases following islet transplantation, but the rate of change is slower than that of the immunoglobulins. Furthermore, unlike the localization of IgG, IgM and complement, the mesangial thickening, although demonstrating marked improvement, remains slightly greater than control levels (Fig. 1) (7).

In parallel with the mesangial lesions, the urinary albumin excretion rate returns to control levels (Fig. 1) (8). Contrastingly, the thickness of the GBM does not decrease to control levels, but rather continues to increase in a manner identical to that in untreated diabetic rats (Fig. 1). The process of GBM thickening has been monitored for 13 months of diabetes (6 months following islet transplant); it is not known whether a longer period following islet transplantation is needed to affect the GBM thickness. This observation must be qualified with the work of Rasch (6) in diabetic rats demonstrating the effect of good control with insulin in diminishing the rate of the development of GBM thickening. Similarly, Cohen and Khalifa (10), working with diabetic rats treated with insulin early in the disease, documented diminished (nearly to normal levels) incorporation of labeled amino acids into glomerular proteins. Both of these reports emphasize the salutary effects of insulin on the synthesis of GBM. However, GBM thickening, once established in the rat, may not return to control levels due to a very slow turnover of GBM constituents. Amelioration of diabetes could be precluded from showing its effect on GBM thickness within the short life span of the rodent. It will probably be necessary to examine the reversibility of GBM thickening in a species more long-lived than the rodent.

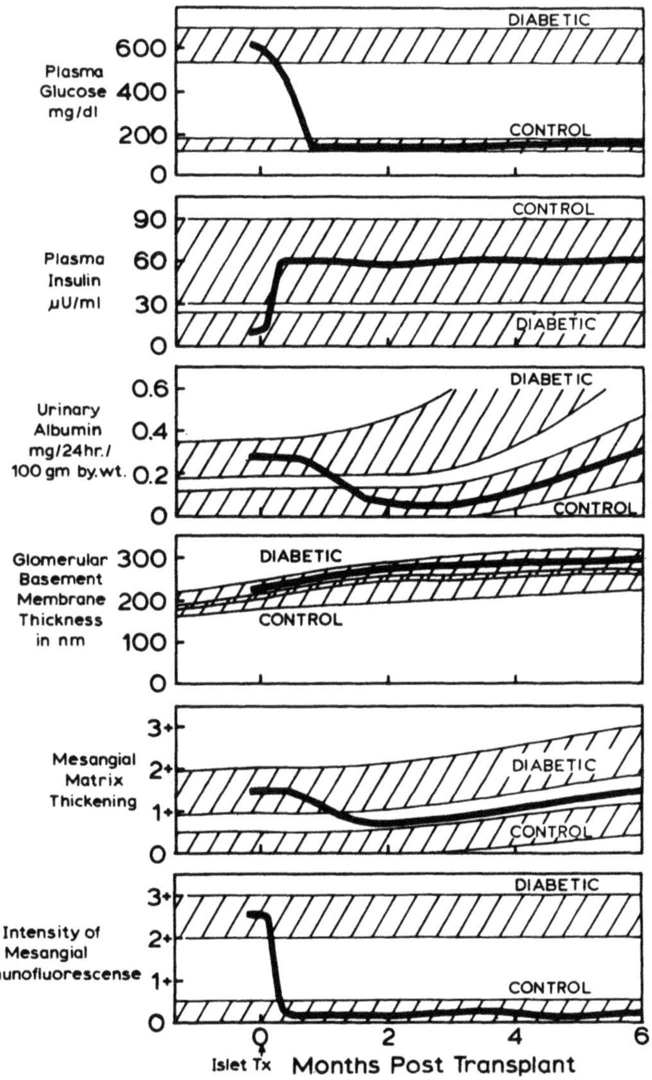

Fig. 1. The effect of islet transplantation on several functional and morphologic parameters altered in the diabetic rat.

Although GBM thickness does not diminish following islet transplantation, the dramatic improvement in albuminuria despite the presence of continued GBM thickening questions the importance of the GBM thickness, per se, in influencing permselectivity of the glomerular capillary wall. Thus the reversal of other abnormal parameters affecting glomerular function in the diabetic subject (notably the increased intracapillary pressures) may be critical in the normalization of urinary albumin excretion rate following islet transplantation.

Correlative observations to those following renal transplantation in man and islet transplantation in the rat were provided by renal transplantation in the rat model (7). Diabetic kidneys transplanted to normal recipients demonstrated marked improvement in the light and immunofluorescent microscopic mesangial lesions, supporting the observation with islet transplantation (7). As with human studies, transplantation of a normal kidney to a diabetic recipient produced diabetic glomerulopathy in the previously normal kidney, emphasizing the importance of diabetic environment in causing diabetic nephropathy.

OTHER FACTORS AFFECTING THE DEVELOPMENT OF DIABETIC GLOMERULOPATHY

Inherent in all the experiments summarized above is the importance of reversing or improving the metabolic state of diabetes. Although glucose intolerance and its associated metabolic sequelae probably initiate the process of diabetic glomerulopathy, other factors (e.g. changes in glomerular capillary pressure alluded to above) may enhance or diminish the rate of its development. Increased glomerular capillary pressure in diabetic rats has been effected first by clipping the renal artery, reducing flow to the clipped kidney and exposing the unclipped kidney to hypertension and enhanced glomerular capillary pressure (11); and secondly, by unilateral nephrectomy and subsequent increased GFR/nephron (12). In both instances the kidney exposed to the increased pressure (the unclipped kidney in the first experiment, the remaining kidney following uninephrectomy) develops, as compared to kidneys in intact diabetic rats, enhanced mesangial deposition of immunoglobulins and complement and mesangial matrix thickening. In the clipped kidneys of diabetic rats, mesangial matrix thickening and deposition of IgG, IgM and complement, although greater than that in kidneys from diabetic rats with 2 non-manipulated kidneys. A similar observation has been made in a diabetic man whose course was complicated by hypertension accompany unilaterial renal artery stenosis (13). The kidney exposed to hypertension showed marked diabetic glomerulopathy while the kidney with the stenotic renal artery revealed little change attributable to diabetes.

Uninephrectomy or clipping a renal artery in normal rats does not cause glomerular lesions similar to those of diabetes. The diabetic state must be present before uninephrectomy can enhance the mesangial lesions. However, uninephrectomy does increase the loss of albumin in the urine (Fig. 2) ((8), suggesting that changes in glomerular capillary pressure significantly affect this functional alteration commonly seen in diabetes. After 4 months of diabetes or uninephrectomy, the effect of uninephrectomy alone or albuminuria exceeds that of diabetes alone (Fig. 2) (8). Frank proteinuria in the diabetic patient frequently accompanies the onset of renal failure. The substantial albuminuria seen with uninephrectomy may signal important functional alterations in the nephron. Although albuminuria in uninephrectomized-diabetic rats receiving islet transplants returns to levels similar to uninephrectomized controls (8), the level of albumin excreted still exceeds that in intact diabetic animals and represents a significant functional alteration.

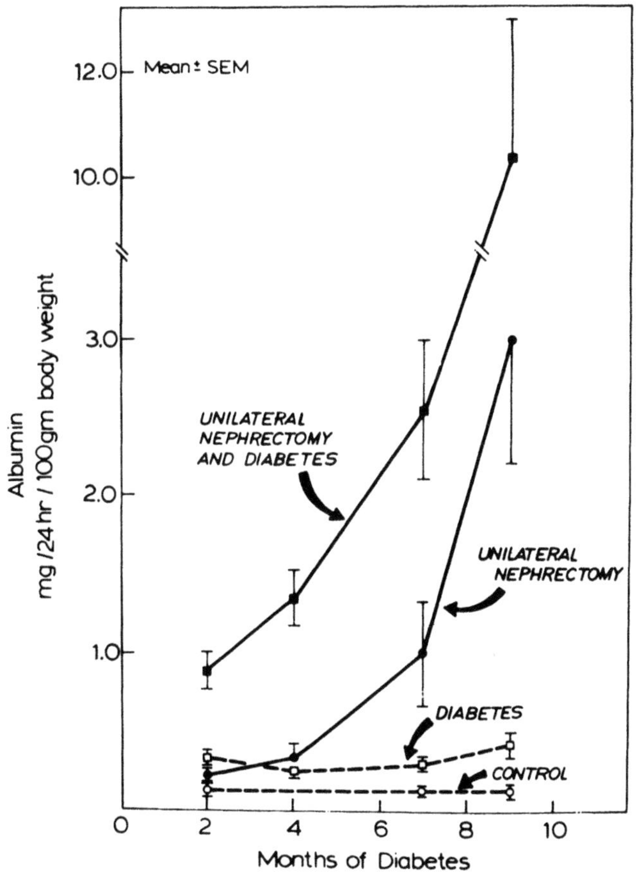

Fig. 2. The progression of albuminuria in control, diabetic, uninephrectomized and uninephrectomized-diabetic rats. (From reference 8, with permission.)

Whether viewed by functional or morphologic changes, uninephrectomy or clipping of the renal artery in the rat, within a short period of time, significantly perturbs the progression of diabetic glomerulopathy. Azar (14) has demonstrated increased glomerular capillary pressure in diabetic rats with 2 kidneys, documenting in diabetic subjects the presence of a factor known to enhance diabetic glomerulopathy. The question of the clinical significance of these observations to man may be approached through the careful monitoring of alterations in GFR and indirect indices of glomerular capillary pressure as they affect the development of diabetic glomerulopathy. Mogensen (4) emphasized that amelioration of only slight hypertension in diabetic patients with early renal failure prolonged the life of their functionally impaired kidneys. Although the uninephrectomy experiments in the rate described above were of short duration, the elevated GFR/nephron without accompanying increases in blood pressure produced dramatic morphologic and functional changes. Perhaps in diabetic man the documented small, but continuing, increases in GFR (4) and filtration fraction (together suggestive of increased glomerular capillary pressure) may over a period of years accelerate diabetic glomerulopathy, a developing process fundamentally dependent upon the metabolic alterations of diabetes. Thus the minor changes in renal physiology established early in diabetes may prove significant over the 10-20 years necessary for the function of the diabetic kidney to become severely impaired.

REFERENCES

1. *Osterby, R. and Gundersen, H.J.G. (1975). Diabetologia 11, 225*
2. *Osterby, R. (1975). Acta med. scand. Suppl. 574, 1*
3. *Mauer, S.M., et al.(1976). Diabetes 25, 709*
4. *Mogensen, C.E. (1976). Diabetes 25, 872*
5. *Gundersen, H.J.G., et al .(1978) Diabetes 27, 432 (abstract)*
6. *Rasch, R. (1977). Diabetologia 13, 426 (abstract)*
7. *Mauer, S.M., et al.(1976). Diabetes 25 (Suppl. 2), 850*
8. *Mauer, S.M., et al. (1978). Diabetes 27, 959*
9. *Steffes, M.W., et al.(1975). J. Lab. Clin. Med. 85, 75*
10. *Cohen, M.P. and Khalifa, A. (1977). Biochimica et Biophysica Acta 500, 395*
11. *Mauer, S.M., et al.(1978). Diabetes 27, 738*
12. *Steffes, M.W., et al.(1978). Diabetes 27, 25*
13. *Berkman, J. and Rifkin, H. (1973). Metabolism 22, 715*
14. *Azar, S. -Submitted for publication*

Supported by grants from National Institutes of Health (HL 06314 and AM 17697)

DISCUSSION

Invited Discussant: H. WEHNER - *Glomerular lesions (glomerulosclerosis and exudative lesions) in streptozotocin-diabetic rats are reversible by islet transplantation. The morphometric studies at our institution showed that 10 weeks after transplantation the mesangium had regressed to nearly normal size.*

The glomerular lesions in streptozotocin-diabetic rats are similar to those seen in humans after long-term diabetes mellitus (Mauer, S.M., et al. 1976 Diabetes Suppl. 2, 850; Wehner, H. 1977, Munch. med. Wschr. 119, 489). (Tab. 1).

TABLE 1

Glomerular changes in streptozotocin-diabetic rats and in diabetic humans.

Glomerular lesions	Diabetic Humans	Streptozotocin Diabetic Rats
Nodular glomerulosclerosis	+	(+)
Diffuse glomerulosclerosis	+	+
Basement membrane thickening	+	+
Exudative lesions	+	+
Aneurysms	(+)	(+)
Adhesions	(+)	(+)
Storage of glycogen	(+)	+

If absolute control of glycemia were possible, some of the factors involved in vasculopathy could be alleviated. Multiple daily insulin dose and islet transplantation seem to delay the diabetes associated changes in the retinal and glomerular vasculature. The purpose of our study (in collaboration with W. Kosters, M. Strauch and Methchild Staudenmeir) was to test the effect of islet transplantation on the glomerular lesions. The subjects were 100 days old highly inbred male Lewis rats. Diabetes was inducted by i.v. injection of 65 mg streptozotocin/kg. Seven months after induction of diabetes, 63 underwent islet transplantation (Kosters, W. 1974, Habilitationsschrift, Heidelberg). Pancreatic islets were isolated by a modification of LACY'S AND SHIBATA'S methods. Rats were injected with 600-800 islets in the portal vein. The blood glucose was determined, using the hexokinase method. The kidneys were stained with PAS, HE and sections o.5-1.o u in thickness were silver impregnated after MOVAT. The morphometric studies were performed as a blind study. For mesangial area, we used the point counting technique (Wehner, H. 1974 Veroffentl. Path. 95, 1).

After injection of streptozotocin, all animals developed hyperglycemia of more than 450 mg/100 ml. Transplanted animals became normoclycemic within 72 hours after receiving the isograft. The light microscopic findings in streptozotocin diabetic rats 7 months after induction are listed in Table 2.

TABLE 2

Renal lesions in streptozotocin-diabetic rats

1. Nodular glomerulosclerosis
2. Diffuse glomerulosclerosis
3. Mesangial cell proliferation
4. Basement membrane thickening
5. Glomerular aneurysms
6. Fibrinoid caps
7. Glomerular adhesions
8. Glycogen storage (not in the macula densa!)
9. Interstitial nephritis (rare)
10. Tubular adenoma (in one case)

The most frequent lesion (100%) in the diabetic group was diffuse glomerulosclerosis. Classic nodules were observed in 37% (Table 3).

TABLE 3

Glomerular changes in age-matched nondiabetic, diabetic and transplanted rats.

Glomerular lesions	Normal controls n=19	Diabetic rats Untreated n=35	Diabetic rats Transplanted n=19
Nodular glomerulosclerosis	Ø	37.1%	5.0%
Diffuse glomerulosclerosis	57.9%	100.0%	30.0%
Exudative lesions	Ø	97.1%	65.0%
Hypercellularity	15.8%	51.4%	15.0%
Aneurysms	10.6%	22.8%	10.0%
BM-thickening	Ø	14.3%	10.0%
Adhesions	5.3%	11.4%	10.0%

Kidney sections taken 10 weeks after islet transplantation showed a marked reduction or an almost complete reversal of the lesions described (Table 3). The morphometric studies of the mesangial area showed a significant increase of the mesangium of 13.4% in comparison with age-matched controls - 8%. After transplantation (10 weeks), the mesangium had regressed to nearly normal size of 9.2% (Table 4).

Table 4

Morphometric analysis of mesangial area.

	Mesangial area (%of total glomerular area)
Normal rats (n=22)	8.09
Diabetic rats untreated (n=37)	13.38
Diabetic rats transplanted (n=19)	9.18

These studies demonstrate that glomerular lesions in streptozotocin diabetic rats correspond to the glomerular changes in humans after longstanding diabetes mellitus (Weil, R., et al (1976) Arch. Path. Lab. Med. 100, 37). Islet isotransplantation partly reverses diabetic glomerular lesions. *(This study was supported by the Deutsche Forschungsgemeinschaft (We 468/9)).*

M. COHEN: *Just a comment and then a speculatory point: The lack of improvement in the thickness of the base of a membrane is not necessarily equitable with a lack of response to improvement of the metabolic control. The turnover of basement membrane, particularly the collagenous portion of the membrane, is extremely slow, on the order of 100 to 200 days. So, the six month period, during which you were following these animals, may not be sufficient to get adequate turnover. The question is: You implied that thickened basement membrane may have nothing to do with the proteinuric process. Are you also implying that it has nothing to do with, or has little to do with, the renal failure and ultimate demise of the patient? Is proteinuria versus elevation or deterioration of creatinine clearance, etc.?*

M. W. STEFFES: *We feel that, to demonstrate any kind of reduction, we'd have to go to a longer lived animal than the rat. With regard to the other comment: we really don't know all these data. These results have made us wonder what is diabetic glomerulopathy? Where are we going? What is the process which really leads to the end stage, which Dr. Deckert talked about earlier, in terms of what does lead to changes in some people and not to others? I truly don't know what the process is. I do think that glomerular basement membrane, whether it is peripheral or in the mesangium, certainly has a process, which is an important part in the development of glomerulopathy. However, the point I want to emphasize is that, even though many of us will continue to use basement membrane thickness to look at the change in the kidney, the fact is that islet transplantation probably reduces the changes in the vascular dynamics of the animal.*

J.R. WILLIAMSON: *Did I understand that, although basement membrane thickening was non-reversible, the mesangial accumulation was? I wonder if you have any electron microscopy on the mesangium? Does this simply reflect cellular atrophy? Is the increase in mesangial mass accounted for by an increase in cellular cytoplasm, or is this extracellular material? It wasn't clear to me if insulin levels in these animals were completely restored to normal. The reason I raise this question is because I'm sure you are aware of recent studies by Scharp et al. (Diabetes 27 (Suppl. 2): 435, 1978) in which it was found that, even though animals who had received islet cell transplants had normal glucose tolerance tests, ocular permeability was not restored to normal unless the insulin response to a glucose tolerance test was also normal.*

M.W. STEFFES: *With regard to mesangium, we are in the process of attempting to measure the mesangial volume by electromicroscopy.*

J.R. WILLIAMSON: *Is the increased mesangium actually cellular cytoplasm, or is it extracellular material?*

M.W. STEFFES: *We just don't know yet. With regard to the insulin levels in both diabetic and un-nephrectomized diabetic animals in this experiment, the insulin levels only were less than the normal range. They clearly were not normal for rats. No question about it. Yet, the parameters were changed, the way we would expect, from previous experiments, in which we obtained normal levels. So, the insulin levels may not be a factor in our view. These were simply morning insulin levels.*

P.L. POFFENBARGER: *I would like you to clarify the model you are using with respect to compensatory renal growth. Compensatory renal growth, as I understand it, is primarily a process involving enlargement of the nephron unit, proximal renal tubular cell hyperplasia and hypertropy, with the total number of glomeruli in the kidney not altered. I don't think we know a great deal about the effect of unilateral nephrectomy on mesangium and basement membrane turnover. Now, because of that lack of information and because you are using it in a diabetic model to study that process, I had trouble understanding how to put those two unknowns together with respect to your data. Also, what is the timing of unilateral nephrectomy with respect to the induction of streptozotocin diabetes?*

M.W. STEFFES: *Well, the timing is within two weeks of diabetes. With regard to glomerular basement membrane, I could tell you that it is essentially the same in diabetic and un-nephrectomized diabetic ani-*

mals. The glomerular volumes are markedly larger in the un-nephrectomized diabetic animals, so that would make the absolute mesangial volume greater in those animals than in the diabetic. Now, in terms of the effect of un-nephrectomy itself, what you are getting at is that we just have larger glomerular with the increase in volume. It is certainly relevant to what's going on here. However, the same process goes on in diabetic man, where the glomerular volume increases remarkably early in the disease, and continues on until very late in the disease. One thing I didn't mention is the fact that islet transplantation will diminish the glomerular volumes acutely within two months in these animals, both diabetic and un-nephrectomy diabetic.

P. L. POFFENBARGER: *Excuse me, I want to clarify one final thing: Doesn't streptozotocin in diabetes affect the compensatory renal growth process?*

M. W. STEFFES: *No, it accelerates, in terms of glomerular volumes. In short, the glomerular volumes in the un-nephrectomized diabetic animals, at six months of diabetes, are bigger than even the un-nephrectomized animals.*

E. PFEIFFER: *In our laboratory, rats were made diabetic. Then, after four months, one kidney was removed for histological examination and then intraportal injection of islets was performed. After four months, the rat was sacrificed and the other kidney was examined. The conclusion was that, as long as the transplantation was performed up to six months after institution of diabetes, a remarkable influence, an improvement in the diabetic condition of the kidney was obtained, and this suggests that complete normalization of blood glucose is effective in that respect.*

A. LERNMARK: *Regarding the number of islets, I wonder if dry preservation would be helpful? In our hands, we found the same as you, that there is about 20% activity of frozen islets in terms of insulin biosynthesis. However, what we found was that, upon thawing the islets, they break up into individual cells. So, I wonder what the recovery is of islets after they are frozen and thawed?*

C. HELLERSTROM: *Yes, that was a problem on our hands at the beginning, too. However, when we switched from slow thawing to quick, we had a 100% recovery of intact islets, so they did not break up into cells. Of course, it is impossible to answer how many islets are required. As a starting point, I think one should regard the old observation of about 1 to 2 gms. of endocrine tissue in the pancreas. Each islet we obtained is about 4 micrograms wet weight. If we assume that we should end up with about 10% of the total endocrine pancreatic mass, this would mean between 25 and 50,000 islets.*

A. NOTKINS: *We prevented the development of virus-induced diabetes by islet transplants. In our system, the SWR mice and their beta cells are susceptible to infection, while the C57 black and their beta cells are resistant. We decided to transplant the C57 black beta cells into the SWR mice to see if that would prevent the development of viral-induced diabetes. The problem with the experiment is that, if you do this transplant, you must cross a major histocompatability barrier. Since we couldn't do that, we took the F1 beta cells instead. The F1 mice are also resistant to infection. You can transplant their beta cells into the SWR mice with minimal rejection. The experiment then was to to put F1 beta cells into SWR mice and, as control, SWR beta cells into SWR mice, then infect them. We did that, and the SWR mice with the SWR beta cells came down with diabetes, while the ones that got the F1 beta cells either did not or came down with only a minimal amount of diabetes. The major reason for this experiment was to find more evidence that the beta cells were actually resistant to infection, but we were also able to prevent the development of diabetes by this transplant.*

M. de GASPARO: *Are you sure that the changes in the kidney are not due to the toxic effect on the kidney?*

M. W. STEFFES: *On the streptozotocin experiments and normal kidney transplanted in the diabetic recipients, we obtained the lesions just as quickly as with streptozotocin. These were kidneys that never saw streptozotocin.*

H. LEBOVITZ: *Are we now trying to transplant and develop all of this methodology for a group of people who already have a basic disturbance? I would be very much interested in hearing comments from Dr. Notkins and others on what they thought was the potential, given this new concept, about the etiology of the various types of insulin dependent diabetes.*

A. NOTKINS: *Regarding viruses, it is really premature to worry about that problem. I think, once the viral infection is over, the transplant would then be successful. Later, if you are dealing with a persistent viral infection, then, of course, you really could be in trouble. However, we don't have any evidence of that at the present time. In terms of the autoimmune response, I think that could be a serious problem if you do have islet cell antibody which would play a pathogenic role. Then, if you put in a new transplant, you could very well react with that transplant. I believe it has to be shown definitively that this islet cell antibody actually is pathogenic, and not just epiphenomenon.*

M. W. STEFFES: *Islet transplantation is not goint to cure diabetes in the diabetic population. It's going to allow us to make some observations in man the way we have in rats, but I think the hope for the future is probably in the mechanical devices.*

SUBSTITUTION OF ISLET-CELL FUNCTION WITH "OPEN-LOOP" INSULIN INFUSION SYSTEMS

K.D. Hepp*, R. Renner, M. Franetzki and H. Mehnert

It is still not entirely clear to what extent the late complications of diabetes depend upon the quality of metabolic control. However, more recent studies have provided strong arguments for a causal relationship (1,2). It also became increasingly evident how inadequate in fact is our therapy with diet and subcutaneous insulin injections (3). This has encouraged investigations on new avenues of treatment, with the aim to restore physiological metabolic regulation. Two major lines of approach are transplantation of islets or the whole pancreas, and replacement of B-cell function by technical devices. In the field of the "artificial B-cell", feedback-controlled ("closed-loop") and "open-loop" or programmed infusion systems are currently under study. Clinical use of glucose-controlled infusion systems showed surprisingly good results. Using blood glucose as the controlling index, even unstable diabetics can be brought into a physiological range, and a number of other substrates and hormones appear to follow suit. These devices are fairly large and can be used only at the bedside for a limited number of days. The ideal device all groups have in mind is an implantable miniaturized system. At present, the weak spot of this concept is the glucose sensor. Electrochemical (4) or enzyme-electrode (5) sensors are not at a stage where they can permanently function in blood or tissue or even serve as control for the potentially dangerous infusion of highly concentrated insulin solutions.

Open-loop systems without the problematical sensor are feasible and less complicated. In 1974, Slama et al. reported their results with a portable pump system in relatively mild diabetics and found no change in comparison to multiple daily injections of regular insulin (6). Further studies from other groups showed a marked improvement in the control of stable and unstable diabetics as compared to conventional subcutaneous insulin treatment (7-10).

TABLE 1. Metabolic control as mean blood glucose (MBG) and mean amplitude of glycemic excursions (MAGE) under conventional insulin therapy and during continuous preprogrammed infusion (bedside apparatus) in 7 stable and 10 unstable diabetics. (Data from (8).

	MBG* (mg/dl)	p**	MAGE* (mg/dl)	p**
Stable diabetics				
pre-infusion period	184.7 ± 16.9		119.2 ± 13.8	
infusion period	131.1 ± 8.2	<0.05	79.1 ± 10.5	<0.0125
post-infusion period	168.5 ± 12.1	<0.05	95.6 ± 6.1	<0.0125
Unstable diabetics				
pre-infusion period	254.0 ± 18.4		187.9 ± 19.1	
infusion period	167.5 ± 10.7	<0.005	126.9 ± 15.1	<0.05
post-infusion period	214.0 ± 12.7	<0.01	158.3 ± 18.9	<0.05

*Mean ± SEM **paired comparison

PRE-PROGRAMMED INTRAVENOUS INFUSION WITH A BEDSIDE APPARATUS

In 1973, we began our cooperation with medical engineers of the Siemens Corporation in Erlangen. Our first experiments were performed with a bedside apparatus, consisting of 24-hour control unit and a commercial infusion pump. The infusion pattern was set on a crossbar distributor using short-circuiting plugs (7,8).

Our aim was to imitate the daily recurring rhythm of a physiological secretion pattern while keeping the diet constant. The infusion profile was adjusted individually to the actual requirements of each patient. The total amount of insulin on the first day was based on the previous insulin requirement, but was corrected during the course of the infusion according to the actual need. After subtraction of a basal rate between 0.4 and 1.2 U/h, the remaining units were distributed in peaks according to the size of the meals. Table 1 shows a comparison of 2-3 days of conventional therapy before and after the infusion period with 2-3 days of preprogrammed continuous intravenous application. In both groups, the stable and unstable diabetics, significant differences were observed in the mean blood glucose level (MBG) and the mean amplitude of glycemic excursions (MAGE), which was used as an index for instability (4).

FIXED PROFILE AND PATIENT-OPERATED CONTROL OF PORTABLE MINIATURIZED INFUSION SYSTEMS

The next step was the development of a miniaturized system which could be carried on the body without impairment of the patients' normal activities, including periods of exercise (17). The unit consisted of an insulin reservoir and a pump which was strapped to the patient's arm and an electronic control device which could be operated by hand (Figure 1). Special insulin preparations (100-1000 U/ml) were developed in the laboratories of the Hoechst Corporation.

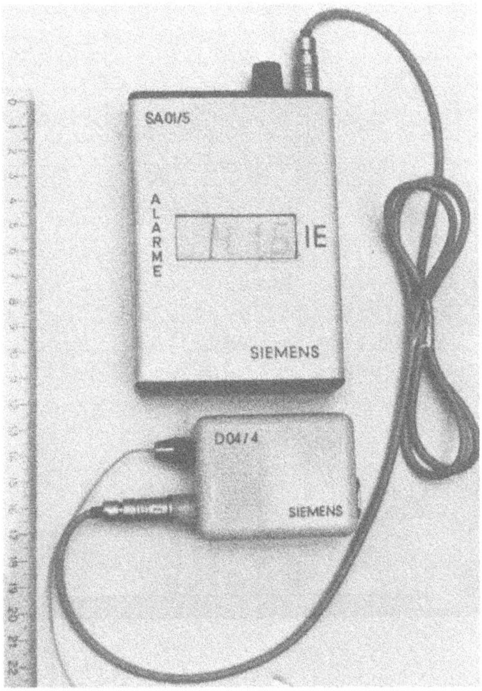

Fig. 1. Portable pump and reservoir connected with control unit with readout for cumulative insulin dose and alarms.

Figure 2 shows results with such a patient-operated system in a 19 year old diabetic. Further development consisted of a programmable control unit which could be connected with a console where, again with the help of a cross-bar distributor, a fixed program was composed. The results on an 18 year old unstable diabetic are illustrated in Figure 4. Strenuous exercise had remarkable little influence on metabolic control. Under the strict dietary regimen of the metabolic ward both systems, patient-operated and fixed program, were comparable. Of special interest were data obtained from the

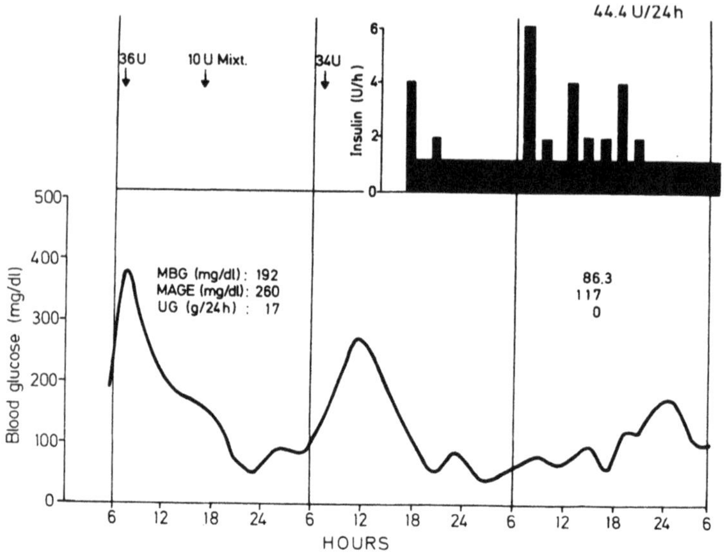

Fig. 2. Continuous insulin infusion (patient-operated) in a 19 year old diabetic. Basal rate, 1.2 U/h plus additional 1 h-pulse at meals (total: 44.4 U/24 h). Previous therapy: 36-10 U 30/70% regular/NPH. Blood glucose was determined at 1-2 h intervals.

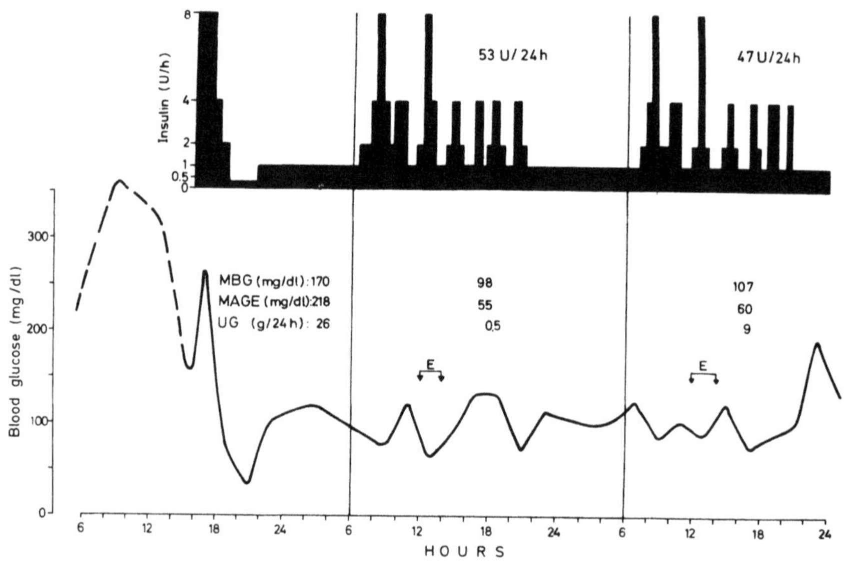

Fig. 3. Pre-programmed insulin infusion in an 18 year old unstable diabetic. Exercise periods are marked "E".

therapy of a 46 year old brittle patient who was suffering from frequent severe hypoglycemias and in whom even multiple injections of regular insulin had failed. Her mean blood glucose of 301 mg/dl with a MAGE of 265 and urine glucose of 114 g/24 h (3 days of pre-infusion period) dropped to a MBG of 161 mg/dl, a MAGE of 129 and a mean urine glucose of 2 g/24 h (7 days of patient-operated infusion) without hypoglycemic reactions. The longest infusion was carried out for 5 weeks with excellent results.

The current problems with these infusion systems are fibril formation in concentrated insulin solutions with clogging of pump and catheter, electronic failures and the occurrence of sterile phlebitides in peripheral veins. However, such open-loop systems provide valuable information as a basis for the development of implantable devices without, and perhaps eventually with, the still problematical glucose sensor.

In a limited number of cases, the current system may already be suitable for clinical use as well as for studies on the relationship between metabolic control and late complications. Our data and those of other groups, working with similar devices, indicate at least better results than what can be currently achieved with conventional subcutaneous insulin injections.

REFERENCES

1. *Raskin, P.H., (1978). Metabolism 27, 235.*
2. *Spiro, R.G., (1976). Diabetologia 12, 1.*
3. *Molnar, G.D. and Reynolds, C., (1977). Horm. Metab. Res. Suppl. 7 (Kruse-Jarres, J.D. and Molnar, G.D. eds.) 148.*
4. *Chang, K.W., et al., (1973). Trans. Amer. Soc. Artif. Intern. Organs 19, 352.*
5. *Updike, S.J. and Hicks, G.P. (1967). Nature 214, 986.*
6. *Slama, G., et al., (1974). Diabetes 23, 732.*
7. *Hepp, K.D., et al., (1975). Diabetologia 11, 349.*
8. *Hepp, K.D., et al., (1978). Klin. Wochenschr.*
9. *Genuth, S. and Martin, P., (1977). Diabetes 26, 571.*
10. *Pickup, J.C., et al., (1978). Brit. Med. J. 1, 204.*

NEWER INSULIN DELIVERY SYSTEMS: CONTINUOUS SUBCUTANEOUS INSULIN INFUSION

J. C. Pickup*, H. Keen, J. A. Parsons,
and K. G. M. M. Alberti

The quest for new methods of administering insulin has been primarily stimulated by the practical difficulty of achieving long periods of strict blood glucose and major intermediary metabolites control with conventional insulin injection therapy. Until such conditions can be realized it is clearly impossible to demonstrate unequivocally the relationship between diabetic control and chronic tissue changes, such as microangiopathy.

In recent years two approaches, islet tissue transplantation and the so-called "artificial pancreas", have been explored as possible means of achieving normoglycemia. Although islet cell transplantation is effective in animals it has, as yet, proved unsuccessful in human studies. Glycemia-controlled insulin delivery systems ("the artificial pancreas") are extremely effective in controlling blood sugar in the short-term in both animals and man but protracted normoglycemia seems to be precluded by the size and complexity of the machinery (i.e. it is not portable and completely reliable). Moreover, the intravenous route of insulin delivery is associated with thrombosis and infection when used in the long-term. This also applies, at least in theory, to portable intravenous infusion systems without servo-control (1,2,3).

We have recently been exploring a new delivery system, continuous, dual-rate, subcutaneous insulin infusion (CSII) using a portable syringe pump (4,5). Initial studies show that CSII is capable of maintaining strict diabetic control for more than 3 months under domestic conditions in ambulant, insulin-requiring diabetic patients.

Fig. 1 shows the syringe pump (the Mill Infuser; Muirhead Ltd., Beckenham, Kent, U.K.) fitted to a patient. The pump (6) has been

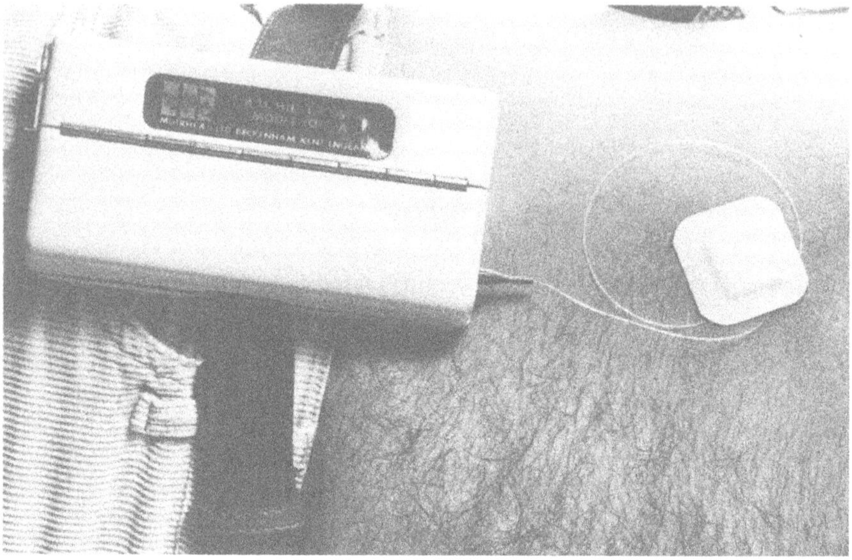

Fig. 1. Specially adapted, dual-rate Mill Hill Infuser worn by a patient. The nylon delivery cannula is implanted in the subcutaneous tissue of the abdominal wall.

adapted by us to deliver at 2 rates, 50 uL/hr and 400 uL/hr. The latter rate is activated 30 min. before meal-times by pressing a guarded button, the rate automatically returning to 50 uL/hr after 17 min. Actrapid insulin is delivered from the 2 or 3 ml pump syringe through a nylon cannula (internal diameter less than 0.2 mm) which is implanted in the subcutaneous tissue of the abdomen. The infuser is worn on a belt around the waist or in a shoulder harness.

Our early clinical experience of blood glucose control by CSII over 24 hours has been described (4). More recently, we have examined long-term domestic use of SCII and have shown that blood levels of the major intermediary metabolites, lactate, pyruvate, 3-hydroxybutyrate and alanine are returned to approximately the non-diabetic state after 24 hr of CSII (5).

Table 1 showns the mean plasma glucose, M-value and range in 6 patients treated by conventional insulin therapy (both once and twice daily insulin) and after 3-4 days of SCII under Metabolic Ward conditions (i.e. fully ambulant but confined to hospital). The known duration of diabetes in these patients was 3-23 years. Control, as assessed by either mean plasma glucose, M-value or range of these values was improved in all patients except No. 6. This patient was a truly "brittle" diabetic with completely unpredictable swings in blood glucose on conventional therapy (soluble insulin three or four times daily), unrelated to food or exercise. We now have experience in the control by CSII of several of these brittle patients. What-

Table 1. Comparison of plasma glucose and M-values in patients on their conventional regimen and during CSII.

	Mean plasma glucose (mmol/l) and range			Mean M Value and range		
#	CT	FID	P	CT	FID	P
1	14.3 (7.2-21.3)	8.2 (2.7-12.2)	< 0.01	142 (9.4-316)	32 (0.02-85)	< 0.01
2	12.0 (4.0-18.3)	6.0 (4.0-11.1)	< 0.01	81 (11-233)	28 (0.01-63)	< 0.01
3	10.9 (4.2-22.4)	8.4 (2.3-12.6)	< 0.02	79 (0.01-348)	36 (0.2-94)	N.S.
4	6.1 (0.8-20.3)	6.5 (3.1-8.8)	N.S.	85 (0.01-433)	8.4 (0.2-26)	< 0.05
5	13.2 (3.8-27.6)	5.5 (2.3-8.3)	< 0.01	109 (0.4-481)	6.5 (0.14-28)	< 0.01
6	11.8 (2.2-28.0)	12.9 (3.4-25.2)	N.S.	125 (0.01-511)	129 (0.1-429)	N.S.

= case number, CT = conventional treatment, FID = final infusion day. M value = mean amplitude of glycemic excursion.

ever is the nature of the unpredictability (variations in either subcutaneous absorption of insulin and/or endogenous insulin secretion, for example) it does not seem to be significantly improved by CSII, at least using the present comparatively simple strategy of high-rate increases before meals. However, it is a rare type of diabetes (7) and it still remains the case that most diabetics are suitable for random allocation to strict control by CSII.

Fig. 2 shows plasma glucose control in a patient studied for 3 consecutive days on conventional treatment (mean ± S.D. plasma glucose 17.7 ± 4.4 mmol/l) followed by 5 consecutive days of CSII under conditions of normal daily activity at home and work (physiotherapy student). The mean (± S.D.) plasma glucose on CSII was 6.9 ± 2.9 mmol/l.

Patients have now undergone domestic CSII for up to 3 months. They monitor diabetic control by measuring blood glucose with "Dextrostix", adjusting the daily insulin dose according to the results. No cannula site infection or palpable lipodystrophy has yet occurred, even when the same cannula has been used at the same subcutaneous implantation position for 2 months.

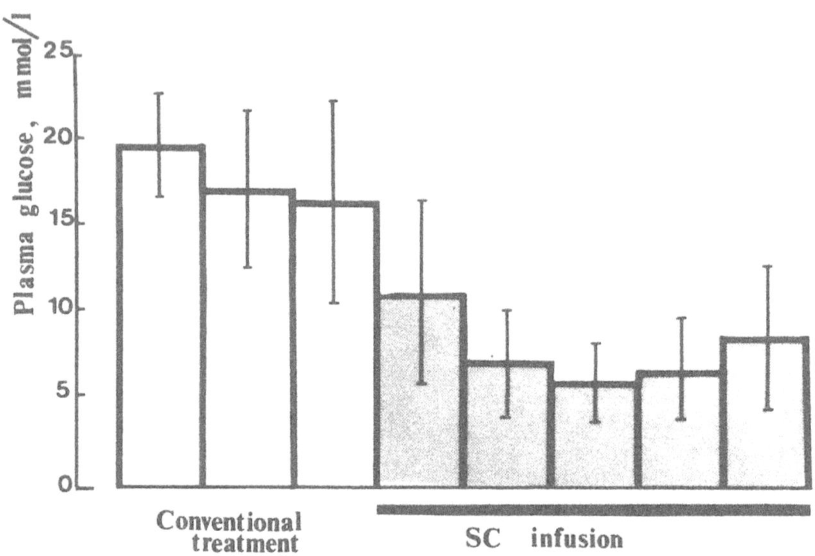

Fig. 2. Mean plasma glucose in a patient on conventional therapy (isophane insulin 40 U, soluble insulin 4 U in the morning) and during CSII. Measurements of blood glucose were made 4 times daily (either Dextrostix or glucose oxidase autoanalyzer). First 3 bars, mean ± S.D. plasma glucose on conventional therapy; shaded bars, mean ± S.D. plasma glucose during 5 days of CSII (not confined to ward).

In the first week of infusion it is commonly found that improved control is achieved using the same or even 20% less daily insulin than on conventional therapy. In one patient infused for 3 months the daily insulin dose fell from 92 U to about 40 U. One may speculate that decreasing insulin dose could be due to less enzymatic destruction of the low volumes of insulin infused, more physiological distribution with mean-time peaks of insulin, or fall in circulating antibodies due to change to monocomponent insulin.

In summary, CSII promises to provide a system suitable for maintaining long-term strict diabetic control and consequently for testing the hypothesis that diabetic microvascular disease can be retarded, arrested or reversed by these conditions.

REFERENCES

1. *Deckert, T., and Lorup, B., (1976). Diabetologia 12, 573.*
2. *Genuth, S., and Martin, P., (1977). Diabetes 26, 571.*
3. *Renner, R., et al., (1977). Diabetologia 13, 427.*

4. *Pickup, J.C., et al., (1978a). Brit. Med. J. 1, 204.*
5. *Pickup, J.C., et al., (1978b). Diabetologia 15, 261.*
6. *Parsons, J.A., et al., (1977). Lancet 1, 77.*
7. *Tattersall, R.B., (1977). Clinics in Endocrinology and Metabolism 6, 403.*

We thank the British Insulin Manufacturers for support. Mr. Roger Blows adapted the Mill Hill Infusers and Mr. K. Kilbourn, Mr. E. Regina, Mr. M. Stimmler and Miss S. A. Wolfman provided skillful technical assistance. The enthusiastic cooperation of our patients and the staff of the Metabolic Ward at Guy's Hospital is gratefully acknowledged.

DISCUSSION

E. PFEIFFER: *I think everything is going quite nicely and comfortably, as long as blood glucose determinations are done by the patient himself.*

M. de GASPARO: *Everyone knows that, if you leave a bottle of insulin on the shelf, it stays stable. Now, if you take a bottle of regular insulin, it is a clear solution, and if you roll gently, slowly and continuously, this bottle becomes gummy. Is that a problem you observed, Dr. Hepp?*

K. D. HEPP: *Yes, this is quite true. This is our major problem right now. It is probably fibrill formation, although we still don't exactly know what the chemistry is. Apparently, no manufacturer has tried to just take a bottle of insulin and gently shake it at a given, or warmer, room temperature, but this is probably what clogs up our machines in some cases.*

R. CAMERINI-DAVALOS: *Am I right in assuming that Dr. Pickup's system is more practical for the time being?*

K. D. HEPP: *For the moment, certainly, yes.*

H. LEBOVITZ: *Does the sodium insulin cause the same problem as the zinc insulin?*

K. D. HEPP: *Well, we have left the insulin chemistry entirely up to our partners in the industry, who are very touchy about it.*

T. DECKERT: *How many of these patients still have endogenous insulin production? You express control as mean blood glucose concentration. How often have you taken the postprandial blood glucose in these patients? If you take many samples during the night, then you have very nice mean blood glucose determination. But, if you take a lot after the meals, this might not be so. Dr. Pickup, I should like to pose a special question. How many minutes, after increasing the basal insulin rate from 50 to 400 microliters per hour, will you have the maximum increase in plasma insulin concentration?*

K. D. HEPP: *What we did is either monitored glucose continuously with an autoanalyzer or intermittently at 1 to 2 hour intervals. The longest was 2 hours and we had done studies beforehand to assure that, within that intermittent sampling, we do not overlook important swings.*

J. PICKUP: *In our initial studies, when patients were in-hospital, we measured the blood glucose every half an hour and then, sub-*

sequently, every hour, while they were ongoing 5 days of continuous subcutaeous insulin. We tried to express control in as many ways as possible, not only mean blood glucose which, of course, disguises the swing, but also the range. As far as the endogenous insulin production is concerned, we measured the peptide in our first batch of 15 or so patients who were in-hospital, and there is absolutely no difference in the control which can be achieved in those who got C-peptide and those who didn't. As far as the timing of the pharmokinetics of insulin absorption is concerned, this is actually very important, and we're currently looking into this. All I can say is that we have only measured total circulating insulin, which is not free, because all of our patients have antibodies which show peaks at about 1½ hours. It is rather sooner that you would expect from a single subcutaneous injection.

G. M. REAVEN: *A question for both Drs. Hepp and Pickup: Have you measured or compared levels of other hormones which are frequently abnormal in these patients - growth hormone, cortisol, epinephrine, etc.?*

K. D. HEPP: *We haven't done systematic studies. We are currently doing that, so I can't show you any data.*

J. PICKUP: *I've measured glucagon during the first 24 hours of continuous subcutaneous insulin infusion, and it remained high. It doesn't change.*

H. LEBOVITZ: *Dr. Pickup, how much maintenance does your instrument have in the chronic patients, the ones that have been on for 3 months? In other words, how often do the subcutaneous catheters have to be changed? Does the patient come to the hospital to have it changed? How reproduceable is the instrumentation over a period of three months?*

J. PICKUP: *I think that the cannula can be left in place for at least two months. It rather depends on whether the patient pulls it out or not. Our only method at the moment of securing it is just to wind the tube around and stick it down with tenacious plaster. Some of our patients pull it out about every fourth night. Therefore, that is the average time for replacement, although on the basis of two or three patients, who have had it in for 1 to 2 months, nothing very much happens in the way of deterioration in control, infection or lipodystrophy. I think one might find that it could be kept in for quite a long time. As far as the pump going wrong is concerned, it does do that, mainly because of the complicated electronics involved. It goes wrong, I suppose, about once every six weeks or so. We always have a backup pump. The actual insertion of the cannula is done in the hospital. It's a 10 minute procedure, very minor, and I would envisage that the patients could have that done at home, which is what we intend to do with a district nurse.*

R. CAMERINI-DAVALOS: *Are we to understand that the subcutaneous tissue does not react abnormally in any way with this type of device? Also, if we have problems, is it really with the mechanical device rather than with the patient's acceptance? Is that correct?*

J. PICKUP: *Yes, that is about it. We've only used nylon cannulas so far, which seem to be quite biocompatible. I've only recently received ethical permission to do biopsies of the implantation site, so that information will have to wait awhile, but I imagine there will be some kind of tissue reaction.*

SUBSTITUTION OF ISLET CELL FUNCTION BY MECHANICAL DEVICE: EXTRACORPOREAL ARTIFICIAL PANCREAS

E. F. Pfeiffer*, W. Kerner and
W. Beischer

Up to now, conventional insulin therapy, irrespective of the many ways selected to adjust insulin dosage, has failed to reestablish a normal correlation between insulin and blood glucose concentration.

Five years ago, we started to reestablish normoglycemia in diabetics by technical means (1-2). The artificial endocrine pancreas, developed at the University of Ulm in collaboration with Mr. A. H. Clemens from Life Science Instruments, Miles Laboratories, Inc., Elkhart, Ind. (USA), is a Glucose-Controlled-Insulin-Infusion System (GCIIS), similar to the system developed independently by Albisser et al (3). Blood is continuously drawn into a double lumen catheter, permitting mixture of blood and heparin at the tip of the intravenous catheter, permitting extracorporeal heparinization. The GCIIS consist of:

1) A glucose analyzer, continuously measuring and monitoring glucose in blood.
2) A pump system for insulin and glucose delivery.
3) A microcomputer, calculating the infusion rate each minute for insulin and dextrose.
4) A printer/plotter, registering each minute real time, mean glucose concentration of the previous minute, amount of infused insulin and dextrose per minute, and total insulin used from the beginning.

Whereas the first generation consisted of a combination of bulky machines, the last version already is a single model of TV-size (4), as shown in Figure 1. This new device is now available on the market under the trade name BIOSTATOR. In this apparatus, a glucose analyzer with an enzyme electrode is employed. However, instead of measuring oxygen depletion, it measures polarographically one of the reaction products, hydrogen peroxide, thus eliminating a second reference electrode. This system is operating well, reducing the blood loss to 50 ml/24 hours and the delay between withdrawal of the blood and the insulin infusion to less than 1 minute.

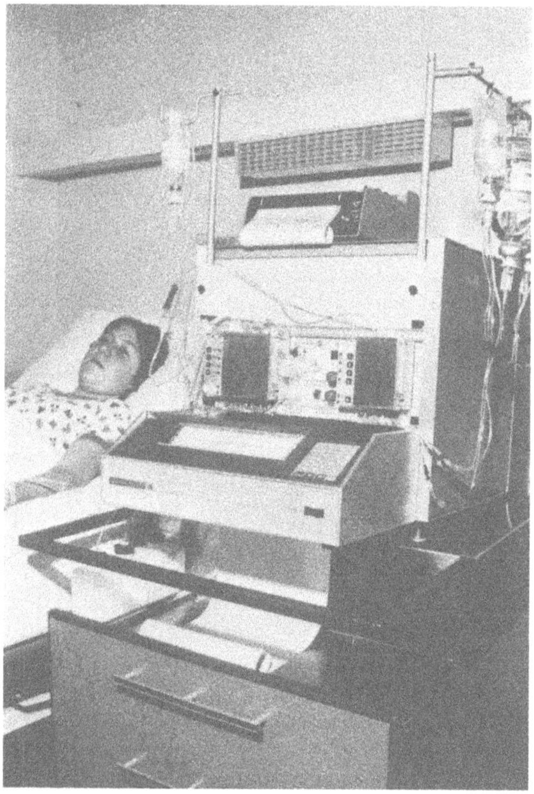

Fig. 1. Latest version of the artificial endocrine pancreas.

EXPERIMENTAL CLINICAL STUDIES

Experiments with perfused isolated rat pancreas have demonstrated a biphasic type of insulin secretion following administration of glucose. However, this experiment is artificial, because the pancreas is perfused by fluids containing constant glucose concentrations and the pancreas does not respond to its own insulin secretion. On the other hand, simple static control of insulin release, based only on absolute glucose concentrations, cannot solve the problem. This has been shown by Kadish in 1964 (5), who infused insulin or dextrose, when blood glucose was above or below present values. Calculations employed for developing the so-called algorithms have been described recently (4-6). The need to select proper algorithms can be shown in the case of two oral glucose loads, which were performed in a juvenile diabetic using different algorithms. A delay in insulin infusion in response to blood glucose increase requires much more insulin without normalizing the blood sugar pattern. Rapid infusion of insulin, on the other hand, though with smaller amounts, better compensates for the glucose infused. Similar results were obtained during 24 hour blood glucose regulation (7) (Fig. 2a,b).

THE INFLUENCE OF RENORMALIZED EXOGENOUS INSULIN APPLICATION ON ENDOGENOUS INSULIN SECRETION

The automatized insulin infusion by the artificial endocrine pancreas favorably influences the "residual secretory capacity" of the B-cell. Endogenous insulin secretion, estimated by measuring the C-peptide in circulating blood, increases, while exogenous insulin is administered for the control of fluctuations in blood glucose (8). The same action must be ascribed to the sulfonylureas, if the Langerhans' islets still respond to these anti-diabetic drugs. Treatment with sulfonylureas for 2 weeks duration in a maturity onset diabetic patient resulted not only in smaller requirements of insulin from the artificial endocrine B-cell, but also produced further increase in C-peptide concentrations (Figure 3).

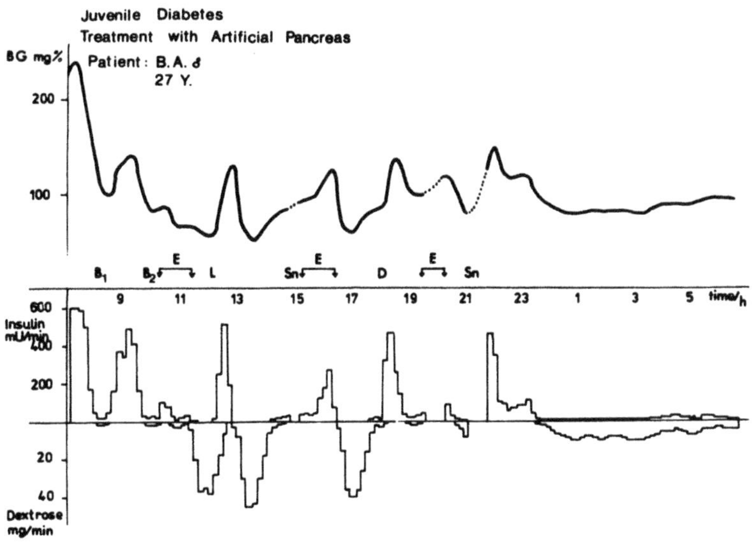

Fig. 2a

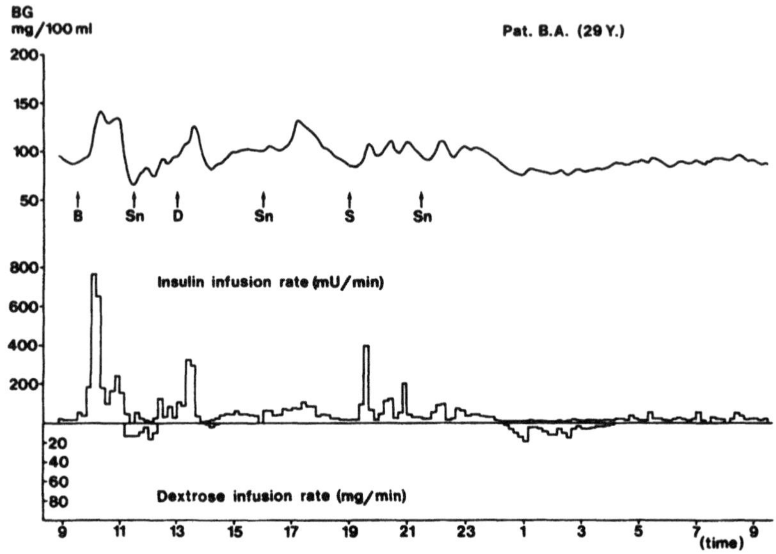

Fig. 2b

Fig. 2a and 2b. Blood glucose concentrations and insulin/dextrose infusion rates over 24 hours in a juvenile diabetic, using different types of algorithms for insulin infusion control (a: first type of algorithms; b: more recent algorith.)

NORMALIZATION OF EXOGENOUS INSULIN INFUSION AND BLOOD GLUCOSE CONCENTRATION, AND SECRETION OF DIABETOGENIC HORMONES

In insulin dependent diabetics, plasma concentration of several diabetogenic hormones, and parameters of lipid metabolism under conventional insulin therapy, were studied. These results were compared to the values obtained after a 3 days' complete blood glucose normalization with the artificial endocrine pancreas. Rapid renormalization of lipid metabolism was easily established in all patients examined. Also, renormalization of glucagon secretion was seen. Inconsistent results were observed when growth hormone concentration was compared. Renormalization of arginine reduced glucagon secretion could also be demonstrated (9).

THERAPEUTIC APPLICATIONS

The four main indications for the artificial endocrine pancreas in emergency situations in diabetes in the hospital are: 1) precoma and diabetic coma, 2) in operative and non-operative delivery of the pregnant diabetic, 3) in surgery on diabetics (and also in total pancreatectomy), 4) in surgical and non-surgical treatment of hyperinsulinsim.

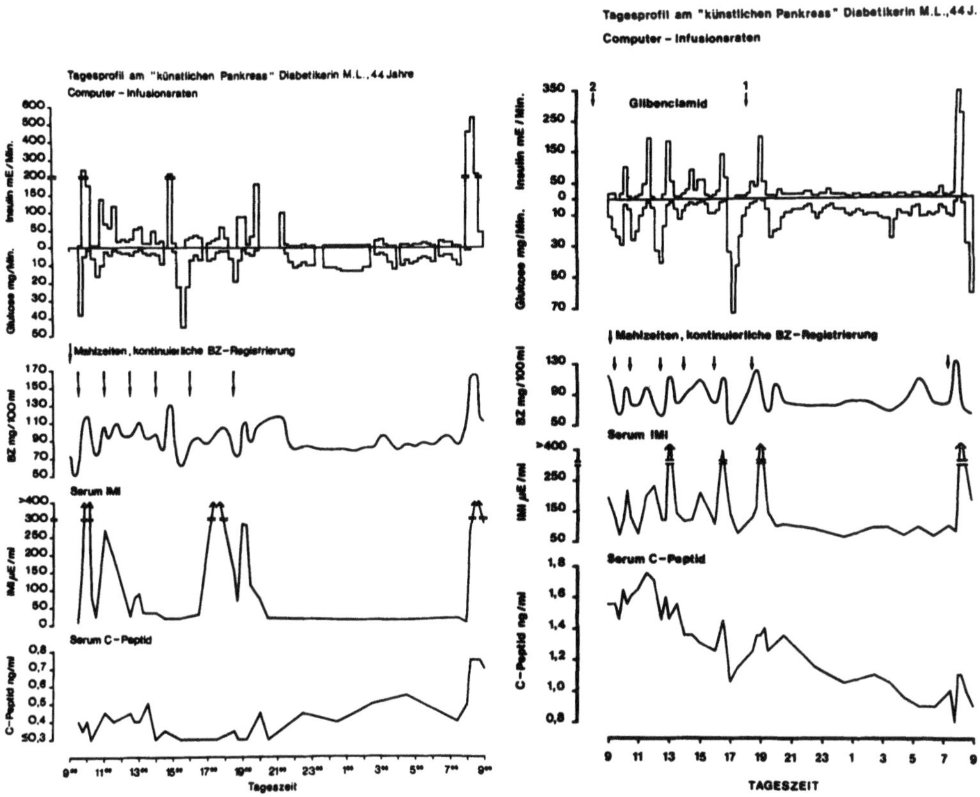

Fig. 3. Blood glucose concentration, insulin/dextrose infusion rate, serum insulin concentration and serum C-peptide concentration over 24 hours in an adult-type diabetic patient before (left side) and during (right side) treatment with glibenclamide.

1) Precoma and Diabetic Coma

Automated insulin therapy of precoma and coma diabeticum has been used in about 30 patients, the first being 89 years old (1). It consisted of an initial continuous infusion of insulin at maximum rate, i.e., of 600 mU/min; when blood glucose declined, the quantities of insulin infused were rapidly reduced, thus preventing hypoglycemic reactions. When necessary, there was automatic dextrose infusion during this stage. Because of automatic exclusion of hypoglycema, we did not aim at handling our coma cases with the lowest possible insulin doses (10). At present, insulin infusions commence with 200 mU/min., followed by a steady decline adjusted to fall in blood sugar concentrations (Fig. 4).

2) Complicated Diabetes, Related Surgery and Gynecology

Further experience has been gained during complicated diabetes-related surgery, including Caesarean section. The application of the apparatus is exemplified by Fig. 5 in a 70 year old patient. After overnight blood glucose control, operation commenced the next day with normal blood glucose concentration. He was maintained under control until the second day after the operation. The artificial pancreas proved to be especially useful in 7 patients with pancreatic non-endocrine tumors following complete duodeno-pancreatectomy. The patients were placed under control by the apparatus for 6 days and could be infused with high caloric glucose containing fluids without any complications regarding blood glucose homeostasis.

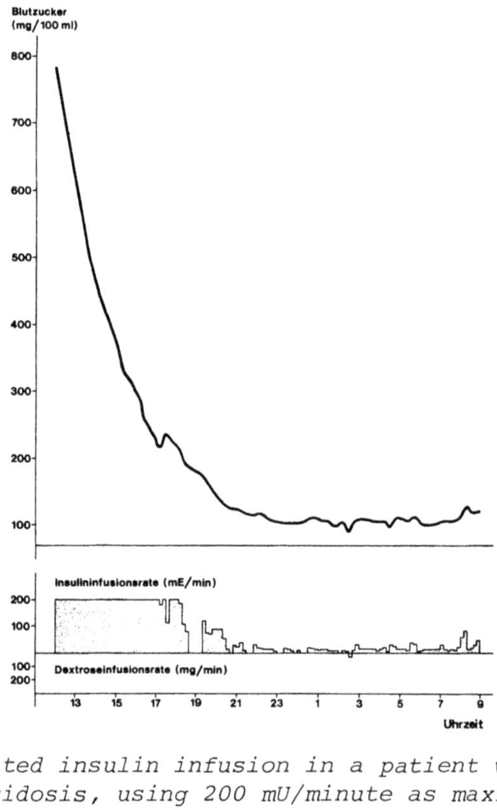

Fig. 4. Automated insulin infusion in a patient with diabetic ketoacidosis, using 200 mU/minute as maximum insulin dose.

3) Hyperinsulinism

Not only hyperglycemia but also hypoglycemic episodes of a certain magnitude due to islet and other carcinoma might be treated successfully. In one case, for more than 4 days, glucose values were stabilized around 70 mg% by automatic glucose-controlled infusion by an average of 10 g of dextrose per hour (12).

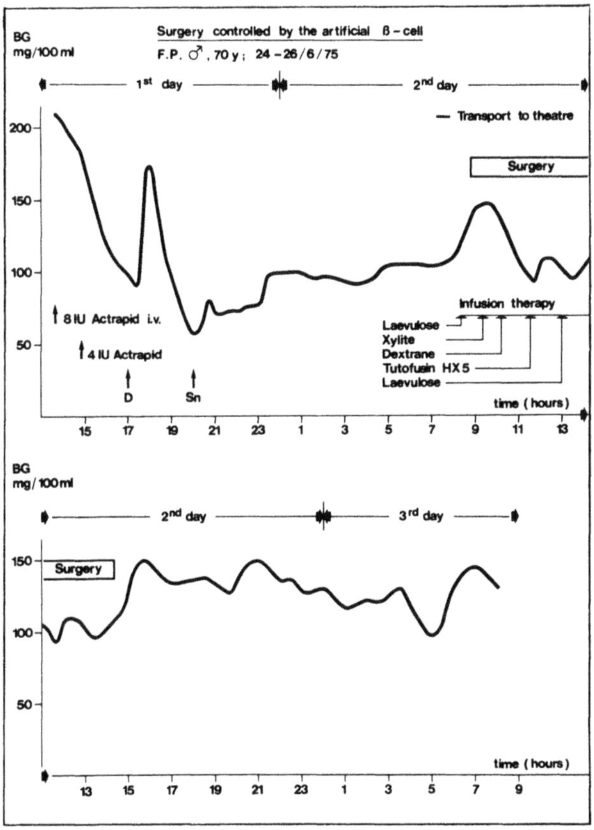

Fig. 5. Blood glucose concentrations regulated by feedback-controlled insulin infusion with the artificial endocrine pancreas during surgery in a diabetic patient.

CONCLUSION

We are far from an implantable artificial endocrine pancreas, which could thereafter relieve diabetics of the daily subcutaneous injections. Now, an extracorporeal artificial endocrine pancreas is available which, even under emergency situations, provides normalization of blood glucose better than had been achieved by the best methods previously.

Further development will aim at the expansion of the automatic control of other parameters (e.g. minerals, oxygen and pH) by creation of a multichannel machine appropriate for use in the intensive care unit and in the operating room. Furthermore, we must design some kind of a "home pancreas" the trained diabetic can use in his own surroundings (home and at work) for weeks or even months. Various combinations of automatic, semi-automatic and preprogrammed versions of those mechanical insulin infusion systems must be designed.

The development of the artificial endocrine pancreas, without any doubt, has improved the prospects for diabetes therapy. Perhaps only the combination of treatment by the artificial pancreas and transplantation of human islets or cultivated beta-cells will represent the means to cure diabetes mellitus and to prevent its complications.

REFERENCES

1. *Pfeiffer, E.F. et al. (1974). Horm. Metab. Res. 6, 339.*
2. *Pfeiffer, E.F. et al. (1974). Die Naturwissenschaften, 61, 455.*
3. *Albisser, A.M. et al. (1974). Diabetes, 23, 389.*
4. *Clemens, A.H. et al. (1977). Horm. Metab. Res. Suppl. Ser. 7, 23.*
5. *Kadish, A.H. (1964). Amer. J. Med. Electronics, 3, 82.*
6. *Kerner, W. et al. (1976). Horm. Metab. Res. 8, 256.*
7. *Kerner, W. et al. (1977). IX. Karlsburger Symposium uber Diabetesfragen, Bd. II.*
8. *Pfeiffer, E.F. et al. (1977). Horm. Metab. Res. Suppl. Ser. 7, 95.*
9. *Schock, D. et al (1978). Diabetologia 15 (Abstra.) 268.*
10. *Kerner, W. et al. (1977). Dtsch. Med. Wschr. 102, 1500.*
11. *Kerner, W., et al. (1978). Acta Endocr. Suppl. 215, 63.*
12. *Beischer, W. et al. (1975). In: Neunte Lebertagung der Sozialmediziner, Bad Mergentheim (in press).*

GLYCEMIC NORMALIZATION USING A PREPROGRAMMED INSULIN DELIVERY DEVICE IN UNRESTRAINED DIABETIC DOGS

A. M. Albisser*, Y. Goriya, A. Bahoric and
E. B. Marliss

Glycemic normalization in diabetes mellitus is an important goal. Until the advent of the artificial endocrine pancreas (1) and the transplantation of pancreatic tissue, no sure method existed for restoring to diabetic subjects a normal glycemic profile. Problems which prevent these methods from being made available for clinical use include the lack of a glucose sensor for the artificial device and the risk of immunological incompatibility of the graft with its host.

To circumvent the need for a sensor, several groups (2-4) have developed programmable open-loop insulin delivery devices. These include only a pump, an insulin reservoir and a flow-rate controller. They do not depend on a glucose sensor. Studies, usually of a short-term nature, were undertaken to explore the feasibility of glycemic normalization using these devices and preprogrammed waveforms of insulin delivery. In most cases the resulting glycemic control was variable and unpredictable, albeit improved compared to subcutaneous insulin therapy.

Using basal insulin delivery and superimposed square waves we showed that the glycemic responses to glucose infusion in anaesthetized pancreatectomized dogs could be consistently normalized. Hyperinsulinemia accompanied this glycemic normalization with peripheral (5) but not with portal (6) insulin delivery. These findings were extended to a more physiological model in long term studies up to one year in duration (7). In these studies a portable, open-loop insulin delivery device (4) was used to infuse insulin peripherally according to a simple preprogrammed waveform. This waveform included a constant basal rate given in the post-absorptive period and a single pulse of 7x basal for 7h in the post-prandial period. With this method of treatment, fasting euglycemia and a near normal response to a mixed meal were achieved, although a mild hyperglycemic rebound was frequently observed following the end of the meal pulse. In the light of the encouraging results obtained in these studies using the open-loop method of treatment, we deciced to explore the extent to which complete glycemic normalization can be achieved by a more complex waveform of insulin delivery in conscious diabetic dogs fed their usual diet.

MATERIALS AND METHODS

The methodological details of 1) the central vein catherization and pancreatectomy, and, 2) the management of diabetic dogs have been previously described (1,7). A schematic representation of the portable insulin delivery system is shown in Fig. 1.

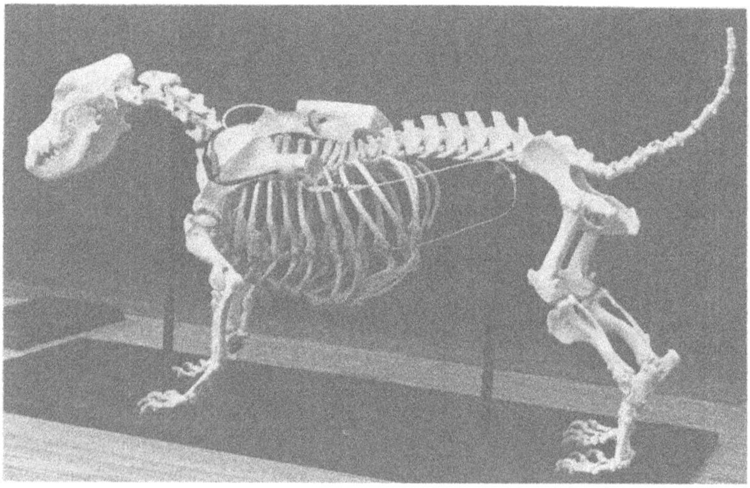

Fig. 1. The portable insulin delivery system. Insulin reservoir and pump are carried in a pocket on one side while the battery-pack and flow-rate controller are carried in another pocket on the other side of a vest-like jacket (not shown) which the dogs wear. The infusion catheter is in the vena cava with access from a superficial vein. The catheter extends through the skin and enters the pocket in which the pump is carried. Total weight is 520g.

Experimental Protocols to Establish the Meal Response in Normal and Diabetic Dogs.

a. Normal Dogs

Six healthy dogs served as normal controls. Their glucose and insulin responses to standard diet were obtained from the analysis of blood samples drawn via an indwelling sampling catheter hourly for 24 hours starting at -1h. The 620g meal contained 33% protein, 30% fat and 37% carbohydrate and was presented at time zero and always eaten within 5 minutes.

b. Diabetic Dogs

Waveforms of meal insulin delivery were studied in a pilot series of experiments. According to these preliminary studies a meal infusion of seven times basal (7 x B) over 7h and a further infusion of (7/3 x B) for 2¼h in the post-prandial period resulted in normal glycemias in the diabetic dogs. Their glycemic and insulin responses were then assessed in the same way as above. Four diabetic dogs were studied repeatedly and the results reported are only from dogs who ate all the food within 5 minutes of its presentation. Blood samples for plasma glucose and IRI levels were taken as before but only for 13 hours following the meal and then one final 23 hour sample the next morning.

RESULTS

a. Meal Response: Normal Dogs (Mean ± SEM)

The 24 hour profile of plasma glucose and IRI concenterations of normal dogs fed the standard diet are shown in Fig. 2. Plasma glucose levels were flat without significant rise or fall throughout the day and remained within the range of 83 ± 5 to 96 ± 2 mg/dl. Post-prandial plasma IRI levels rose from basal levels of 11 ± 2 uU/ml to a peak of 44 ± 11 uU/ml at 3 hours but remained significantly above the fasting levels for 15 hours and returned to fasting levels thereafter.

b. Meal Response: Diabetic Dogs (Mean ± SEM)

Starting from normoglycemic levels of between 86 ± 7 and 104 ± 11 mg/dl in the fasting state, post-prandial plasma glucose concentrations during the meal insulin infusion remained essentially unchanged and within the normal range throughout the meal insulin infusion (Fig. 2). Values ranged from 79 ± 9 to 106 ± 14 mg/dl over the 9¼h meal infusion. Euglycemic fasting levels of 89 ± 13 mg/dl were observed the next morning.

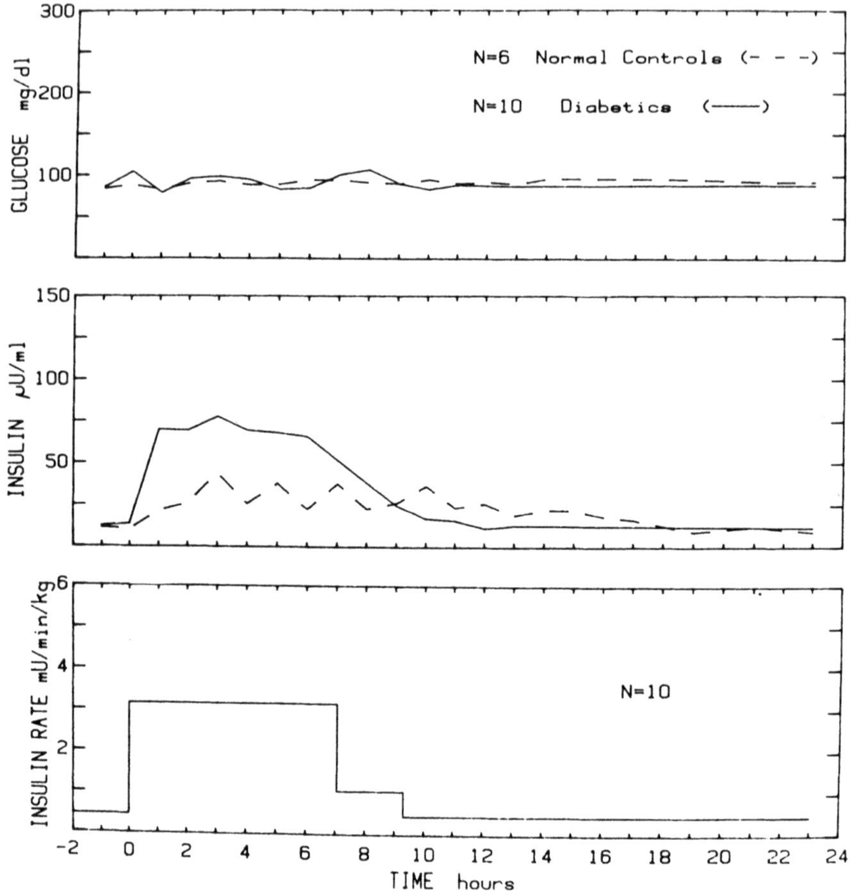

Fig. 2. The glucose and insulin responses of unrestrained healthy controls and pancreatectomized dogs to their usual diet (620g) presented at time t=0 (about 0900 a.m.). Approximate meal composition: 33% protein, 30% fat, 37% carbohydrate. Intravenous insulin treatment was according to the waveform in the lower panel (meal pulse is 7 times basal for 7h and 7/3 basal for 2¼h).

Fasting plasma IRI concentrations were 12 ± 1 μU/ml and rose during the first meal insulin pulse to levels which ranged from 52 ± 8 to 78 ± 8 μU/ml. Following the end of the first pulse of the meal infusion, IRI levels fell gradually to basal values over 3h and remained in this range throughout the remainder of the experiment. The basal infusion rate was 0.45 ± 0.03 μU/kg/min and was enhanced to 3.16 ± 0.21 μU/kg/min for 7h and then lowered to 1.05 ± .07 in μU/kg/min for 2¼h in the post-prandial period. Mean body weight was 12.6 ± -/5kg.

c. Comparison of Diabetics vs Normal Controls

There were no significant differences in glycemias between the normal controls and infused diabetics at any time during the course of the experiments. Fasting IRI levels in the diabetics were not significantly higher than normal. However, during the first meal infusion in the post-prandial period, the IRI levels were significantly higher than normal. During the second pulse of the meal infusion, IRI levels fell to normal by 9h and remained below normal thereafter, the differences being significant only at 10 and 12h.

DISCUSSION

It was remarkable that the fasting blood glucose levels of the healthy laboratory beagle did not rise following the ingestion of a standard mixed meal. Insulin levels rose and oscillated between 2 and 4 times the fasting values while remaining elevated for what appeared to be a very prolonged post-prandial period. Notwithstanding the amount of this single meal or the rapidity with which it was ingested, the glucose and insulin responses observed in the dog are notably different from those observed in normal man. These studies on the normal animals provided the criteria for glycemic control in the diabetics.

Fasting euglycemia and an normoglycemic response to the usual diet were easily restored to pancreatectomized dogs treated with a simple preprogrammed waveform of insulin infusion which was enhanced above basal for 9¼h during the post-prandial period. The animals used in this study received a single daily mixed meal of fixed composition,the calculated caloric content of which was 1300Cal based on data from the manufacturers. Meal absorption was prolonged some 9h in both the diabetic and normal dogs. In this regard it has been reported that gastric emptying of small volumes of solids in the dog was only completed in 3-4h (8).

Despite the 37% carbohydrate content of the food, no glycemic excursion was observed in the normals (Fig. 2). In diabetic dogs studied previously without enhanced meal insulin, the effects of this absorbed carbohydrate on the plasma glucose were clearly evident (7). In order to normalize the glycemia during meals, in addition to the basal insulin given, 14.5 Units of additional insulin were needed. In the present study, 15.3 Units were required with meals to reduce to normal the glycemic excursion in these diabetic dogs (body weights were not significantly different).

Post-prandial plasma IRI levels rose 2 to 3 times higher than in normal dogs. Normoglycemia in the diabetic dogs was thus accompanied by peripheral hyperinsulinemia. Reducing either the rate or the duration of the meal insulin pulse results in a glycemic excursion which is greater than that seen in the healthy controls. This relative hyperinsulinemia appears due to the peripheral route of insulin delivery (5,9). It has been shown in anesthetized pancreatectomized dogs given glucose infusions with both closed-loop (artificial *B*-cell) and open-loop (preprogrammed) insulin delivery that normal peripheral insulin levels are observed when insulin is delivered portally (6) but not when it is delivered peripherally (5). These findings imply the necessity of portal insulin infusion in the treatment of diabetes mellitus.

Whether the mild meal-associated peripheral hyperinsulinemia obtained in these studies is harmful in the long term remains to be established. Further clinical studies with diabetic patients are proceeding.

REFERENCES

1. *Albisser, A.M., et al. (1974). Diabetes 23:389.*
2. *Deckert, T. and Lorup, B. (1976). Diabetologia 12:573.*
3. *Service, J.F. (1978). J. Lab. Clin. Med. 91:480.*
4. *Albisser, A.M., et al. (1978). Med. Prog. Technol. 5:187.*
5. *Botz, C.K., et al. Submitted to Diabetologia.*
6. *Albisser, A.M., et al. Diabetologia, in press.*
7. *Albiser, A.M., et al. (1978). Diabetes 27 (Suppl 1) 439.*
8. *Hinder, R.A. and Kelly, K.A. (1977). Am. J. Physiol, 233:E335.*
9. *Botz, C.K., et al (1976). Diabetes 25:691.*

This work was conducted as a research project in the Artificial Pancreas Program at The Hospital for Sick Children in Toronto, and benefited in part from the financial support of The Juvenile Diabetes Foundation, The Juvenile Diabetes Research Foundation, The Medical Research Council of Canada, The Pfizer Company of Canada, and the Kroc Foundation.

We are grateful for the enthusiastic cooperation and energetic help of Mr. H. L. Tang for the insulin assays, Mr. W.S. Jackman for the pumps and reservoirs, Mr. R. T. Ferguson for the battery-packs and flow-rate controllers, Ms. H. Nielsen for assistance in the care of the animals, and Ms. I. Gibson for preparation of the manuscript.

DISCUSSION

Invited Discussant: A. H. CLEMENS: *The flow scheme of the glucose monitor extends the useful range of the glucose sensor up to 1000 mg/dl and permits a rapid push-button controlled two-point calibration of the glucose analyzer without disconnecting the double-lumen catheter from the patient. A convenient glucose addition calibration procedure assures the accurate readout of a true whole blood glucose concentrations instead of plasma values, without the need for concurrrent hematocrit measurements. A carefully controlled correlation study confirmed that the whole blood glucose values measured by the BIOSTATOR glucose analyzer compare very favorably against the hexokinase/glucose -6- phosphate dehydrogenase National Glucose Reference Method (Fig. 1).*

Throughout the evolution of glucose controlled insulin infusion since 1964 a variety of feedback control schemes and control algorithms had been proposed and several of these had actually been used for closed-loop glucose regulation in man. Most of these control algorithms incuded a procedure for the calculation of a "predicted" glucose value originally proposed to compensate for the analyzer lag time, because it had become clear from earlier studies that an excessive delay between the blood withdrawal and the glucose readout would introduce a significant error in the closed-loop control. The predicted glucose value was an extrapolation of the last measured value by the rate of change recorded over the previous few minutes. It was subsequently found that if a predicted glucose value was calculated beyond the glucose difference to compensate for the analyzer lag time, a "quasi" derivative effect could be achieved to mimic a first phase insulin release.

Although the glucose regulation achieved with an early set of control algorithms (Ewart, T.G., et al 1973 In: A.S. Iberall, A.C. Guyton; Proceedings of the American Physiological Society, p. 509) was a significant improvement over conventional insulin therapy, the resulting glucose curve typically resembled that of a maturity-onset diabetic with a delayed glucose peak and a subsequent overshoot into the hypoglycemic range (Kerner, W., et al. 1976 Hormone & Metabolic Research, 8 (4): 256).

In order to more systematically investigate the glucose control dynamics, we found it necessary to develop control algorithms which permitted a optimization of the dynamic first phase insulin response to a rise in glucose levels independently of the optimization of a down regulation of the insulin release in response to a fall in glucose levels (Kerner, W., et al. 1976 Hormone & Metabolic Research, 8 (4): 256).

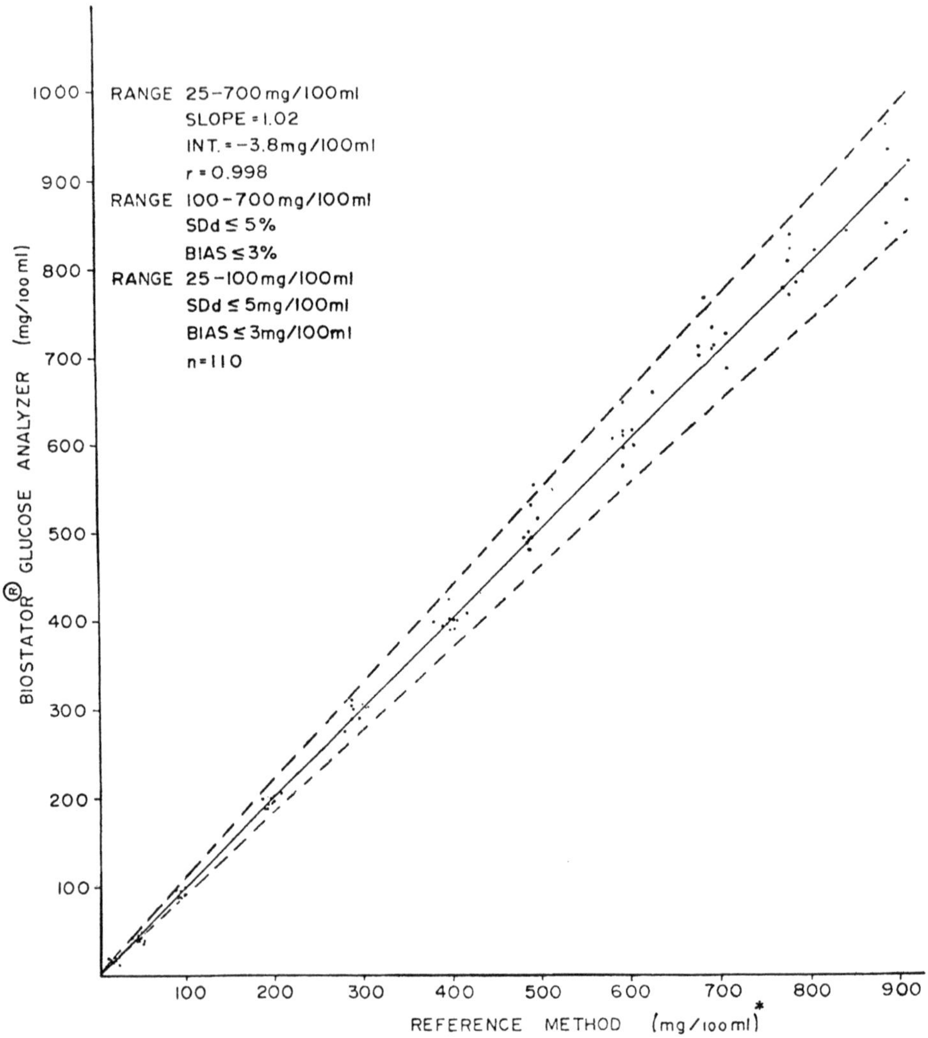

Fig. 1.

In order to use control constants which were physiologically more meaningful we replaced the "tangens hyperbolicus" with a biquadratic control function for proportional or static control of insulin release (Clemens, A.H., et al 1977 Proceedings of a Workshop-Conference, March 1976, Freiburg (Germany). Hormone & Metabolic Research, suppl. series #7, p. 23). In this new algorithm, RI became the control constant for the required basal insulin release at BI, the desired basal glucose level, and QI the adjustment for the slope of the control curve. The static insulin infusion rate then became

$$IR = RI \left(\frac{G - BI}{QI} + 1 \right)^4$$

More recently, the power of the static control equation was reduced to a quadratic function

$$IR = RI \left(\frac{G - BI}{QI} + 1 \right)^2$$

in order to further reduce the insulin release at hyperglycemic levels, and to increase the infusion rate slightly above and decrease it immediately below BI for improved stability at this selected basal glucose level.

Investigations into the timing of a physiologic insulin response to a glucose challenge revealed that the first phase (dynamic) insulin release from the BIOSTATOR system slightly preceded the appearance of the C-peptide in a normal subject (Pfeiffer, E.F., et al 1975). This indicated that the overall BIOSTATOR system's response time of less than two minutes no longer necessitated the calculation and use of a predicted glucose value on irder to compensate for the analyzer and/or sytem's lag time. Instead, we now were able to apply a true derivative function to the dynamic control mode.

In its simplest form, the dynamic insulin infusion rate became

$$IR = K \times \frac{dG}{dt} \text{ , or } IR - K \times m$$

Following the earlier mentioned rationale, we continued to use separate constants for the control of the insulin release in response to a rise (KR) and a modulation of the insulin infusion in response to a fall (KF) in glucose concentration.

In order to reduce any "noise" sensitivity of the system, we introduced a least square regression line fit through the last five glucose values instead of a straight G averaging over the last four minutes. We also expanded the basic equation for the dynamic control into

$$IR = KR \text{ or } KF \times m \times (GY-BI)$$

to prevent any "dynamic" insulin release in response to actual or apparent changes in blood glucose concentrations below BI, i.e., the desired blood glucose level. GY is the last measured glucose value, corrected to fit the regression line.

Studies with the BIOSTATOR GCIIS have shown that the exogenous insulin requirements largely depend upon the subject's weight, his insulin sensitivity and any remaining endogenous insulin release capacity. The basal insulin release rate (RI) for an insulin dependent diabetic with no residual beta cell function and a "normal" insulin sensitivity is approximately 2mU per minute per 10 kg body weight. During these studies it was also found necessary to adapt the magnitude of the dynamic insulin response to the subject to be controlled, not unlike the necessity to adjust the basal insulin release RI for static control to the individual subject's requirements. If one factors RI into the dynamic control algorithm

$$IR - K \times m\ (GY-BI) \times RI,$$

the KR and KF values need no longer be individualized. The insulin release for an insulin dependent diabetic (Operating MOde 3) now becomes the simple addition of operating modes 1 plus 2, or

$$IR = RI\ \left[\left(\frac{GY-BI}{QI} + 1\right)^2 + KR \times m\ (GY-BI)\right]$$

for a rising blood glucose and

$$IR = RI\ \left[\left(\frac{GY-BI}{QI} + 1\right)^2 + KF \times m\ (GY-BI)\right]$$

for a fall in a glucose concentration.

The evolution of the control algorithms for closed-loop insulin infusion has, thus, changed from a qualitative glucose regulation in the early (1974) model to a quantitative glucose control (1975-1977) and, more recently, to a fine tuning of the insulin release, while maintaining optimized glucose regulation.

Although an automatic infusion of dextrose (Pfeiffer, E.F., et al. 1977 Proceedings of a Workshop-Conference, March 1976. Freiburg (Germany). Hormone & Metabolic Research, suppl. series #7, p. 95), or glucagon (Marlis, E.B., et al 1977 Diabetes Vol. 26, #7, p. 663) to counteract a hypoglycemic reaction to a hyperinsulinemia is no longer necessary, we have maintained the feedback-controlled dextrose infusion for the treatment of insulinomas and for metabolic studies involving glucose clamping above the physiologic blood glucose level, or to counteract preprogrammed exogenous insulin infusions.

LIST OF PARTICIPANTS

Asterisks denote invited speakers
Daggers denote invited discussants

Ambjorn Agren
Histological Department
University of Uppsala
Uppsala, Sweden

*K. George M.M. Alberti
Department of Clinical Biochemistry
Royal Victoria Infirmary
Newcastle upon Tyne, NE1 4Lp
England

*A. Michael Albisser
Biomedical Research
The Research Institute
The Hospital For Sick Children
Toronto M5G 1X8, Canada

C. E. Aldinger
Department of Pharmacology
Pfizer Central Research
Groton, Connecticut 06340

*James W. Anderson
Department of Medicine
Veterans Administration Medical Center
University of Kentucky College of Medicine
Lexington, Kentucky 40507

Arne Andersson
Histological Department
University of Uppsala
Uppsala, Sweden

Susan Bacon
Nuffield Orthopaedic Center
Oxford, England

*Jose Barbosa
Department of Medicine
University of Minnesota
Minneapolis, Minnesota 55455

W. Beischer
Department of Medicine I
Center of Internal Medicine
Pediatrics and Dermatology
University of Ulm
Ulm, Germany

Lynn J. Bennion
Phoenix Clinical Research Section
National Institute of Arthritis, Metabolism and Digestive Diseases
National Institutes of Health
Phoenix, Arizona 85016

Peter H. Bennett
Epidemiology and Field Studies Branch
Southwestern Field Studies Section
National Institute of Arthritis, Metabolism and Digestive Diseases
National Institutes of Health
Phoenix, Arizona 85016

Margaret C. Blanks
Diabetes and Atherosclerosis Research
The Upjohn Company
Kalamazoo, Michigan 49001

David M. Brown
Department of Laboratory Medicine and Pathology and Department of Pediatrics
University of Minnesota
Minneapolis, Minnesota 55455

*Rafael A. Camerini-Davalos
Division of Diabetes and Metabolism
Department of Medicine
New York Medical College
New York, New York 10029

Kirsten Capito
Department of Biochemistry A
Panum Institute
University of Copenhagen
Copenhagen, Denmark

*Sven Carlstrom
Department of Medicine
University Hospital of Lund
S-221 85 Lund, Sweden

Mei Chen
Veterans Administration Medical Center
Division of Clinical Pharmacology
University of Washington
Seattle, Washington 98108

Myra M. Chern
Department of Laboratory Medicine and Pathology
University of Minnesota
Minneapolis, Minnesota 55455

Sung C. Choi
Department of Biostatistics
Medical College of Virginia
Richmond, Virginia 23298

Morten Christy
Steno Memorial Hospital
Gentofte, Copenhagen, Denmark

†A. H. Clemens
Life Science Instruments Division
Miles Laboratories, Inc.
Elkhart, Indiana 46514

*Rex S. Clements, Jr.
Diabetes Research and Training Center
Department of Medicine
University of Alabama
School of Medicine
Birmingham, Alabama 35202

Michael C. Cloutier
Department of Internal Medicine
Division of Endocrinology and Metabolism and the Metabolism Research Unit
The University of Michigan
Ann Arbor, Michigan 48109

F. Coce
Institute for Diabetes
Endocrinology and Metabolic Diseases
"Vuk Vrhovac"
University of Zagreb
41000 Zagreb, Yugoslavia

†Margo Panush Cohen
Wayne State University
School of Medicine
Detroit, Michigan 48207

*Torsten Deckert
Steno Memorial Hospital
Gentofte, Copenhagen, Denmark

*Marc M. de Gasparo
Department of Research
Division of Pharmaceuticals
Ciba Geigy
CH-4002 Basle, Switzerland

Paul de Herdt
Department of Research
Division of Pharmaceuticals
Ciba Geigy
CH-4002 Basle, Switzerland

H. Dies
Section of Diabetes and Lipid
Metabolism
National Institute of Nutrition
Mexico 22, D.F.

Theodore Ehrenreich
Department of Pathology
New York Medical College
New York, New York 10029

*Stefan S. Fajans
Department of Internal Medicine
Division of Endocrinology and
Metabolism and the Metabolism
Research Unit
The University of Michigan
Medical School
Ann Arbor, Michigan 48109

Henry C. Fawthorp
Endocrinology and Metabolism
Biochemical Research
McNeil Laboratories
Fort Washington, Pennsylvania
19034

Mark N. Feinglos
Division of Endocrinology
Department of Medicine
Duke University Medical Center
Durham, North Carolina 27710

R. Femenic
Institute for Diabetes,
Endocrinology and Metabolic
Diseases
"Vuk Vrhovac"
University of Zagreb
41000 Zagreb, Yugoslavia

J. Figueroa
Section of Diabetes and Lipid
Metabolism
National Institute of Nutrition
Mexico 22, D.F.

Eunice V. Flock
Phoenix Clinical Research Section
National Institute of Arthritis,
Metabolism and Digestive
Diseases
National Institutes of Health
Phoenix, Arizona 85016

Manfred Franetzki
Department of Medical Engineering
Siemens A.G.
Erlangen, Germany

*Norbert Freinkel
Center for Endocrinology,
Metabolism and Nutrition
Department of Medicine and
Biochemistry
Northwestern University Medical
School
Chicago, Illinois 60611

*George C. Gerritsen
Diabetes and Atherosclerosis
Research
The Upjohn Company
Kalamazoo, Michigan 49001

F. J. Gomez-Perez
Section of Diabetes and Lipid
Metabolism
National Institute of Nutrition
Mexico 22, D.F.

*Sebastiano Grasso
Department of Morbid Anatomy
University of Catania
Catania, Italy

Richard F. Hamman
Department of Epidemiology
Johns Hopkins School of Hygiene
and Public Health
Baltimore, Maryland

Bernard Hanover
Department of Medicine
Division of Diabetes and Metabolism
New York Medical College
New York, New York 10029

*Carl J. Hedeskov
Department of Biochemistry A
Panum Institute
University of Copenhagen
Copenhagen, Denmark

*Claes Hellerstrom
Histological Department
University of Uppsala
Uppsala, Sweden

Ann C. Henderson
University of Texas Medical Branch
Galveston, Texas 77550

*K. Dietrich Hepp
3rd Medical Department and Diabetes Research Unit
Schwabing City Hospital
Munich, Germany

Andre Herchuelz
Laboratories of Experimental Medicine and Pharmacology
Universite Libre de Bruxelles
1000 Brussels, Belgium

P. K. Ho
Department of Medicine
Division of Diabetes and Metabolism
New York Medical College
New York, New York 10029

T. Derek R. Hockaday
Department of the Regius Professor of Medicine
Radcliffe Infirmary
Oxford, England

Joseph J. Hoet
Unit for Endocrinology and Nutrition
Medical School
University of Louvain
B-1200 Brussels, Belgium

W. J. Irvine
Endocrine Unit
Immunology Laboratories and University Department of Medicine
Royal Infirmary
Edinburgh, Scotland

John Jarrett
Unit for Metabolic Medicine
Guy's Hospital Medical School
London, SE1 9RT, England

*David J. A. Jenkins
Department of the Regius Professor of Medicine
Radcliffe Infirmary
University Laboratory of Physiology
Oxford, England
Department of Gastroenterology
Central Middlesex Hospital
London NW10, England

A. Bennett Jenson
Laboratory of Oral Medicine
National Institute of Dental Research
National Institutes of Health
Bethesda, Maryland 20014

Takahiro Kanatsuna
Department of Medicine
University of Chicago
Chicago, Illinois 60637

*Panayotis G. Katsoyannis
Department of Biochemistry
Mount Sinai School of Medicine
City University of New York
New York, New York 10029

Harry Keen
Unit for Metabolic Medicine
Guy's Hospital Medical School
London SE1 9RT, England

W. Kerner
Department of Medicine I
Center of Internal Medicine
Pediatrics and Dermatology
University of Ulm
Ulm, Germany

Charles Kilo
Department of Medicine
Washington University
School of Medicine
St. Louis, Missouri 63110

*H. P. Krause
Institute of Pharmacology
Bayer Ag
Wuppertal 1, West Germany

Robert Krill
Endocrinology and Metabolism
Biochemical Research
McNeil Laboratories
Fort Washington, Pennsylvania 19034

A. B. Kurtz
Department of Nuclear Medicine
Middlesex Hospital
Hospital Medical School
London, England

Morgens Larsen
Steno Memorial Hospital
Gentofte, Copenhagen, Denmark

*Harold E. Lebovitz
Division of Endocrinology
Department of Medicine
Duke University Medical Center
Durham, North Carolina 27710

*Ake Lernmark
Department of Histology
University of Umea
Umeå, Sweden

Oscar Lozano-Castaneda
Section of Diabetes and Lipid Metabolism
National Institute of Nutrition
Mexico 22, D.F.

*Willy J. Malaisse
Laboratories of Experimental Medicine and Pharmacology
Universite Libre de Bruxelles
1000 Brussels, Belgium

S. Michael Mauer
Department of Pediatrics
University of Minnesota
Minneapolis, Minnesota 55455

D. P. McDonald
Department of Pharmacology
Pfizer Central Research
Groton, Connecticut 06340

Alan K. McKenzie
Department of Internal Medicine
Division of Endocrinology and Metabolism and the Metabolism Research Unit
The University of Michigan
Ann Arbor, Michigan 48109

John R. McRae
Veterans Administration Medical Center
Division of Clinical Pharmacology
University of Washington
Seattle, Washington 98108

Hellmut Mehnert
3rd Medical Department and Diabetes Research Unit
Schwabing City Hospital
Munich, Germany

*Hans Peter Meissner
Department of Internal Medicine
University of Saarland
D-6650 Homburg-Saar, Germany

Stewart A. Metz
Veterans Administration Medical Center
Division of Clinical Pharmacology
University of Washington
Seattle, Washington 98108

*Boyd E. Metzger
Department of Medicine
Center for Endocrinology, Metabolism and Nutrition
Northwestern University Medical School
Chicago, Illinois 60611

J. Philip Miller
Department of Preventive Medicine
Washington University School of Medicine
St. Louis, Missouri 63110

Jørn Nerup
Steno Memorial Hospital
Gentofte, Copenhagen, Denmark

Bo Nilsson
Histological Department
University of Uppsala
Uppsala, Sweden

Richard Nineham
University Laboratory of Physiology
Oxford, England

*Evan Norris
Pfizer Laboratories Division
Pfizer, Inc.
New York, New York 10017

R. Nosadini
Department of Clinical Biochemistry
Royal Victoria Infirmary
Newcastle upon Tyne, NE1 4LP
England

*Abner Louis Notkins
Laboratory of Oral Medicine
National Institute of Dental Research
National Institutes of Health
Bethesda, Maryland 20014

G. Noy
Department of Clinical Biochemistry
Royal Victoria Infirmary
Newcastle upon Tyne, NE1 4LP
England

Takashi Onodera
Laboratory of Oral Medicine
National Institute of Dental Research
National Institutes of Health
Bethesda, Maryland 20014

*Werner Oppermann
Department of Medicine
Division of Diabetes and Metabolism
New York Medical College
New York, New York 10029

G. Palumbo
Department of Obstetrics and Gynecology
University of Catania
Catania, Italy

John A. Parsons
Laboratory for Endocrine Physiology and Pharmacology
National Institute for Medical Research
London NW 7 1AA, England

Sumer Pek
Department of Internal Medicine
Division of Endocrinology and Metabolism and the Metabolism Research Unit
The University of Michigan Medical School
Ann Arbor, Michigan 48109

Gunnar Persson
Department of Medicine
University Hospital of Lund
S-221 85 Lund, Sweden

Birger Petersson
Histological Department
University of Uppsala
Uppsala, Sweden

*Ernst F. Pfeiffer
Department of Medicine I
Center of Internal Medicine
Pediatrics and Dermatology
University of Ulm
Ulm, Germany

*John C. Pickup
Unit for Metabolic Medicine
Guy's Hospital Medical School
London SE1 9RT, England

Per Platz
Tissue-Typing Laboratory of the Blood-Grouping Department
State University Hospital (Rigshospitalet)
Copenhagen, Denmark

*M. J. Peterson
Department of Pharmacology
Pfizer Central Research
Groton, Connecticut 06340

†Stephen Podolsky
Endocrinology and Metabolism Section
Veterans Administration
Out Patient Clinic
Boston, Massachusetts 02108

*Phillip L. Poffenbarger
Department of Medicine and Department of Human Biological Chemistry and Genetics
University of Texas Medical Branch
Galveston, Texas 77550

Margret Preissler
Department of Physiology
University of Saarland
D-6650 Homburg-Saar, Germany

*Thaddeus E. Prout
Greater Baltimore Medical Center
The Johns Hopkins School of Medicine
Baltimore, Maryland 21204

W. Puls
Institute of Pharmacology
Bayer Ag
Wuppertal 1, West Germany

*Gerald M. Reaven
Veterans Administration Hospital
Palo Alto, California 94304

*Alluru S. Reddi
Department of Medicine
Division of Diabetes and Metabolism
New York Medical College
New York, New York 10029

*Francois Regnault
Retinal Diseases Research Group
Cochin Hospital
Paris , 14 ème France

Rolf Renner
3rd Medical Department and Diabetes Research Unit
Schwabing City Hospital
Munich, Germany

*R. Paul Robertson
Veterans Administration Medical Center
Division of Clinical Pharmacology
University of Washington
Seattle, Washington 98108

Arthur H. Rubenstein
Department of Medicine
University of Chicago
Chicago, Illinois 60637

*Pablo Rubinstein
The Lindsley F. Kimball Research Institute of The New York Blood Center
New York, New York 10021

S. Rugola
Department of Obstetrics and Gynecology
University of Catania
Catania, Italy

*J. A. Rull
Section of Diabetes and Lipid Metabolism
National Institute of Nutrition
Mexico 22, D.F.

*Lars Peter Ryder
Tissue-Typing Laboratory of the Blood-Grouping Department
State University Hospital (Rigshospitalet)
Copenhagen, Denmark

J. Sanchez-Gochicoa
Section of Diabetes and Lipid Metabolism
National Institute of Nutrition
Mexico 22, D.F.

Stellan Sandler
Histological Department
University of Uppsala
Uppsala, Sweden

R. Sarges
Department of Medicinal Chemistry
Pfizer Central Research
Groton, Connecticut 06340

Gunnar Sartor
Department of Medicine
University Hospital of Lund
S-221 85 Lund, Sweden

*Peter J. Savage
Southwestern Field Studies Section
National Institute of Arthritis, Metabolism and Digestive Diseases
National Institutes of Health
Phoenix, Arizona 85016

Bengt Schersten
Department of Medicine
University Hospital of Lund
S-221 85 Lund, Sweden

*David E. Schteingart
Department of Internal Medicine
Division of Endocrinology and Metabolism and the Metabolism Research Unit
The University of Michigan
Ann Arbor, Michigan 48109

J. Schulte
Section of Diabetes and Lipid Metabolism
National Institute of Nutrtition
Mexico 22, D.F.

Joanne Scott
Department of Medicine and Department of Human Biological Chemistry and Genetics
University of Texas Medical Branch
Galveston, Texas 77550

Abdullah Sener
Laboratories of Experimental Medicine and Pharmacology
Universite Libre de Bruxelles
1000 Brussels, Belgium

Zdenko Skrabalo
Institute for Diabetes, Endocrinology and Metabolic Diseases
"Vuk Vrhovac"
University of Zagreb
41000 Zagreb, Yugoslavia

Roger Smith
Nuffield Orthopaedic Center
Oxford, England

*Michael W. Steffes
Department of Laboratory Medicine and Pathology
University of Minnesota
Minneapolis, Minnesota 55455

Donald F. Steiner
Department of Biochemistry
University of Chicago
Chicago, Illinois 60637

Louis H. Strugatz
Division of Diabetes and Metabolism
Department of Medicine
New York Medical College
New York, New York 10029

Nicole Suciu-Foca
Departments of Pathology and Surgery
College of Physicians and Surgeons
Columbia University
New York, New York 10027

Arne Svejgaard
Tissue-Typing Laboratory of the Blood-Grouping Department
State University Hospital (Rigshospitalet)
Copenhagen, Denmark

Morgens Thomsen
Tissue-Typing Laboratory of the Blood-Grouping Department
State University Hospital (Rigshospitalet)
Copenhagen, Denmark

Heng S. Tsao
Department of Internal Medicine
Division of Endocrinology and Metabolism and the Metabolism Research Unit
The University of Michigan
Ann Arbor, Michigan 48109

G. Tumino
Department of Pediatrics
University of Catania
Catania, Italy

*Gene F. Tutwiler
Endocrinology and Metabolism
Biochemical Research
McNeill Laboratories
Fort Washington, Pennsylvania 10934

Carlos A. Velasco
Department of Medicine
Division of Diabetes and Metabolism
New York Medical College
New York, New York 10029

Rodolfo S. Victoria
Department of Internal Medicine
Division of Endocrinology and Metabolism and the Metabolsim Research Unit
The University of Michigan
Ann Arbor, Michigan 48109

R. Vigo
Department of Pediatrics
University of Catania
Catania, Italy

*Mladen Vranic
Department of Physiology
University of Toronto
Toronto, Ontario, Canada M5S 1A8

†H. Wehner
Pathologisches Institut
D-7630 Lahr, Klostenstr.
19, Germany

†*Joseph R. Williamson
Department of Pathology
Washington University
School of Medicine
St. Louis, Missouri 63110

Thomas M. S. Wolever
University Laboratory of
Physiology
Oxford, England

Ji-Won Yoon
Laboratory of Oral Medicine
National Institute of Dental
Research
National Institutes of Health
Bethesda, Maryland 20014

INDEX

www.ingramcontent.com/pod-product-compliance
Ingram Content Group UK Ltd.
Pitfield, Milton Keynes, MK11 3LW, UK
UKHW051449290926
15471UKWH00008B/1093
* 9 7 8 1 4 6 1 5 9 1 1 1 5 *